Nurses on the Front Line
When Disaster Strikes, 1878–2010

1878–2010

D0061888

Barbra Mann Wall, PhD, RN, is a nurse historian known for her studies on women and health care institutions and for her focus on Catholic hospitals and oral histories of retired nurses. Her recent work addresses the history of disaster nursing in the Southwest and the way people interpret disasters of the past. She is Associate Professor and Associate Director of the Barbara Bates Center for the Study of the History Nursing, University of Pennsylvania School of Nursing, with previous faculty positions at Purdue and Duke Universities. She is widely published, with 19 refereed journal articles, 4 chapters in books, and 2 books, one of which, *Unlikely Entrepreneurs: Catholic Sisters and the Hospital Marketplace, 1865–1925* won the 2006 Lavinia Dock Award for Best Book, American Association for the History of Nursing (AAHN). Her newest book, *American Catholic Hospitals: A Century of Changing Missions and Markets*, is in press with Rutgers University Press. Dr. Wall is a member of Sigma Theta Tau, the American Associations for the History of Nursing and Medicine, the Council for the Advancement of Nursing Science, and more. She presents at major international and national nursing and women's research meetings and is the recipient of numerous research and program grants, from four to six figures.

Arlene W. Keeling, PhD, RN, FAAN, is the Centennial Distinguished Professor of Nursing and directs the Center for Nursing Historical Inquiry at the University of Virginia. She also chairs the Department of Acute and Specialty Care. She is immediate past president of the American Association for the History of Nursing and now second Vice President. Dr. Keeling is widely published with 26 peer-reviewed journal articles, 2 books, and 11 chapters in books, along with numerous book reviews and commentaries. In 2007, she received the Lavinia Dock Award (AAHN) for her book *Nursing and the Privilege of Prescription*. Most recently she led a team of historians in writing the history of the American Association of Colleges of Nursing. She is the recipient of numerous research grants and is a member of Sigma Theta Tau and the American Academy of Nursing. A noted academic, Dr. Keeling presents internationally at major nursing and historical meetings.

Nurses on the Front Line
When Disaster Strikes,
1878–2010

Barbra Mann Wall, PhD, RN
Arlene W. Keeling, PhD, RN, FAAN

Editors

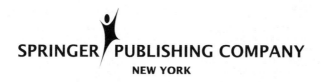

SPRINGER PUBLISHING COMPANY

NEW YORK

Springer Publishing Company, LLC
11 West 42nd Street
New York, NY 10036
www.springerpub.com

Acquisitions Editor: Allan Graubard
Production Editor: Gayle Lee
Cover Design: Steven Pisano
Project Manager: Amor Nanas
Composition: Manila Typesetting Company

ISBN: 978-0-8261-0519-6

E-book ISBN: 978-0-8261-0520-2

11 12 13 / 5 4 3 2

The author and the publisher of this Work have made every effort to use sources believed to be reliable to provide information that is accurate and compatible with the standards generally accepted at the time of publication. Because medical science is continually advancing, our knowledge base continues to expand. Therefore, as new information becomes available, changes in procedures become necessary. We recommend that the reader always consult current research and specific institutional policies before performing any clinical procedure. The author and publisher shall not be liable for any special, consequential, or exemplary damages resulting, in whole or in part, from the readers' use of, or reliance on, the information contained in this book. The publisher has no responsibility for the persistence or accuracy of URLs for external or third-party Internet Web sites referred to in this publication and does not guarantee that any content on such Web sites is, or will remain, accurate or appropriate.

Library of Congress Cataloging-in-Publication Data
Nurses on the front line : when disaster strikes, 1878–2010 / [edited by] Barbra Mann Wall, Arlene Keeling.
    p. ; cm.
    Includes bibliographical references.
    ISBN 978-0-8261-0519-6
    1. Disaster nursing — United States — History. I. Wall, Barbra Mann. II. Keeling, Arlene Wynbeek, 1948-
    [DNLM: 1. Disasters—history—United States. 2. Nurse's Role—history—United States. 3. History, 19th Century—United States. 4. History, 20th Century—United States. 5. History, 21st Century—United States.
    WY 11 AA1]
    RT116.N87 2010
    610.73'49—dc22

                                                                            2010026537

Printed in the United States of America by Hamilton Printing.

Contents

PART II

Contributors

Patricia A. Connor Ballard, APRN-BC, MSN, PhD, Director of the Inova Learning Network, Inova Health System, Falls Church, VA

Patricia D'Antonio, PhD, RN, FAAN, Associate Professor of Nursing and Division Chair, Family and Community Health, University of Pennsylvania School of Nursing, Philadelphia, PA

Julie A. Fairman, PhD, RN, FAAN, Professor of Nursing and Director of the Barbara Bates Center for the Study of the History of Nursing, University of Pennsylvania School of Nursing, Philadelphia, PA

Jonathan Gilbride, MSN, RN, Pediatric Nurse Practitioner, New York, NY

Marie E. Kelly, MSN, RN, Nursing Informatics Specialist, Children's Hospital of Philadelphia, Philadelphia, PA

John C. Kirchgessner, PhD, RN, PNP-BC, Assistant Professor of Nursing, St. Johns Fisher College, Rochester, NY, and Assistant Director, Center for Nursing Historical Inquiry, The University of Virginia, Charlottesville, VA.

Deanne Stephens Nuwer, PhD, Associate Professor of History, University of Southern Mississippi, Hattiesburg, MS

Teresa M. O'Neill, PhD, RNC, MN, APRN, Professor of Nursing, Our Lady of Holy Cross College, New Orleans, LA

Patricia M. Prechter, EdD, RN, MSN, Professor of Nursing, Associate Vice President and Dean for Academic Affairs, Chair of the Department of Nursing and Allied Health, Our Lady of Holy Cross College, New Orleans, LA; Col. (retired) Louisiana Army National Guard, State Chief Nurse and Deputy Commander, Louisiana Medical Command

Deborah A. Sampson, PhD, MSN, FNP-BC, CS, Assistant Professor, Boston College Connell School of Nursing, Chestnut Hill, MA

Audrey Snyder, PhD, RN, ACNP, CEN, FAANP, FAEN, Assistant Professor, University of Virginia School of Nursing, Charlottesville

Fusun Terzioglu, PhD, MSc, RN, Associate Professor and Vice President of the Nursing Department, Hacettepe University, Ankara, Turkey

Jean C. Whelan, PhD, RN, Adjunct Assistant Professor of Nursing and Assistant Director of the Barbara Bates Center for the Study of the History of Nursing, University of Pennsylvania School of Nursing, Philadelphia

Preface

Just before 5:00 p.m., January 12, 2010, a violent earthquake (magnitude 7.0) struck the Haitian capital of Port-au-Prince, leveling the entire city.[1] According to a photographer on the scene, "It was general mayhem": buildings crumpled, shantytown homes destroyed, tens of thousands injured and dead.[2] As the chaos unfolded, newscasters broadcast the disaster on television and the Internet, often over broken and intermittent satellite links. The desperate need was first for water and relief supplies, and second for heavy equipment to move tons of rubble. Doctors and nurses who could treat devastating injuries and administer lifesaving antibiotics and intravenous fluids were also in high demand, as were volunteer aid workers and military personnel.

The earthquake and the effects of the aftershocks were far reaching. The capital's main hospital had crumpled, and makeshift treatment centers were soon overwhelmed. Roads were completely destroyed or blocked with traffic and rubble, complicating relief and evacuation efforts. By January 17, despite assistance from countries all over the world, 300,000 Haitians and visitors were living in the streets and in temporary camps throughout the region. According to the United Nations Secretary General, it was the worst humanitarian crisis in decades.[3] By February 12, Haitian officials estimated that 230,000 people had died.[4]

The scenes depicted on the continuous TV and Internet newscasts showed helicopters dropping food packages to survivors, cargo planes being unloaded in the only available airport, Red Cross workers dispensing food and water, and emergency rescue teams digging out those who were still alive. The images were reminiscent of those broadcast in other recent disasters, including the September 11, 2001, terrorist attack on New York's World Trade Center, the Sumatra tsunami in 2004, and Hurricane Katrina in 2005. They were also typical of those depicted on the front pages of newspapers over a century ago when an earthquake devastated San Francisco in 1906.[5]

Storms and fires also wreak havoc with communities, killing and injuring people and leaving others homeless. Take, for example, one 2009 Internet news report documenting the effects of a series of disasters:

> In little more than one week, a series of horrific natural disasters has carved a swath of destruction from the tiny island of Samoa west to a massive section of Southern India. . . . Typhoon Ketsana hit the Philippines on Saturday, September 24, 2009, dumping a month's worth of monsoon rain in twelve hours. Wednesday, September 30, a series of earthquakes rocked Sumatra in Indonesia, and Samoa and Tonga in the South Pacific. Later that week monsoon rains in Southern India caused flooding worse than any seen in that country in at least sixty years. Current reports say as many as 2.5 million people have been affected by the floods.[6]

A few days later, another Internet news account reported that a fire in the San Bernardino National Forest, driven by winds of 40 miles per hour, destroyed homes in southern California and threatened others, driving residents to evacuation centers in nearby towns.[7]

In addition to natural and human-made disasters, epidemics of infectious diseases periodically sweep through a country or the world, causing widespread illness and numerous deaths. In the spring of 2009, for example, H1N1 influenza erupted in Mexico and quickly became pandemic. Meanwhile, avian influenza (H5N1) looms on the horizon as a threat to the world community, and gushing oil in the Gulf of Mexico destroys an entire ecosystem.

DISASTER PREPAREDNESS

Since September 11, 2001, when New York's World Trade Center collapsed after a terrorist attack, the United States has placed an increasing emphasis on disaster preparedness. Recently, schools have developed nursing programs for disaster preparation, and nursing faculty have published textbooks on the subject. In her book *Disaster Nursing and Emergency Preparedness*, author Tener Goodwin Veenema observed that because nurses constitute the largest sector of the health care workforce in the United States, they will "certainly be on the front lines of any emergency response."[8] Indeed, nurses have been on the front lines of disaster response throughout history—triaging patients, providing immediate care in emergency rooms, administering requisite vaccines to the community, and providing psychological support.

What nurses did in the past can inform disaster preparations for today. As nurse historian Ellen Baer asserts, "The historian investigates past experience, examining assumptions, attitudes, interests, and points of view so that past events can be carefully understood, present possibilities accurately assessed, and future interventions appropriately undertaken."[9] In order for nurses' experiences in past disasters to be useful today, however, they must be made explicit. Unfortunately, nurses' work in disasters is often overlooked in the news coverage at the time and in the history books. After all, caring for the sick and injured is what nurses do routinely. This book attempts to fill that gap by recognizing the nursing contributions in past disasters—essentially providing historical evidence to inform disaster policies for the future.

The book is more than a simple narrative. It examines and analyzes, within the historical context of the period, the nurses' roles in responding to specific disasters from the late nineteenth through the early twenty first centuries. Disasters that occurred in various regions in the United States, Canada, Turkey, and Haiti are examined. Thus, the book provides a window on nurses and their activities in many different disaster scenes, examining their work in the context of different times and places. Natural disasters such as earthquakes and hurricanes and those caused by unexpected accidents or intentional or unintentional human error are highlighted.

The nurse's role as part of a community response is specifically analyzed. It will be shown that the ways in which nurses responded to disasters often were framed by a desire to restore stability in the aftermath of a chaotic event. Analysis of the nurses' actions supports historian Patricia D'Antonio's thesis that nurses worked as members of families and communities.[10] They responded with improvised activities at the local and national scenes in collaborative efforts with others. At the same time, the book demonstrates that disasters temporarily unraveled stable gendered, social, racial, geographical, and professional boundaries.

The book's significance thus is threefold. First and foremost, it documents the nursing experience in several major disasters that occurred from 1878 to the present, filling a gap in health care history. Nurses are primary contact persons with patients, whether during calamitous events or routine day-to-day care in hospitals, homes, outpatient and public health facilities, government agencies. Because of their unique role with patients, they are in a position to participate in all aspects of the disaster response, including evacuation, triage, physical and psychological care at the scene and afterward, case finding, screening measures, vaccinations, and disease surveillance. Second, it is important that nurses have a clear understanding of what to expect during disasters. This book illuminates lessons learned from previous calamities for use in disaster preparation today. Finally, it argues for not forgetting the roles of race, class, and gender in any model for disaster response. The book shows that, while traditional categorizations of race, class, and gender blurred during disasters and often ruptured altogether, these resumed after the crisis passed.

While the disasters that make up the book are organized chronologically and geographically, themes are identified that cut across time and place. These include (1) improvised activities at the local and national scenes; (2) cooperation and collaboration among previously established professional and social networks; (3) leadership and courage; (4) spontaneous community support; (5) restoration of order out of chaos; (6) the creation of healing narratives; and (7) the crossing of cultural, geographical, and professional boundaries in response to the crisis. Yet disasters are not tidy; conflicts occurred that also will be discussed. Patricia D'Antonio and Jean C. Whelan's opening chapter introduces each of the disasters. Following that, the book uses numerous case studies that demonstrate how nurses' roles at the local level intersected with the American Red Cross, the American Nurses Association, the U.S. Public Health Service, the military, and other federal and state organizations, and how this intersection changed over time.

The book also highlights policy implications of the different disasters, particularly focusing on the federal government's response. Before 1950, the federal government provided negligible assistance to communities suffering from a disaster. Local and private voluntary agencies such as the American Red Cross took primary responsibility.[11] It was not until 1950, after a series of hurricanes hit the East Coast, that the Disaster Relief Act became the first permanent disaster law passed by Congress. The Alaska earthquake, described in chapter 10, was one of the first single disasters to directly lead to policy legislation: the Alaskan Earthquake Assistance Act in 1964. After the Federal Disaster Relief Act of 1970, the federal government assumed the role as the primary provider of funds and expertise to deal with disasters. The Federal Emergency Management Agency was not established until 1979.[12]

REMEMBERING DISASTERS

Some caveats are in order. All of the disasters in this book provided the impetus for reflection by health care workers, survivors, and organizations in the form of letters, memoirs, oral histories, newspaper stories, and professional publications that are preserved in accessible archives. Many of the sources, however, are recollections of eyewitnesses who reconstructed the events, which involved creating a version of the past.[13] Sometimes people "remember" not only what they did but what they wish they had done, or what they believed they were doing at the time. Furthermore, in many stories, time allows the interviewees to "rewrite" events in their own minds, and they recall what they now think their actions were.[14] Thus, their memoirs, letters, and publications only tell a partial story. While they help reconstruct a representation of the past, some of their views need to be corroborated by other sources, such as newspaper accounts or official Red Cross reports. Still, these stories can serve as important sources for historians interested in the experiences of people who typically do not leave written documents.[15]

In addition to the simple telling of the story, the ways writers, journalists, filmmakers, city leaders, and survivors themselves *interpret* and *commemorate* disasters are important. Indeed, how "people apprehend, feel, and process . . . [or] narrate . . . calamities," helps them "make sense of that which seems most senseless." In this respect, the book contributes to theoretical formulations on disasters by Kevin Rozario, who argues that, when buildings are destroyed, "it is necessary not only to manufacture new material structures but also to repair torn cultural fabrics and damaged psyches."[16] As the case studies in this book show, people not only rebuilt physical structures after the disasters but also constructed stories that facilitated emotional and psychological recovery. Their reactions were historically grounded in the writers' own circumstances and purposes for writing. If one keeps these issues in mind, these sources can provide insights into how specific groups of people constructed meaning in their lives and work.

After disasters, nurses, doctors, and other health care professionals performed feats of dedication and self-sacrifice. Yet viewing disasters through the lens of history shows that disasters occur not in a vacuum but within a complex social and political context. Each of the disasters represented in this book occurred in a particular time and place that informed local responses. History's contribution to disasters brings complexity and context to debates over what are appropriate and inappropriate responses. In considering this complex social and political context, each chapter concludes with discussion questions that raise contextual and ethical issues. Contextual issues include an analysis of nursing leadership within a specific time period and a consideration of the disciplinary boundaries of nursing in that period. Ethical issues include nurses' duty to care, their struggles with triaging dilemmas, and the experience of moral distress. As one considers these questions, it becomes increasingly clear that time and place matter; that historical context does indeed shape the community response to any disaster.

NOTES

1. http://www.nytimes.com/2010/01/13/world/americas/13haiti.html
2. Ibid.
3. U.N. Secretary General, MSNBC newscast, January 17, 2010.
4. Mead Over, "Death Toll From Haiti's Earthquake in Perspective," http://blogs.cgdev.org/globalhealth/2010/02/death-toll-from-haiti%E2%80%99s-earthquake-in-perspective.php (accessed March 11, 2010).
5. For a definition of disaster, see Tener Goodwin Veenema, *Disaster Nursing and Emergency Preparedness* (New York: Springer Publishing, 2007), 4–5.
6. Liz O'Neill and Michael Hill, "Seeking Survivors after Asian-Pacific Catastrophes," http://crs.org/indonesia/earthquakes-typhoon&?utm_source=google-grant&utm_medium, p. 1 (accessed October 15, 2009).
7. "Southern California Forest Fire Destroys 3 Homes," October 15, 2009, http://www.cbsnews.com/stories/2009/10/04/ap/national/main5361617.shtml
8. Veenema, *Disaster Nursing and Emergency Preparedness*, 4.
9. Ellen D. Baer, "Introduction," in *Enduring Issues in American Nursing*, eds. Ellen D. Baer, Patricia D'Antonio, Sylvia Rinker, and Joan E. Lynaugh (New York: Springer Publishing Company, 2001), 8.
10. Patricia D'Antonio, "Nurses—And Wives and Mothers: Women and the Latter Day Saints Training School's Class of 1919," *Journal of Women's History* 19, no. 3 (2007): 112–136. See also Patricia D'Antonio, *American Nursing: A History of Knowledge, Authority, and the Meaning of Work* (Baltimore: Johns Hopkins University Press, 2010).
11. G.A. Kreps, "The Federal Emergency Management System in the United States: Past and Present," *International Journal of Mass Emergencies and Disasters* 8, no. 3 (1990): 281. C. B. Rubin, ed., *Emergency Management: The American Experience, 1900–2005* (Fairfax, VA: Public Entity Risk Institute, 2007).

12. Rutherford H. Platt, *Disasters and Democracy: The Politics of Extreme Natural Events* (Washington, DC: Island Press, 1999), 12–15.
13. P. Hamilton, "The Oral Historian as Memorist," *Oral History Review* 32, no. 1 (2005): 11–18; D. Pollock, ed., *Remembering: Oral History as Performance* (New York: Palgrave Macmillan, 2005): and Barbra Mann Wall, Nancy Edwards, and Marjorie Porter, "Textual Analysis of Retired Nurses' Oral Histories," *Nursing Inquiry*, 14, no. 4 (2007): 279–288.
14. Alessandro Portelli, *The Battle of Valle Giulia: Oral History and the Art of Dialogue* (Madison: University of Wisconsin Press, 1997).
15. M. Confino, "Some Random Thoughts on History's Recent Past," *History & Memory* 12, no. 2 (2001): 29–55; and P. Winn, "History and Memory: Perspectives on the Past," transcript of audio clip available at http://www.learner.org/channel/courses/worldhistory/unit_transcript_2.html (accessed August 31, 2006).
16. Kevin Rozario, "Making Progress: Disaster Narratives and the Art of Optimism in Modern America," in *The Resilient City: How Modern Cities Recover From Disaster*, eds. Lawrence J. Vale and Thomas J. Campanella (New York: Oxford University Press, 2005), 32.

Acknowledgments

The American Nurses Foundation through Grant 2008-003, generously supported the research for chapter 3, "The San Francisco Earthquake and Fire, 1906: 'A Lifetime of Experience'"; chapter 7, "The 1921 Tulsa Race Riot and the 'Angels of Mercy'"; and chapter 8, "The New London, Texas, School Explosion, 1937: 'Unparalleled Disaster.'"

Chapter 5, "Nurses' Response Across Geographic Boundaries in the Halifax Disaster, December 6, 1917: Border Crossings," was supported by the Barbara Brodie Nursing History Fellowship, Center for Nursing Historical Inquiry, University of Virginia School of Nursing, Charlottesville, Virginia.

Portions of the following articles were used with permission from the publishers: Barbra Mann Wall, "Healing After Disasters in Early Twentieth-Century Texas," *Advances in Nursing Science*, 31, no. 3 (2008): 211–224; Julie A. Fairman and Jonathan Gilbride, "Gendered Notions of Expertise and Bravery," *Journal of the History of Medicine and Allied Sciences* 58, no.4 (2004): 442–449; and Patricia D'Antonio and Jean Whelan, "Moments When Time Stood Still: A Look at the History of Nursing During Disasters," *American Journal of Nursing* 104, no. 11 (2004): 66–72. Portions of the following book were used with permission from the publisher: Deanne Stephens Nuwer, *Plague Among the Magnolias: The 1878 Yellow Fever Epidemic in Mississippi* (Tuscaloosa: University of Alabama Press, 2009).

The authors also acknowledge the Sisters of Charity of the Incarnate Word, Villa de Matel Archives, Houston, Texas; and the Sisters of Providence, Providence Archives, Mother Joseph Province, Seattle, Washington.

Introduction

Patricia D'Antonio and Jean C. Whelan

As the horrors of September 11, 2001, unfolded in New York City, suburban Virginia, and rural Pennsylvania, the little comfort there was to be had came from knowing that hundreds, if not thousands, of our fellow nurses, physicians, and other rescue and relief workers had mobilized to care for the victims and their families. Their brave and heroic work served their patients and their professions well. As they triaged and treated individuals, calmed and comforted families, and coordinated the flow of material aid and other kinds of assistance, these nurses carried on a tradition of disaster relief that reminds us all just what it means to be a professional.

Yet, historically, formally trained nurses had to prove their worth in disaster relief. Conventional wisdom had long held that in the chaos and confusion of disasters, sheer brawn was better than brains; only men possessed the courage to risk possible death, and women's responsibilities lay just with their immediate families. These histories about nursing in disaster relief, then, are more than just chronicles of bravery, compassion, and skill: They also tell a story about the growth and evolution of a profession. In honor of those who nursed the victims of September 11, 2001, we remember other moments when nurses came to the aid of those stricken by disasters. Part I of this book examines historical disasters, while part II looks at nursing in contemporary disasters.

Part I begins with the yellow fever epidemic of 1878. In midsummer of that year, yellow fever, a terrifying disease endemic to tropical climates, with no known cause, few effective treatments, and an extraordinarily high mortality rate, was developing in the lower Mississippi valley. In chapter 1, Deanne Stephens Nuwer describes this epidemic, the expanded role played by nurses, and the role that race played in this racially reactionary society. Provisions and financial aid came from a variety of sources, both within the state and without. Still, as efforts to contain this outbreak failed, local relief efforts were overwhelmed. Among those who nursed in Mississippi's yellow fever epidemic were religious orders of women, such as the Sisters of Charity, who had a long history of helping the poor in Mississippi. Of the 12 sisters who nursed in the epidemic, 6 died.

Another group of nurses came from the Howard Association, a benevolent organization with roots in New Orleans. Both Black and White women and men worked as nurses for the Howard Association. Separate facilities existed for Whites and Blacks, but the Howards helped provide needed provisions and medical and nursing care for all. If not for these nurses' services, suffering would have been much greater.

In chapter 2, Barbra Mann Wall explores the work of nurses after September 8, 1900, when a monstrous hurricane completely destroyed the barrier island of Galveston, Texas. Winds of over 125 miles per hour pushed waters from both the Gulf of Mexico and Galveston Bay together in a storm surge that left 6,000 to 8,000 dead and 25,000 homeless. The hurricane was the worst single disaster in American history. Wall asserts that nurses worked not only as clinicians in hospitals and community health areas but also as members of their families and communities. These workers included Clara Barton, the founder of the American Red Cross, who traveled to Galveston in what would become her last relief mission to personally deliver aid to the survivors. Barton's recollections also spoke to the savage toll disasters exacted on both survivors and relief workers. Galveston had to burn fires day and night for weeks to control the spread of diseases caused by decaying human corpses and animal carcasses. As Barton remembered, "that peculiar smell of burning flesh, so sickening at first, became horribly familiar within the next two months, when we lived in it and breathed it, day after day."[1]

In actions typical of Barton's policy of restarting local work, she helped revive the area's economy by providing strawberry plants to farmers who had been accustomed to supplying the earliest strawberries to northern markets. The hurricane had washed away every plant, and no money was available to buy more. Barton resigned from the Red Cross in 1904, and the following year the agency reorganized to begin actual nursing and medical services during wartime and disaster.

In chapter 3, Barbra Mann Wall and Marie E. Kelly bring together the dramatic experiences of nurses and other health care workers who witnessed the terrible events of April 18, 1906, when an earthquake struck San Francisco. San Francisco was already infamous throughout the country and the world for its repeated earthquakes and fires. But when the "Great Earthquake," as it would become known, finally struck the city at 5:13 on the morning of April 18, 1906, the subsequent "Seventh Great Fire" destroyed whatever remained standing. More than 250,000 people were left homeless, and recent estimates suggest 3,000 died from earthquake- and fire-related causes. The magnitude of relief needs overwhelmed the combined resources of both the U.S. Army and the American Red Cross. San Francisco's Chinese communities found their needs ignored. And there simply were not enough trained nurses available to assist the sick and wounded.

Wall and Kelly examine sources that have not been previously noted in historical literature on disasters. They draw from materials published in 1906 and 1907 in the form of letters and written reminiscences by nurses who were present at the time. These documents articulate the meanings of the experiences to nurses themselves and the implications for nursing's image of itself as a caring profession.

The San Francisco earthquake brought significant structural changes in the way nursing organized formal disaster relief efforts. The American Red Cross worked with the American Nurses Association to expedite a reorganization plan that had been established in 1905. Local nursing organizations joined forces with area Red Cross chapters; new standards for nursing volunteers met professional criteria; and, most important, the Red Cross created its National Committee on Nursing Service under the leadership of Jane Delano, then superintendent of the Army Nurse Corps and president of the American Nurses Association. Delano died in 1919 while visiting American nurses assisting French war relief efforts, but the Red Cross nursing service she established served her country in war, disasters, and emergencies through the twentieth century.

Mining disasters in the early twentieth century were horrendously common, with 18 coal mine disasters in 1907 alone. What still ranks as the country's worst mining disaster is the Monongah coal mine explosion of that year, in which 361 men and boys died. In chapter 4, John Kirchgessner illustrates how miners overcame class and ethnic conflicts in the response to the Monongah disaster. Descriptions of several workers who either died or barely escaped the disaster are powerful, and he relates how the unwritten Miners' Code guided the response team such that no one was left behind. This disaster stirred the country to give greater attention to safety conditions for miners, and it led Congress to create the Bureau of Mines.

Ten years later, on December 6, 1917, during World War I, a harbor collision and subsequent explosion devastated the North American seaport city of Halifax, Nova Scotia. In chapter 5, Deborah A. Sampson analyzes how and why nurses crossed geographic boundaries to provide care amid chaos. Nurses from Halifax, other parts of Canada, and the New England states worked together in hospitals, dressing stations, and damaged homes. Indeed, Halifax and different areas in New England shared a heritage of refuge, collaboration, and cooperation. The chapter illustrates the interrelatedness of American and Canadian nursing history and culture and serves as an example of collaboration typical of Canada-U.S. relations.

Chapter 6, by Arlene W. Keeling, shows how nurses in Boston played a critical role in the 1918 influenza pandemic that spread around the globe—it was the most devastating pandemic in recorded world history. Ironically, the parades and parties that celebrated the end of World War I in November 1918 ultimately provided, in their crowds of tightly packed people, further fuel for the influenza fire. When in the winter of 1919 the pandemic finally subsided, 20 to 40 million people lay dead worldwide. In the United States alone, influenza claimed over 675,000 lives. In response, the average life span of Americans decreased by 10 years, because most victims were between the ages of 20 and 40.

Nurses helped prevent the further spread of influenza and reduced the severity of the pandemic. They taught individuals, families, and communities the key principles of respiratory hygiene, hand washing, disinfection of household utensils, and the critical importance of wearing gauze masks in public. Of course, nurses also cared for those stricken. Many, however, found themselves in the uncomfortable position of enforcing a legally binding quarantine or period of isolation on often unwilling patients.

The influenza pandemic had many heroes and heroic stories. The unacknowledged heroes of the pandemic, however, were the student nurses who provided almost all the nursing care delivered in American hospitals. Most stayed by their patients' bedsides despite pleas from family and friends that they see to their own safety. Untold hundreds of American student nurses died.

The Tulsa Race Riot of 1921 was not only one of the most violent racial confrontations in America, but it has also been one of the most marginalized. Attempts by members of Tulsa's African American community to protect one of their own from a lynching erupted into a night of violence that left 300 dead, hundreds more wounded, and the entire African American neighborhood of Greenwood destroyed. Some White entrepreneurs exploited the situation by taking photos and selling them as postcards. The story of the Tulsa Race Riot has only recently become part of our national history. In chapter 7, Barbra Mann Wall shows how the American Red Cross quickly sent nurses and physicians to Tulsa to treat and care for all the survivors, regardless of race. As a result, Black Tulsans referred to them as the "Angels of Mercy." A legacy of its work after the 1921 race riot was that the Red Cross became the top responder to both natural and human-made disasters across the country.

On March 18, 1937, a natural gas leak in a school in New London, Texas, caused an immense explosion while school was in session. More than 300 children and 14 teachers died, making it the worst catastrophe to take place in a U.S. school building. In chapter 8, Barbra Mann Wall examines survivors' narratives and the city's commemoration activities that took place after this disaster as means of healing and restoration. Survivors revealed the great difficulty and pain of reconstructing an event and the guilt that they survived while others did not. Narratives also illustrated pride that the people rebuilt the school, a memorial, and a museum. Wall asserts that part of the nurse's role is to help survivors of disasters to establish meanings and thereby regain control over their lives and futures.

Wall also argues that contextual factors of time and place shaped the ways in which people made sense of their disaster experiences. She interprets the different experiences of people within a framework of "place" that includes not only the influence of geography but also culture, economics, class, race, and religion. In addition to describing nurses' work for survivors, Wall describes a significant policy change that occurred after the school disaster. Survivors successfully petitioned the state legislature to require that a malodorant be used in all gases so that future leaks could be detected.

In chapter 9, Patricia A. Connor Ballard describes the Cocoanut Grove nightclub fire of 1942. On the evening of November 28, 1942, a busboy at Boston's popular Cocoanut Grove nightclub accidentally set fire to some decorative bunting. Within seconds, the entire club erupted in flames. Within minutes, 492 people lay dead, and as many were injured in what was then the worst fire in recorded history. Boston's hospitals were overwhelmed not only with critically burned survivors but also with distraught friends and families.

Critical care nurses credit the immediate aftermath of the Cocoanut Grove fire as one of the seminal events in the development of their specialty. Massive numbers of burn victims tested not only their triage skills but also their ability to manage and maintain fluid volumes, shock, skin integrity, structural alignments, and pain control. Also, in the inevitable panic and pandemonium of the fire's aftermath, nurses and physicians discovered the power of attending to the emotional as well as physical needs. Our understanding of normal grief reactions came directly from Erich Lindemann's work with the survivors and the families of the Cocoanut Grove fire. Less well known is how nurses learned to care for the caretakers. Stories abound of nurses and others working for hours in emergency rooms and then seeking temporary respite among less draining chores in their hospital's laundries and kitchens.

The Great Alaska Earthquake occurred on Good Friday, March 27, 1964. All across south central Alaska, buildings collapsed, huge fissures opened in the ground, and tsunamis directly led to 131 deaths. The earthquake caused property damage of more than $750 million and was felt as far away as the Gulf of Mexico. In chapter 10, Barbra Mann Wall analyzes what has been viewed as a competent disaster response as nurses worked in hospitals, mass shelters, and public health programs in Anchorage and coastal areas of Kodiak Island, Seward, and Valdez that were heavily damaged. Specifically, she focuses on Providence Hospital in Anchorage and public health agencies in the state.

After the earthquake, priorities included preservation of life, restoration and maintenance of utilities and communication, and reestablishment of order. Wall explores nurses' work in both inpatient and public health facilities such as shelters and immunization clinics, and the role that gender played in their responses. She shows that widespread panic did not occur as nurses provided leadership, screening measures, triage, vaccinations, and disease surveillance. Furthermore, the Alaska earthquake directly led to policy legislation with the passage of the Alaskan Earthquake Assistance Act in 1964.

Part II opens with chapter 11, in which Julie A. Fairman and Jonathan Gilbride analyze the gendered nature of disaster responses through the "hospital stories" of a nurse who worked in a burn unit on September 11, 2001. Told by a nurse who is male, the stories demonstrate scientific and technical language, "a militarist sense of preparation for war." The authors argue that, during disasters, policies and protocols no longer applied as expediency and patients' needs took priority. Traditional boundaries between health professionals blurred as professionals focused on "getting the job done."

In chapter 12, two nurses who lived through the destruction of Hurricane Katrina and worked in shelters during and after the hurricane tell their own stories: Teresa M. O'Neill, who volunteered at a shelter west of New Orleans, in Gonzales, Louisiana; and Patricia M. Prechter, a colonel in the Louisiana National Guard who nursed at the New Orleans' Superdome. They recount their days leading up to the hurricane, the storm itself, and their work in its aftermath. Hurricane Katrina was one of the deadliest hurricanes in our nation's history. It struck New Orleans on the morning of August 29, 2005, causing a storm surge that breached the city's levees and floodwalls and caused massive flooding. It also destroyed other cities on the Gulf of Mexico coast, along with 150 miles of coastline. More than 1,800 people died.

The authors show how nurses responded to a need, whether dictated by military command or through a desire to be of service during the disaster. This chapter also illutrates the expansion of nurse's roles as they participated in diagnosis, prescription, and treatment, and they made significant differences in medical and nursing outcomes. They were proud to represent nursing and were prepared to face the many challenges they encountered, including threats to their own safety. At the same time, the authors caution readers about the contingency of hurricane planning, and they call for flexibility and organization, the hallmarks of experienced nurses, in implementing disaster plans.

Like the other chapters in part II, chapter 13, by Audrey Snyder, Fusun Terzioglu, and Arlene W. Keeling, is not a history. Many histories on the Turkey and Haiti earthquakes of the early twenty first century will be written in the years to come. This chapter instead examines the aftermath of earthquakes at the international scene as thousands of homeless people congregated in tent cities. These camps created not only public health risks but also psychological challenges when individuals were cut off from their main means of support.

The book's concluding chapter, by Barbra Mann Wall and Arlene W. Keeling, reflects on common themes. The chapters gathered in this book show that, indeed, contextual factors of time and place influenced both the methods and efficacies of disaster responses.

NOTE

1. Clara Barton, "To the People of the United States," 1900 Storm Online Manuscript Exhibit, Red Cross Records, MSS #05-000, p. 18. http://www.gthcenter. org/exhibits/storms/1900/Manuscripts/RedCross_7/index.html (accessed July 5, 2006).

Part I

CHAPTER 1

The 1878 Yellow Fever Epidemic in Mississippi:"For God's Sake, Send Us Some Nurses and Doctors"

Deanne Stephens Nuwer

For God's sake, send us some nurses and doctors. All down with fever. We are destitute.[1]

On September 4, 1878, citizens in Holly Springs, Mississippi, telegraphed Governor John Stone requesting more nurses and physicians. City officials had just declared a yellow fever epidemic in the city. In the late nineteenth century United States, the appearance of yellow fever was a cause of major concern. Because of its virulence, the yellow fever epidemic of 1878 was particularly challenging. Its cause was unknown, plus it spread extensively through the South. From July to October, 1878, 28% of the stricken individuals in Mississippi died. Blacks also contracted the fever, although only 7% died. There is no consensus explanation for this disparity, although possible exposure to the disease in Africa may have provided Blacks with some inherited resistance. Mistakenly thought to be immune to the disease, many Blacks nursed the ill in Mississippi, alongside Whites and Catholic sisters.

Although three nurse training schools based on the Nightingale model had been established in the 1870s in New York, New Haven, and Boston, nurses, for the most part, trained with others who practiced rudimentary nursing skills or learned by trial and error in hospital settings. Such was the case with nurses who helped tend the sick in multiple yellow fever epidemics across the South in the mid- to late-nineteenth century.

Particularly challenging to the medical and civilian population was the yellow fever epidemic of 1878 because of its extensive swath of infection. Examination of the 1878 yellow fever epidemic in Mississippi reveals a microcosmic view of the epidemic as it played out through the South and highlights the significant roles nurses played in this catastrophe.

By 1878, Mississippi had a long history of efforts to control the dreaded contagion by establishing quarantines early. In 1799, lawmakers in the state prohibited vessels or immigrants with a contagious disease such as yellow fever from entering the then-U.S. territory. Later, officials added a $2,000 fine or 12-month prison sentence to those individuals who knowingly brought a contagious disease into the region. Efforts to curtail the spread of diseases continued after Mississippi entered the Union in 1817 and culminated with the creation of the Mississippi State Board of Health in 1877.[2] Nonetheless, regardless of the measures taken to curb its spread, yellow fever regularly appeared in the state, particularly among the populations who lived along the river and in railroad towns where people migrated, seeking safety during times of an outbreak.

Once a person contracted yellow fever from an infected *Aedes aegypti* mosquito carrier, the disease caused a horrific response that usually appeared within four days. The stricken person exhibited a high fever often soaring to 102° and 104°, flushed face, bloodshot eyes, and shaking chills. Repeatedly, victims complained of severe back and extremity pain. Accompanying these symptoms was severe damage to the liver, kidneys, and heart. Death resulted in the more serious cases from renal failure, heart failure, toxemia, and internal infections. Mild infections of the disease often go undiagnosed because yellow fever can appear to be a simple cold with flu-like symptoms. Recovery in this case begins within a week or two after contracting the disease. A full convalescence for severe cases requires complete bed rest and stringent nursing care, often for several weeks.[3]

During the 1878 yellow fever epidemic, private relief organizations, including those that provided nursing care, assumed the overwhelming responsibility of caring for those citizens stricken with the fever. Mississippi health officers were unable to provide the necessary funds to ensure adequate nursing treatment because of economic problems and political constraints. The newly created Mississippi State Board of Health (1877) simply could not cope with the crushing numbers of cases as it lacked money and the means to enforce its suggestions; it was basically an advisory board in its early stages. Therefore, parochial and private groups stepped in to fill the vacuum.

CATHOLIC SISTER NURSES

The Sisters of Charity religious order had a history of helping Mississippians prior to the yellow fever epidemic of 1878. They had been active during the Civil War, particularly in the area around Holly Springs.[4] When officials announced yellow fever in Holly Springs, Sisters of Charity quickly requisitioned the Marshall County Courthouse and turned it into a hospital. The beds for yellow fever patients were simple straw piles that could be easily swept out to clean. Father Anacletus Oberti, the local priest from St. Joseph's Catholic Church, directed the 12 sisters. These volunteer nurses exhibited remarkable devotion toward their patients. They labored long hours under the guidance of Howard Association doctors, many of whom were physicians from outside of Mississippi (see p. 4). One contemporary described the nursing work the sisters administered in the following manner: "Like angels of mercy, they hovered over the loathsome spot day and night, caring not who the patient might be if only his life could be spared. One by one these sisters fell until six of them, with the faithful priest, Father Oberti, lay dead".[5] A single monument marks their collective grave in Holly Springs. Doctor Swearingen, the Howard Association doctor who worked alongside the sisters at the courthouse hospital, was so moved by Sister Corinthia's devotion to her patients and her self-sacrificing manner that he scratched a tribute to her on a wall in the courthouse hospital following her death. The epitaph remains there to this day.[6]

The Sisters of Charity in Holly Springs labored unceasingly to nurse the sick and dying, Black and White. According to one account, they "took charge of the main hospital and did not shrink from anything and did not spare themselves from the work of mercy."[7]

Another religious order that provided nursing care to Mississippians in 1878 was the Sisters of Mercy. Founded in 1831 by Catherine McAuley, an Irish Catholic laywoman who wanted to help the economically poor, this order lived and worked in Vicksburg during the 1878 epidemic. The Vicksburg facility had been established in 1860 and was part of the original foundation of this Irish order when it spread to the Americas, which eventually came under the umbrella of the Sisters of Mercy of the Americas, St. Louis Regional Community. The foundation's early ministries focused on health care and education. The sisters also were instrumental in providing nursing care to both Confederate and Union soldiers during the Civil War, as the siege of Vicksburg was a pivotal battle that witnessed thousands of causalities on both sides.[8]

The model of individual attention and hygienic measures provided to Civil War soldiers was also the standard for tending to yellow fever victims in 1878 Vicksburg. St. Paul's Catholic Church remained open as a refuge for those with the disease in the city. The sisters would also go to patients' homes and care for the sick. During the epidemic, Sisters of Mercy were also active in Arkansas, Missouri, and Louisiana as they helped to relieve the suffering of those people stricken with yellow fever.[9]

The Sisters of Mercy were some of the few remaining citizens in Vicksburg in October 1878 because the city was virtually a town of death. Only doctors, nurses, and health officials traveled there to help the sick and dying. Father John McManus and his assistant, Father John Vitolo, both died of yellow fever along with four Sisters of Mercy during the epidemic. One, Sister Mary Regis, was from Copiah County, Mississippi, and had just entered the convent on February 23, 1878. Sister Mary Bernadine Murray was also a recent arrival to the convent, having entered less than a year before, on December 21, 1877. Both of these new sisters worked tirelessly ministering to the suffering citizens of Vicksburg, until they, too, lay among the dead. Another member of the order, Sister Mary Vincent, traveled to Meridian, Mississippi, with a small group "to bring peace and comfort to the parting soul" of all who died of yellow fever. She was unable to complete the trip between Vicksburg and Meridian because of the shotgun quarantine in place on the railroad line. The conductor of the train forced the sisters to disembark 10 miles from Meridian at the small village of Chunky, since the train could not enter Meridian. The sisters received warm hospitality at Chunky until they finally made their way back to Vicksburg. Sister Mary Vincent lived through the 1878 epidemic.[10] Nurses such as the Sisters of Mercy and the Sisters of Charity were needed throughout Mississippi during this epidemic as communities continued to struggle with overwhelming numbers of cases and fatalities. Further north, the city of Holly Springs was no different.

THE HOWARD ASSOCIATION NURSES

A major charitable organization that played a key role during the 1878 epidemic was the Howards. The group first began operating in New Orleans as the Young Men's Howard Association when 30 civic-minded men created this charitable society after the 1837 yellow fever epidemic in that city. Throughout the following years, including the Civil War upheaval, the group did not alter its vision—to help victims in epidemic outbreaks. During the 1878 epidemic, the organization arranged for physicians and nurses to travel to locales with yellow fever so that they could administer medicines to the sick and provide critical nursing attention to the victims. The organization hired nursing personnel with no regard to gender or race. Often the nurses and doctors were from areas outside of the epidemic's swath of infection. With nursing care and all necessities provided by the Howards, most people treated by them survived.[11]

As noted at the beginning of this chapter, by September 4, city officials had declared yellow fever an epidemic in Holly Springs and requested more nurses and doctors. Governor John Stone was unable to respond, but the Howard Association alerted the citizens in Holly Springs that 10 more nurses were on their way to their city. The Howards also informed the city's officials that if they required other vital supplies, that organization would send them upon request. One of the Howard Association doctors, R. M. Swearingen of Texas, assumed control of the Marshall County Courthouse Hospital after his arrival. He worked with the Sisters of Charity and Father Oberti. Many citizens in Holly Springs hailed the Howard volunteers who had come from surrounding states such as Louisiana, Texas, and Kentucky as heroes, and others in the city would no doubt have suffered immeasurably more if local doctors and nurses had been their only source of care, as many of the local medical community had succumbed already to the contagion.[12]

Some of the volunteers who came to help Mississippians were not as responsible as others. Instances where physicians misbehaved and where nurses acted with a distinct lack of propriety are not commonplace but do exist. For example, the Howards recruited a group of nurses from Washington, DC, to send to Southerners stricken with the disease. While traveling south, these preprofessional nurses apparently engaged in "the most reckless style of kissing and hugging on the [railroad] cars after Louisville [Kentucky]" and "decent people" observed "an event approaching the most abandoned exploits of bacchanals" on the platform of a Pullman sleeper near Colesburg, Kentucky. These "naughty nurses" continued to drink champagne and indulge in "promiscuous lovemaking" for the duration of the trip.[13] Evidently, not all medical and nursing personnel were beyond reproach.

While the nurses from Washington, DC, misbehaved on their trip to the South, an assistant male nurse named S. Thomas of Martin, Tennessee, robbed a patient under the care of Mrs. Laborde, the head nurse in a private household in Holly Springs. When law officers arrested Thomas, he attempted to swallow the money rather than be caught with the evidence. His trick did not work, however, and officials locked the thief in the Holly Springs jail. Mrs. Laborde worried that all of the excitement would cause her patient to relapse.[14]

Although many Mississippians across the state offered their services unselfishly, citizens had no choice but to rely upon volunteers, most of them from other states, to ameliorate the effects of the epidemic. The volunteers from organizations like the Howards and other benevolent charities brought with them needed manpower and provisions such as teas, herbs, disinfectants, and clean clothes and bedding. With a state board of health that had no legislative power and little monetary backing, Mississippi found itself completely helpless in an epidemic of this magnitude. Fortunately for Mississippians and other Southerners affected by the epidemic, those organizations that buttressed the South during this yellow fever outbreak were overwhelmingly upright and sincerely interested in helping those in dire need.

Religious vows and devotion to humanity motivated many who provided aid to the yellow fever victims. During the epidemic, caretakers acted as medical consultants, hospital administrators, and nurses. Their responsibilities often spanned 24-hour shifts, frequently with no relief. Many of these people died while performing their duties.

As challenging as caretaking was in Mississippi during the epidemic, racial issues complicated outreach to the Black community in the state even more. The government showed little competence in helping White folk and seemed to ignore Blacks completely. The Black population had less access to organized charity and often was the brunt of flagrant disregard in meeting medical needs during the epidemic. However, instances of interaction in nursing care exist and attest to humanitarian efforts on the part of the Blacks.

With a history of caregiving, Black women demonstrated compassionate efforts to care for Whites and others during the epidemic. Noted historian of nursing Linda E. Sabin states in reference to caregiving by Blacks that in the antebellum South and during the Civil War, "while externally powerless in the world of slavery, these women [slave nurses] had considerable internal power within a family that was dependent upon them."[15] Historian Drew Gilpin Faust also concludes that it was African American women who were the primary nurses during the Civil War.[16] Any cooperation between the races during this time was remarkable, however, in light of the turmoil of the Reconstruction years and the Democrats' return to power in Mississippi and the South.

CROSSING GEOGRAPHIC BOUNDARIES TO HELP

Some Blacks remained in communities to help others, including Whites, during the epidemic. Others, volunteering from different states, came to Mississippi to aid those in need. A large group of Blacks volunteered as Howard nurses to accompany a prominent White physician of Chattanooga, Tennessee, to Vicksburg, a stricken Mississippi River town. James Busby Norris was an esteemed physician who was in charge of the nurses. The Vicksburg Howards, under the guidance of W.M. Rockwood as president and W.A. Fairchild as secretary, welcomed the doctor and his nurses into the city on September 3. Sixteen nurses accompanied Norris, half of whom were Black men. Sabin asserts that men never made up the majority of nurses, and that Black men nurses always had a subservient role under the direction of either a White male or female if they cared for people outside of their own communities. According to Sabin, 74 males were volunteer nurses during the 1878 yellow fever epidemic, and 20 of those died. Also, an additional 126 male volunteers provided community care as assistants to medical personnel. Sabin postulates, "The traditional female domestic role of caring for the sick was transferred to the public male domain when entire communities, commerce, and property were at stake." Certainly, White males had to demonstrate their commitment to the community as providers and protectors of those who were perceived as helpless—women, children, and the elderly—while Black males were more free to volunteer for other reasons besides social expectations.[17]

Included in the cadre were the following Blacks: John J. Marshall (first listed as Joseph J. Marshall), Asa Peacock, Eldridge Massingale, John Johnson, Woodson Ellington, Paul Miller, Johan A. Logan, and Gus Williams. These particular community care nurses may have volunteered because of the high wages being offered. They probably found the opportunity economically appealing. All of the nurses were "experienced" and had already had yellow fever. On their trip to Vicksburg, the party traveled on a special train of the Alabama Great Southern Railroad line, and each nurse received a yellow ribbon badge with "Chattanooga Yellow Fever Nurse" printed on it.[18]

It is significant that 50% of the nurses accompanying Norris to help the city of Vicksburg were Blacks. Were these nurses allowed to ride in the same railroad cars as the eight White caregivers? Did these nurses receive some of the basketsful of food that local Chattanooga businessmen gave to the party to tide them over on their long trip south? Were these Tennessee Black nurses treated differently than those in Mississippi under the new Democratic regime? These questions are pertinent to the understanding of the role of Black male nurses and their evolution as caregivers, but research reveals no answers.[19] However, the spirits of volunteerism and self-sacrifice on the part of these nurses undoubtedly deserve attention. One contemporary praised the group when he noted: "The Doctor and these nurses deserve the highest credit for the step they propose taking. They go into the midst of a plague, the ravages of which are more terrible this year than ever before. They do this for the sake of suffering humanity, risking their lives for the good of others."[20]

Newspaper accounts and personal recollections reveal an apparent appreciation for those Blacks who helped minister to others. One such example involves Bob Reed of Water Valley, Mississippi. Reed remained in Water Valley during the yellow fever epidemic and exemplified interracial health care efforts. Reed was an elderly Black man who had assumed he was immune to yellow fever as he had survived a previous yellow fever bout in Natchez years earlier. When officials declared an epidemic in Water Valley, Reed began to help "both White and Colored patients." He oversaw the daily nursing regimen of feeding, bathing, shaving, and administering enemas to people with the disease. He also assisted in the burial of the dead. Reed was obviously invaluable during the town's yellow fever epidemic, as adequate numbers of nurses to attend to the sick were not available, since so many of the town's citizens fled the pestilence.[21] Reed demonstrated compassion during the extreme times and administered necessary nursing care. He did it as a volunteer.

Communities across Mississippi begged for nurses as the epidemic continued in the state through the fall months. Any nurse would have been welcome in stricken towns. For example, citizens in Greenville, another Mississippi River town, reported that the "Situation is horrible. Four hundred remain and cannot get away; 200 sick; nearly 100 dead. No boats running; telegraph line down for about 10 days; cannot make their wants known; are shut out from the world. For God's sake get nurses, supplies, and money on other boats."[22] Locales throughout the state required more medical aid than could be provided as the epidemic maintained its grip on Mississippi.

Grenada was another city that suffered severely during the 1878 yellow fever epidemic. Remaining officials in that city petitioned the Howards in September to send additional medical personnel to fill the vacuum created by the disease in that town. The city's doctors and nurses had either died by the early fall or were so exhausted that Grenada had virtually no medical coverage. Townsfolk telegraphed Howard Associations in various locations, begging for 25 nurses to come and tend yellow fever victims. The city's officials even offered the exorbitant salary of $5 per day if a nurse answered their plea.[23]

Answering the call, the New Orleans Howards sent two physicians and 16 nurses to Grenada to assist that city's fever-stricken citizens and its one remaining doctor, R.J. Ray. Additionally, Dr. Woolfolk of Kentucky volunteered his professional services but sadly soon appeared on the city's death roll. By the end of September, Grenada's epidemic had run its course. A contemporary newspaper recorded that the citizens of Grenada rejoiced when yellow fever finally abated: "Our people can never forget the open-handed generosity with which their wants have been supplied by North, South, East and West alike."[24]

OVERWHELMING GRATITUDE VERSUS RESUMPTION OF RACIAL DISCRIMINATION

In return for the Howard's relief outpourings, Mississippians not only in Grenada but throughout the state expressed overwhelming gratitude to them in various ways, including tributes. One example was a poem, "The Howards of the South." This work by an unknown author appeared in papers across the nation, from New Haven, Connecticut, to Pascagoula, Mississippi. The verse recounted the "brave hands that bear up nobly the stricken fevered head" and appreciated that the North had sent "her treasure, her silver and her gold, [but] you give your time, your courage and sympathy untold." The *London Standard* also printed a tribute to the brave Howards in which they were immortalized as "the flower and pride of the great English race, on whom a more terrible, more merciless enemy has now fallen." Furthermore, the South's youth, according to the London tribute, "volunteer to serve and die in the plague-stricken cities" and "their sisters and wives, mothers and daughters, are dying and suffering" in towns "desolated by the yellow fever." The article further reported that nurses faced imminent danger and a "martyr's death" when they volunteered to be Howards. Commenting on the generosity of the members of the Howard Association and others, the *Louisville Medical News* contributed its opinion of the general relief effort when that journal printed the following: "The suffering and destruction that resulted excited the deepest sympathy in all parts of the Union. Physicians and nurses hastened from every quarter to the assistance of the afflicted communities."[25] The Howards were especially integral to the healing of Mississippi during the epidemic because of their role in providing needed medical and nursing personnel to the stricken communities.

Although the Howard Associations provided much-needed aid to the majority of infected areas in Mississippi, the nurses hired by the group usually experienced exasperating circumstances as they assisted the sick. Female Howard workers were paid much less than males, and Blacks received the least of all as representatives of marginal groups in nineteenth-century society. Generally poor sanitary conditions and the very nature of yellow fever symptoms made ministering to the sick an overwhelming task. Nursing care compensation probably was not commensurate with the job at hand. Nurses received far lower salaries than physicians, even though both doctors and nurses risked their lives equally to treat the sick. Those physicians hired by the Howards earned $10 per day, with a horse and buggy provided; however, nurses received on the average $4 per day with room and board. Black nurses hired by the Howards fared even worse as they earned only $3 daily with board, certainly highlighting the disparity between the races.

Perhaps as a result of the pay and the frustration that must have accompanied nursing duty, one White nurse stationed at Hernando described her situation when she penned a letter to the Memphis Howard Association that had hired her to work in Mississippi. She stated that she was starving and that she was "broken down for want of food and rest." Apparently, her patient was a taskmaster because she further wrote, "Quinn will die, and he is so aggravating that he may live for two or three days; he has no friends, and no wonder, for a more cantankerous cuss I never met with." She was also unhappy about her location when she stated, "The folks at the rum-mill above are only swine and will not come near me." In a desperate plea for help, she ended her letter by threatening, "I am sick and starving, and in self-defense will have to leave or kill the patient, and I do not like to do either. Come at once or I leave." Obviously, this woman was not typical of the nurses who worked for the Howards or indeed of females of the times; she was not shy about complaining that compensation was not adequate for her demanding nursing job and that her room and board were substandard. The outcome of the situation between Quinn and his nurse remains unknown, and no Quinn appears in Power's or Keating's lists of yellow fever deaths for Hernando.[26]

AFTERMATH

By December, the yellow fever epidemic in Mississippi had run its course for the most part. Local physicians across the state submitted their official case numbers and deaths from their areas to the Mississippi Board of Health. Exact numbers are difficult to establish because of faulty record keeping, hesitancy in recognizing yellow fever, and poor communication. Mississippi reported 4,100 deaths out of an approximate state population of 970,000, essentially 25% of the total deaths nationwide, which totaled 16,296. Within the state, 50 physicians and four members of the Mississippi State Board of Health died. The total number of nurses who died helping patients is indeterminable because of the practice of privately ministering to family members and inaccurate record keeping.[27]

After the 1878 yellow fever epidemic, medical practitioners commonly accepted the portability of yellow fever because its course could be traced along railroad lines and water routes as refugees escaped along these paths. The contemporary germ theory, with fomites as the method of transmission, also became acceptable to the majority of physicians as technological improvements such as more advanced use of the microscope provided further information for an alternate explanation of diseases. The existence of a living causative agent was generally gaining acceptance in the medical community. No longer were miasmic inhalations from swamps or putrid privies believed to be the cause of yellow fever. The medical community, however, still debated about divergent theories of treatment. It would not be until the 1880s that Dr. Carlos Finlay of Cuba experimented with mosquitoes as vectors in yellow fever transmission. By 1905, Finlay's mosquito theory would be proven with the help of Clara Maass, a nurse from New Jersey who volunteered to be bitten by an infected mosquito while she worked with the international team in Cuba attempting to conquer yellow fever. In the experiment to prove the transmission theory, Maass died, and with her death, the mosquito was confirmed as the vector of yellow fever.[28]

CONCLUSION

Nurses played a pivotal role in ministering to patients in the yellow fever epidemic of 1878. After the epidemic, it became apparent that better regulation for medical personnel was needed in Mississippi and the nation. The process of expanding public health efforts in this state would not be easy, but the result of the 1878 epidemic was an emerging public health care program—one that would grow and come into its own in the twentieth century, just as professional nursing training would become a reality in the same time frame. The two movements are inseparable, as public health is dependent upon trained, competent medical personnel with nurses leading the vanguard.

STUDY QUESTIONS

1. Discuss risks nurses took when they worked during epidemics in the 1870s. Compare and contrast these to nurses' experiences with epidemics today. What protections are nurses offered today?
2. Discuss how people living in the South might be more susceptible to a disease such as yellow fever.
3. How might the disaster response differ if the disease were in the Midwest? In the Northeast?

NOTES

1. Governor John Marshall Stone was elected in 1876 and served as the state's first Democratic governor after Reconstruction. Quotation is in Governor John M. Stone Papers, Mississippi Department of Archives and History, Jackson, MS.
2. Felix J. Underwood and R. N. Whitfield, *A Brief History of Public Health and Medical Licensure: State of Mississippi 1799–1930* (Jackson: Mississippi State Board of Health, n.d.), 1–8.
3. Robert Berkow, ed., *The Merck Manual of Diagnosis and Therapy*, 13th ed. (Rahway, NJ: Merck Sharp & Dohme Research Laboratories, 1977), 57–58; Earnest Hardenstein, *The Yellow Fever Epidemic of 1878 and Its Homeopathic Treatment* (New Orleans, LA: J.S. Rivers, 1879), 86.

4. Cleta Ellington, *Christ: The Living Water, The Catholic Church in Mississippi* (Jackson, MS: Mississippi Today, 1992), 170–172.
5. R. M. Swearingen, "Tribute to Sister Corinthia," 1878, Marshall County Museum, Holly Springs, Mississippi; William Baskerville Hamilton, "Holly Springs, Mississippi, to the Year 1878" (master's thesis, University of Mississippi, 1951), 83; Ellington, *Christ: The Living Water*, 169–173. The six Sisters of Charity who died were Sisters Stanislaus, Stella, Margaret, Victoria, Lorentia, and Corinthia.
6. The epitaph to Sister Corinthia reads as follows: "Within this room September 1878 Sister Corintha [sic] sank into sleep eternal among the first to enter this realm of death. She was the last save one to leave. The writer of this humble notice saw her in health gentle but strong as she moved with noiseless steps and serene smiles through the crowded wards. He saw her when the yellow plumed angel threw his golden shadows over the last sad scene and eye unused to weeping payed [sic] the tribute of tears to the brave and beautiful 'Spirit of Mercy.'" This tribute was in the Marshall County Courthouse until 1926, when the courthouse underwent renovation. When the city decided to renovate the building, officials saved the portion of wall with the inscription. The city at that time returned the portion of wall to the Sisters of Charity in Nazareth, Kentucky. When organizers chartered the Marshall County Museum in 1970, the sisters in Kentucky loaded the wall piece onto the back seat of an automobile and drove it to Holly Springs for that city's museum display, thus returning it to its rightful place of origin.
7. *History of Marshall County, Mississippi, A Souvenir Edition Commemorating the Marshall County Centennial Celebration*, (Holly Springs, MS: The Garden Club of Marshall County, 1936); Ellington, *Christ: The Living Water*, 169–173.
8. "Sisters of Mercy Regional Community of St. Louis," http://www.mercync.org/stlhistory.htm (accessed Sept. 20, 2009). See Sister Mary Paulinus Oakes, *Angels of Mercy: An Eyewitness Account of the Civil War and Yellow Fever by a Sister of Mercy: A Primary Source* (Baltimore, MD: Cathedral Foundation Press, 1998) and Robert J. Miller, *Both Prayed to the Same God: Religion and Faith in the American Civil War* (Lanham, MD: Rowman & Littlefield Publications, 2007) for good overviews of the Sisters of Mercy's and the Sisters of Charity's contributions to health care. See also Sister Mary Hermenia Muldrey, *Abounding in Mercy: Mother Austin Carroll* (New Orleans, LA: Habersham, 1988) for the biography of Mother Austin Carroll, who brought nuns all over the South. For a good overview of the battle of Vicksburg, see Michael B. Ballard, *Vicksburg: The Campaign That Opened the Mississippi* (Chapel Hill: University of North Carolina Press, 2004).

9. "Sisters of Mercy Regional Community of St. Louis."

10. J. L. Power, *The Epidemic of 1878 in Mississippi: Report of the Yellow Fever Relief Work Through J. L. Power, Grand Secretary of Masons and Grand Treasurer of Odd Fellows* (Jackson, MS: Clarion-Steam, 1879), 192; Register of Sisters and Loose Paper Collection, Sister Mary Vincent Brown, Private Collection, Sisters of Mercy Convent, Vicksburg, Mississippi; Ellington, *Christ: the Living Water*, 451–452. The Mercy Regional Medical Center in Vicksburg today is the result of the dedication and hard work that the Sisters of Mercy extended during the Civil War, the 1878 yellow fever epidemic, and the years of service to that city. The sisters listed on the death rolls in Vicksburg in 1878 were Sisters Mary Regis Grant, Mary Bernadine Murray, Regina Ryan, and Columba McGrath. The convent that was on the hospital's grounds has been moved to Jackson, Mississippi.

11. Peggy Bassett Hildreth, "Early Red Cross: The Howard Association of New Orleans, 1837–1878," *Louisiana History* 20 (Winter, 1979): 49–75. The Howards became more or less obsolete after the 1878 epidemic because state boards of health and national agencies expanded their roles in public health. The Howards continued to list themselves as a charitable organization in New Orleans directories, however, as late as World War I.

12. Helen Craft Anderson, "A Chapter in the Yellow Fever Epidemic of 1878," *Publications of the Mississippi Historical Society* 10 (1909): 223–229; Governor Stone Papers, MDAH, Jackson, MS; H.W. Walter from J.R. Stoutmayd, September 13, 1878, Sisters of Charity Archives, 1878 File, Nazareth, KY.

13. *The Cincinnati Commercial*, September 17, 1878.

14. New York *Herald*, September 16, 1878.

15. Linda E. Sabin, *Struggles and Triumphs: The Story of Mississippi Nurses 1800–1950* (Jackson, MS: MHA Health, Research and Educational Foundation, 1998), 7.

16. See Drew Gilpin Faust, *Mothers of Invention: Women of the Slaveholding South in the American Civil War* (Chapel Hill: University of North Carolina Press, 1996).

17. Linda E. Sabin, "Unheralded Nurses: Male Caregivers in the Nineteenth-Century South," in *Nurses' Work: Issues Across Time and Place*, Patricia D'Antonio, et al., eds. (New York: Springer Publishing Company, 2007), 58. Sabin gathered her statistics from J.P. Dromgoole, *Dr. Dromgoole's Yellow Fever: Heroes, Honors, and Horrors of 1878* (Louisville, KY: John P. Morton, 1879).

18. *In Memoriam, James Busby Norris, M.D.* (Chattanooga, TN: Crandall & Company, 1879), 7–8.

19. Power, *The Epidemic of 1878 in Mississippi*, 192–193. Listed among the Vicksburg dead were four African-American nurses, three of whom accompa-

nied Norris. "Sept. 9, Peacock, col. 40 y.; Sept 13, John Johnson, col. 26 y.; Sept. 16. Ed. Massengale, 40 y., Chatanooga [sic] nurse." Also, the entry of "Sept. 13, Thomas Edwards, col., 36 y., Chattanooga nurse" appeared. Presumably, Edwards joined the group at a later date. No information surfaced on the other nurses. Obviously, record keeping regarding African American cases/mortality rates was sketchy as the entries do not include Peacock's first name, and officials mistook Massengale's first name of Eldridge as Ed. (Edward?).

20. *In Memoriam, James Busby Norris, M.D.*, 7.
21. Harris Allen Gant, "Yellow Fever in Mississippi, 1878–1905: Personal Recollections, Experiences, Reminiscences, Autobiography and History," *Mississippi Doctor* 13 (1936–37): 23. Apparently Reed lived through the epidemic as his name does not appear in Power's list of fatalities or in J. M. Keating, *A History of Yellow Fever: The Yellow* Fever *Epidemic of 1878 in Memphis, Tenn.* (Memphis, TN: Howard Association, 1879). Keating also compiled lists of yellow fever fatalities in Tennessee and Mississippi. See also Sabin, "Unheralded Nurses," 56.
22. *Pascagoula (Miss.) Democrat-Star*, September 6, 1878.
23. Power, *The Epidemic of 1878 in Mississippi*, 165.
24. *Pascagoula (Miss.) Democrat-Star*, October 1, 1878.
25. *Pascagoula (Miss.) Democrat-Star*, October 11, 1878; "Heroism of the Southern People in War and in Pestilence," quoted from *London Standard* in Power, *The Epidemic of 1878 in Mississippi*, 206–207. *Louisville Medical News*, December 7, 1878.
26. Dromgoole, *Dr. Dromgoole's Yellow Fever*, 76 and 103; Keating, *History of the Yellow Fever Epidemic 1878*, 248–249.
27. Gant, "Yellow Fever in Mississippi," 23–25; Hardenstein, *The Yellow Fever Epidemic of 1878*, 36; *Report of the Mississippi State Board of Health For the Years 1878–1879* (Jackson, MS: Power and Barksdale, 1879), 2–25. For a list of physicians who died in the epidemic, see Mary Lois Ragland and Kathy Ragland Renfroe, comps., *Yellow Fever Epidemic of 1878* (Vicksburg, MS: n.p., 1987), 55. Population statistics are from Ralph D. Cross, ed., *Atlas of Mississippi* (Jackson, MS: University Press of Mississippi), 52.
28. Greer Williams, *The Plague Killers* (New York: Scribner, 1969), 185–208. See John T. Cunningham, *Clara Maass: A Nurse, A Hospital, A Spirit* (Belleville, NJ: Rae Books, 1968) for a biography of this heroic nurse.

CHAPTER 2

The 1900 Galveston Hurricane: "Unspeakable Calamity"

Barbra Mann Wall

Unspeakable calamity been visited upon Galveston, utterly beyond local relief.[1]

With these words, the Associated Press captured the devastation of what was probably a category 4 hurricane that struck Galveston, Texas, on September 8, 1900. By midafternoon of that day, eyewitnesses reported chest-deep flooding around the city and winds that sent roof slates and timbers flying. The peak of the storm hit in the late evening, demolishing more than 3,600 homes, drowning their occupants, and killing others by flying debris. In terms of lives lost, it still ranks as the worst natural disaster in North American history. The huge scale was such that no social class was spared. Using religious and heroic rhetoric, one survivor wrote, "I have passed through the most trying experience of my life. . . . It was surely through God's mercy that I kept my presence of mind all that terrible night and brought my parents through alive."[2]

More recently, on September 13, 2008, the powerful category 2 Hurricane Ike moved onto the Texas Gulf Coast, flattening houses, obliterating entire towns, and claiming 177 deaths in the United States and Caribbean. Of these, 74 were in Haiti and 33 in Texas. Hundreds of people remain missing.[3] Residents of Galveston followed mandatory evacuation orders, and the University of Texas Medical Branch (UTMB) staff evacuated all their patients. Staff credit emergency preparedness plans learned from Hurricane Rita, which hit in September 2005, as helping them prepare for Hurricane Ike.[4] This recent disaster serves as an impetus to look beyond Hurricanes Ike and Rita to see what can be learned from the devastating hurricane of 1900 that nearly destroyed the city, killed between 6,000 and 8,000 people, and left 25,000 homeless. A retrospective view of disasters—the analysis of experiences in the past—is an essential component of preparing the country to face future calamities.

Recent work on disasters has focused on architectural rebuilding of cities after disasters,[5] while other studies have examined cities' resilience to such calamities,[6] public policy,[7] the impact of specific traumatic events on particular individuals and communities, and the media's role in relief.[8] In this chapter, the health care responses after the 1900 disaster are examined through newspapers and the voices of the people who lived through it. These accounts reveal their thoughts and actions as they tried to make sense of catastrophic experiences by sharing them with others.[9] The hurricane is placed within the context of the various forces that shaped Galveston in 1900.[10]

Many variables affect how people handle tragedies, including the scale of the disaster, the depth of social attitudes, and cultural norms prescribing gender roles. Classic sociological research on disasters emphasizes widespread helping behaviors among members of the affected community, and this happened after the Galveston hurricane. Research also shows that conflicts suspend temporarily as residents and organizations try to overcome the challenges the disaster brings, and this also occurred in Galveston in 1900.[11] But other studies have begun to focus on how factors such as poverty, race, and gender influence disaster responses and recovery outcomes.[12] This chapter includes similar analyses, and it supports Patricia D'Antonio's thesis that nurses worked not only as clinicians in hospitals and community health areas but also as members of their families and communities.[13] Thus, this is a story about a community response to a tragedy in which nurses were one part.

The city of Galveston is located on a 27-mile-long barrier island that sits between the Gulf of Mexico and Galveston Bay, and it is from 1 to 3 miles wide. Its geographic location, however, makes it vulnerable to storms. In 1900, it was the wealthiest city in the state, with a deepwater port that served Texas and other states west of the Mississippi River. It competed with New Orleans as the leading cotton port in the nation. Galveston was an architectural treasure with its opera house, large Victorian mansions, electric streetcars, concert arenas, and the lavish Tremont Hotel where Red Cross President Clara Barton eventually stayed.[14] The city also was conspicuous for its alleys and back buildings inhabited by many Blacks. Alley dwellers and front-house residents were all vital parts of the city.[15]

At the same time, racial tensions were evident: In 1900, 106 Black Americans were lynched, primarily in southern and border states.[16] Black men all over Texas had lost voting rights as early as 1895.[17] Furthermore, Jim Crow segregation had been extant in the South since the 1870s, and it had only been four years since the landmark Supreme Court decision *Plessy v Ferguson* upheld the constitutionality of segregation.[18] Thus, any Black person who was ill in Galveston was housed in separate hospital buildings.

EXPERIENCING THE STORM

The only description known to have been written while the storm was raging was an anonymous note by a young woman, likely a nurse, who was employed at John Sealy Hospital and who rode out the storm inside the building. On the morning of September 8, as the tempest escalated, she wrote, "It does not require a great stretch of imagination to imagine this structure a shaky old boat out at sea" (see Figure 2.1). The building rocked as water surrounded it, and the nurse had her "hands full quieting nervous, hysterical women." She wrote, "The scenes about here are distressing. Poor people, trying vainly to save their bedding, & clothing. Methinks the poor nurses will be trying to save their beds in short order." By 3 p.m. she was beginning to want "something to cling to."[19]

Galveston's St. Mary's Infirmary, owned and operated by the Sisters of Charity of the Incarnate Word, was another hospital hit by the storm. During the day of September 8, the sister nurses were doing their usual tasks, ignoring the changes in the weather outside. But when flying slates began crashing windows, they suddenly took notice. From a second-story window, they could see boats on the street where street cars had been running only an hour earlier. After 4 p.m., boats began arriving at the doors and windows of the hospital with refugees and those injured by debris. From 1,500 to 2,000 people sought shelter in the hospital—Black, White, Protestant, Catholic, young and old, rich and poor. By 5 p.m., the hospital was totally dark. The first floor flooded so that everyone moved to the upper floors, all terrorized by the strong winds. Around midnight, the howling wind subsided and the water began to recede.[20] Figure 2.2 shows the extensive damage that St. Mary's Infirmary suffered. Its chapel was ruined.

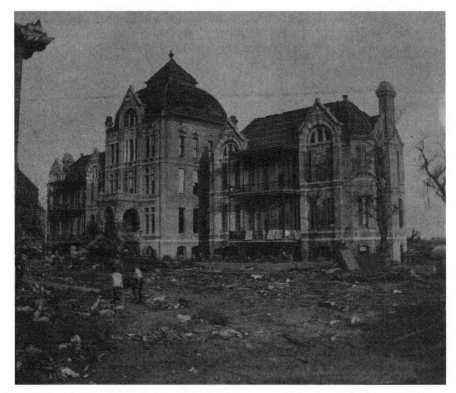

Figure 2.1   John Sealy Hospital, September 1900. G-1771 FF8.3 #1, Courtesy Rosenberg Library, Galveston, TX.

St. Mary's Orphanage, which stood on the beach facing the Gulf of Mexico, was also destroyed. Tragically, 90 children and 10 Incarnate Word Sisters died. The nuns had tried to protect their charges by tying themselves to the children with clothesline, but the 20-foot storm surge collapsed the dormitories and washed the sisters and children out to sea. Later, some of the bodies floated ashore still tied together.[21]

Galveston was devastated. Reflecting on the scene after the storm, Isaac M. Cline, the local forecast official and Section Director, wrote:

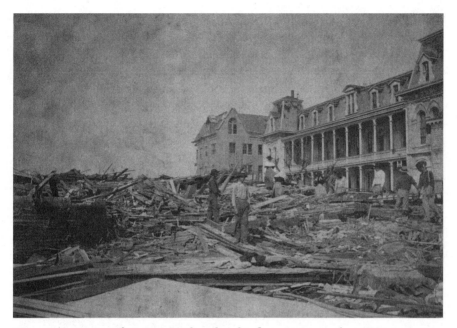

Figure 2.2   Ruins of St. Mary's Chapel and Infirmary, September 1900.
G-1771 FF8.4 #2. Courtesy Rosenberg Library, Galveston, TX.

> Sunday, September 9, 1900, revealed one of the most horrible sights that
> ever a civilized people looked upon. About three thousand homes, nearly
> half the residence portion of Galveston, had been completely swept out of
> existence, and probably more than six thousand persons had passed from life
> to death during that dreadful night. The correct number of those who per-
> ished will probably never be known, for many entire families are missing.[22]

Nurses and other health care workers had to tend to survivors numbed
by the total devastation. One woman wrote that everyone seemed to be
stunned, "and you never see any emotion displayed of any kind. Every one
is perfectly calm! We all seem to have gone through so much."[23] Another,
a visiting salesman who experienced the storm while at the Tremont Hotel,
wrote, "I have not been able to do anything since my experience in Galveston. Every little noise startles me. My nerves are gone."[24]

Many survivors wrote stories of their personal heroism as they recalled
the harrowing afternoon and night of September 8, 1900. They saw houses

floating away with whole families drowned and wagons carrying heaps of dead bodies. Death and destruction were so extensive that it is not surprising that many of the survivors' personal accounts demonstrated a desire to do something positive. Hence, they used heroic language in describing the many lives they saved. For example, one volunteer worker for the police department recalled that, along with two other men, he "brought in a total of forty-three refugees. Every one of them came through."[25] In these cases, "heroes" were the rescuers who saved many people from certain death.

The language of heroism also was evident in writings about St. Mary's Infirmary. Father J.B. Gleissner, a patient during the storm, reminisced in 1938, "In the hallway, I saw a scene of bravery" as some of the sisters "standing knee-deep in the water" were pulling those floating by to a place of safety.[26] Joseph Hawley, a railroad executive, was chair of the Committee on Public Safety and played a key role in the city's recovery. "Every man here has nerve and has tried to do his duty," he wrote. "Instances of courage and heroism are thick."[27]

After the disaster, however, tensions arose between what the media needed for a story and how people saw themselves. Galveston newspaper reporters took a leading role in shaping a myth by ascribing heroic status to physicians. They heralded an intern at St. Mary's Infirmary, Zachary Scott, who, they purported, had saved over 200 lives when he carried patients to St. Mary's main building from the county building a quarter of a mile away. This story dominated historical accounts until many years later, when Scott's own memoir dispelled the heroic legend. John E. Weems, for his 1957 book, *Weekend in September*, had interviewed Scott, who was retired and living in Austin at the time, and quoted him as saying, "There weren't 200 patients in there. Besides, about fifty were ambulatory patients, and they walked over. . . . I didn't carry them. I didn't do it all myself either; I couldn't have. Other men in the hospital helped me."[28] Whether or not Scott ever tried to correct this version of the story at the time is unknown, but eventually it became a source of embarrassment for him. In 1900, the media created an icon that helped lessen the threat of the trauma, whereas Scott's memoir showed a conflicting story. 57 years later, after the community's need for heroes had lessened, it was easier for Scott's more accurate account to be heard and accepted, thus revealing that the past can be recalled and retold in different ways under different times.

Several of the buildings at the UTMB, established in 1891, were damaged but stood intact. Books in the university library suffered severe water damage, and all hospital records from January to June, 1900, were lost. John Sealy Hospital, part of UTMB, survived the storm with no reported deaths, but it was badly damaged. The hurricane also destroyed the Nurses' Home, part of the School of Nursing that had formed in 1894. A writer in a November 1900 issue of a nursing journal gave details: "The nurses saved themselves by wading in water up to their chests to the hospital;"[29] and they were left without clothes other than those on their backs and little water and food.[30] An 1898 graduate from John Sealy School of Nursing, who survived by going to the top floor of the hospital, later recalled, "There were just 21 of us nurses in John Sealy. Three of the girls were afraid and ran away. Two others were drowned. . . . They were out on special duty when the storm hit, and we never saw them again."[31]

The struggle for survival presented ethical dilemmas as well. Initial reports from St. Mary's Infirmary noted that only eight persons escaped alive, but other sources refute this statistic.[32] An undated history of the infirmary quoted a survivor: "Only one life was lost—a crippled girl who bravely bade those who tried to rescue her, to make their escape, deeming their lives more precious than her own."[33] Since efforts were initially taken to save these patients, one might wonder if decisions were made as to who should be rescued and who should be left behind. Did a form of wartime triage take place that night, in which survival efforts favored the hardiest? Did the writer perhaps feel guilty that this woman was not saved, when all others did, in fact, reach safety, thereby assuaging the writer's feelings by creating a story of the woman's heroism? The scant information available about this incident raises more questions than answers.

PROVISIONS FOR RELIEF

Local Response

In 1900, there was no permanent program of federal disaster relief in the United States, and local and private voluntary agencies were the primary responders to disasters.[34] On September 9, socially and politically prominent Galveston men met at the Chamber of Commerce to organize a Central Relief Committee, with men placed in charge of subcommittees such as hospitals, finances, safety, burials, and correspondence. They immediately declared martial law, with the National Guard keeping order, and then commandeered all men to begin the gruesome search for the dead. This decision privileged no social class. Any able-bodied man who refused to work would not be given any food. A central commissary supplied relief stations for each ward. City leaders sent the following Associated Press message to the President of the United States, city mayors, and other public officials: "Unspeakable calamity been visited upon Galveston, utterly beyond local relief. . . . Not one family has escaped serious injury. . . ."[35] The message was no exaggeration.

Attitudes about gender were apparent in the accounts of how the disaster responders organized the division of labor. In a sensationalist account written just after the storm, Paul Lester noted that men steered the boats in a "manly way," while women went about "comforting and trying to ease the fears of the many who had come to [the hospital] seeking safety."[36] One survivor recalled that, during the storm, "rope had been obtained and was cut for use by each man in connection with the women and children he was to look after in case the house went to pieces."[37] Some women, however, had different accounts. Ida Smith Austin spoke of the enthusiasm with which "mere women and even children" heroically dealt with the situation and brought order out of chaos.[38] While most survivors reported men drilling holes in floors to prevent buildings from floating away, one remembered her mother taking an axe and quickly chopping holes in every floor of the house.[39] Thus, while some men demonstrated their commitment to protecting those they perceived to be helpless, such as women and children, many women's descriptions of themselves did not conform to such submissive representations.

As the storm escalated, Black patients from the segregated hospital moved to the main buildings at John Sealy and St. Mary's and mixed with other patients in the White wards, without any recorded problems. Indeed, during this perilous time, racial norms were temporarily lifted. The language used by Louisa Rollfing is significant for what it says about racial boundaries. She recalled that her husband and two Black men "held on together" and were able to get to a grocery store for shelter.[40] Blacks and Whites normally would not be in close physical presence, let alone grasping each other, but this 1932 memoir reflects the writers' choice to show that during the peak of the storm, racial norms were set aside. Other survivors' writings that surfaced after the storm, however, showed that racial prejudice had re-emerged. Many conformed to the dominant view that Blacks were "ghouls," as they reported exaggerated stories of them with flour sacks or pockets filled with jewelry taken from dead persons' fingers and ears, despite written evidence to the contrary. One New York writer claimed that there were no Americans among the ghouls; rather, they were Blacks and poor Whites from southern Europe. These claims led to vigilante-type action as armed volunteers shot suspects on sight.[41]

A graphic lithograph sketch (Figure 2.3) featured debris and dead bodies, while in the left lower corner the stereotypical Black man is being shot for looting. Unfounded stories of criminals cutting off fingers and ears to obtain jewelry were not unusual after disasters. Yet, Jan Harold Brunvand identifies the "cut finger" story as a myth; indeed, an urban legend.[42] In 1901, newspaperman Clarence Ousley investigated rumors and police reports of looting and found that racial status was unknown for most suspects.[43]

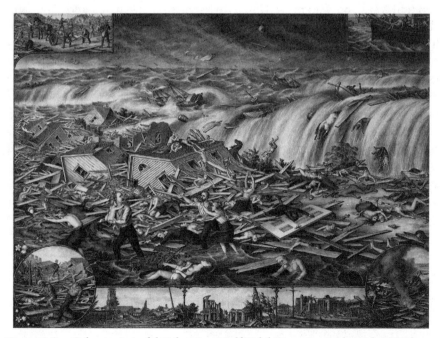

Figure 2.3   Galveston's Awful Calamity—Gulf Tidal Wave, September 8th 1900, by a Chicago publisher. G-1771 FF12.1 #5. Courtesy Rosenberg Library, Galveston, TX.

The wretched image of death and pollution of air and water pervaded accounts of the Galveston storm. By September 10, newspapers were filled with stories about recovering the dead. Identifying the thousands of bodies was a major task; fearful of disease, city authorities decided to dispose of the decomposing corpses by dumping them at sea. But when they washed ashore, the decision then was made to burn the bodies en masse in bonfires throughout the city.[44] Thus, a smoky haze and acrid stench of burning flesh pervaded the Galveston neighborhoods for weeks on end. In addition, salt spray from the storm had contaminated cisterns for rainwater. One traveling salesman wrote his wife that he had no water to drink: "I had to go around to the drugstores and pay 25 cents a pint for mineral water and it cost me $1.50 a day for water to drink. The weather was fearful hot 98 to 99 degrees. Now if I don't have a long spell of fever or rheumatism it will be a miracle."[45]

The disaster response was a collaborative effort. Monetary relief from inter- and intrastate donors began pouring into the city, along with clothing and medical supplies that were channeled through the Red Cross. Steamers brought food and water; the U.S. Army sent soldiers, tents, and food; and the U.S. Marine Service established a hospital camp at nearby Houston. The Galveston Health Department immediately called in men with drays to start clearing the streets of dead animals, refuse, debris, and garbage (see Figure 2.4). Local drugstores distributed medicines and supplies to the indigent sick and injured, while other committees restored water and solicited emergency financial help.[46]

Individual physicians advertised that they would be dressing wounds in their offices. Blacks also played a role. The headquarters of the national Black press in Galveston sent out messages to all the leading Black newspapers to obtain financial assistance. In addition, Namahyoke Curtis volunteered her services in Galveston. Like many women of the day, she was not trained as a nurse, but she had many years of public service, including a stint as a contract nurse with the War Department during the Spanish American War in 1898.[47]

Within five days, mail, telegraph, and water services were restored. Help came from all over the country, including six physicians and 20 nurses from Bellevue Hospital in New York.[49] On September 16, the *Galveston Daily News* reported on the Fifth Ward Hospital:

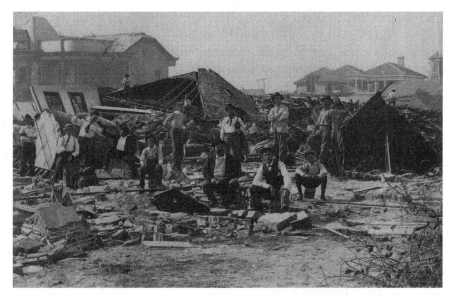

Figure 2.4   Working Men Clearing Debris, September 1900. SC 14 #30.
Courtesy Rosenberg Library, Galveston, TX.

> The Fifth Ward (medical) relief station is established at No. 3 engine
> house, with hospital accommodations for male and female, in the post
> office building, thoroughly equipped for the care of the sick and wounded.
> The station is in charge of Dr. A.F. Sampson, with the following assistants:
> Dr. Harrison of Columbus, Dr. A.R. Kuykendall of Bosque County, Dr.
> A.J. Lielitaki of Houston, Dr. R.H. Cossitt of New York, and trained nurses
> Chas. W. Rogers of New York, Clarence Berghelm of Houston and Miss
> Hinton of Galveston.[50]

The Sick and Injured Committee established dispensaries in different
parts of the city with physicians and trained nurses working in each. The
fact that the *Galveston Daily News* mentioned trained nurses as part of this
relief response is one of the first places that their visibility actually came
to the surface. Still, on September 12, a doctor described only the work of
other physicians when he stated, "The hospitals in Galveston were doing
grand work in caring for the sick and injured, and . . . the doctors of Galveston were working night and day caring for the needy."[48]

Houses that were left standing were filled with the injured, both rich and poor.[51] Care from outsiders should not blind us to the most fundamental response to the disaster: that of family members and neighbors caring for each other. In an oral history, Katherine Vedder Pauls recalls her mother saving the life of a neighbor's infant during the height of the storm:

> My mother took him and saw that there was still a spark of life. She crawled on her hands and knees through the darkness into the northeast room where . . . she pulled a knitted woolen petticoat and a broken bottle of blackberry cordial. . . . She stripped the baby of its wet clothing and wrapped it in the woolen garment and placed the now dry and purring kitten next to the baby's body for warmth.

She instructed the baby's mother to put the cordial "drop by drop into the baby's mouth." Gradually, "the tiny cold body grew warm and soon a wailing infant demanded food."[52]

The Sisters of Charity of the Incarnate Word initially cared for survivors at St. Mary's Infirmary by building a fire in the street, drying water-soaked cookies and crackers found in a damaged grocery store, and feeding them to the patients and refugees. For days they remained in their full habits that had been soaked in the storm.[53] On September 16, the sisters announced that St. Mary's had reopened and that it could take 100 more patients.[54] Hospital records over the next two weeks indicated that most of the injured had fractures and contusions. Thereafter, laborers came with puncture wounds, back injuries, and hand and finger trauma, likely sustained from clearing debris. Beginning in October 1900 and continuing through February 1901, sisters saw patients with dysentery and typhoid fever. In December alone, they admitted 22 cases of typhoid.[55] Survivors remembered a lack of disinfectants and a fear of epidemics, but no widespread disease occurred due to the rapid preventive responses of physicians, nurses, and the Red Cross.

Red Cross Response

There were no specific procedures for notifying the Red Cross of any disaster in 1900, and Clara Barton did not receive the news until September 10.

With funds that had been raised through the *New York World*, she and her staff of three women and five men first arrived at Texas City, just across the bay from Galveston, where tents and kitchens had been set up.[56] Texas City, too, had suffered severe damage from the hurricane. A well-equipped temporary hospital was in operation with surgeons and nurses caring for the injured. Boats came from Galveston filled with the sick, injured, and grieving; patients were lifted off the steamers in chairs and carried by others to the temporary facilities in Texas City or by rail to Houston. Boats also brought women, children, and elderly evacuees; on September 17 one of these steamers took the Red Cross contingent to Galveston.[57]

The 78-year-old Barton personally joined the relief work in Galveston, her last such trip, and her arrival was met with great fanfare. She often insisted on assuming full control of operations, but due to her poor health, she and her staff supplemented the work of the local Central Relief Committee. The Red Cross did compete with the local ward commissaries, however, which eventually turned relief work over to Barton's team. In addition, Barton ensured that White middle-class Galveston women, through their new Red Cross Auxiliary, would provide greater leadership at the distribution stations.[58] This was a significant move. In addition to women becoming co-chairs of ward committees, at Barton's encouragement they also went into the community to assess different needs and arrange for food, clothing, and materials for shelter. While middle-class women had traditionally worked in benevolent societies to provide relief for the poor, this was the first time in Galveston that women became part of the official city relief structure.[59]

Upon Barton and her team's arrival in Galveston, city leaders welcomed them as "Red Cross Nurses," although according to Red Cross Vice-President Ellen Mussey, "the major part of our party were large and stalwart men who knew nothing about sickness, either of themselves or others." One of the physicians informed her that they "needed no nurses," and she replied that she was glad, "as we had none to give him." After a debacle in Jacksonville, Florida, in 1888 when the Red Cross recruited nurses for a yellow fever epidemic, a scandal had developed when some nurses were accused of being drunk. Thereafter, Barton rarely included nurses in her entourage, and they did not accompany her to Galveston.[60]

That no nurses were available came as a surprise to the doctor, however, and he wanted to know what the Red Cross purported to do. When Mussey asked what he needed, he replied that surgical dressings and medical supplies were most in demand. Within 24 hours, she had filled the order.[61] By the 20th of September, two carloads of disinfectants reached Galveston and were turned over to the local health department. Medicines secured by the Red Cross included alcohol, bichloride tablets, collodion (a solution used in surgical dressings), castoria, brandy, and glycerine. Equipment included thermometers and atomizers.[62] Although the Red Cross brought no nurses, trained nurses from New York, Memphis, and elsewhere volunteered in the distribution centers to help with the massive tasks of sorting and distributing clothing, shoes, bedding, and cooking utensils.[63]

Barton's recollections spoke to the savage toll disasters exacted on both survivors and relief workers. She wrote about seeing miles of debris and piles with unburned dead bodies and vile smells of burning flesh. She had been instrumental in organizing the American Red Cross in 1881, and Congress had only recently given it a formal charter as a disaster relief agency on June 6, 1900, with Barton as president. She wanted the Red Cross to become the undisputed leader for emergency relief in the United States, and she used her national reputation as a humanitarian to bring this about.

As Red Cross workers, nurses, and other volunteers distributed donated clothing, they found that much of it was unusable, either too heavy for the climate or too shabby. Mrs. Fannie Ward's Red Cross report noted, "There was hardly a thing in stock for people of the better class. It must be remembered that we were not supplying tramps and beggars, nor the ordinary applicants for charity—but ladies and gentlemen." Red Cross workers bought them what they needed or else gave them money to buy their own clothing.[64]

The Red Cross collaborated with volunteers from various charitable and patriotic societies, including the Women's Relief Corps, the Women's Christian Temperance Union, and the Grand Army of the Republic. It did not dominate the Galveston relief effort. The War Department furnished rations and tents immediately after the disaster and a boat to carry people back and forth to the mainland. The U.S. Navy provided a gunboat for the use of state and city leaders. The Relief Committee itself spent close to $1.3 million for food, building costs, clothing, sanitation and plumbing systems, temporary shelters, and burying the dead. Still, as Marian Moser Jones argues, "Barton's Red Cross provided a powerful, female-led counterpart to the male-led relief committee. It addressed not public needs such as sanitation and public order, but personal needs of survivors," such as clothing and cookware.[65]

Barton worked not only with White city leaders, both men and women, but also with Blacks, in contrast to Whites who had kept Blacks off the relief committees. The following account in the Black-owned newspaper, the *City Times*, offers a picture of how the writer thought about this: "The colored man is good enough to save the lives of the little White babes, White women and even men. . . . and yet in all of that he has not been good enough to even be represented as a committeeman."[66] Although the White newspapers rarely mentioned Blacks except as criminals, several survivors' stories told of Blacks driving carriages that took Whites to safety. This did not escape Louisa Rollfing, who remembered to pay her Black driver and thank him for his "careful driving."[67]

Some Black citizens interpreted the catastrophe using the language of God's judgment. The above writer stated, "God's eye has been over this little sinful place before this destruction, and it is still watching it and the people." J.C. Luke, a Black laborer, said that he was sorry for the great destruction and loss of life, but God worked "in mysterious ways and this is a warning to the people here."[68]

In Barton's report, she portrayed Blacks as "poor, dark figures struggling toward the light."[69] On the other hand, through her numerous experiences with disaster relief, she was attuned to their problems. Earlier, the Red Cross had responded to a hurricane in Port Royal, South Carolina. The fact that most of the survivors were Black led to a paltry response. Comparing the million dollars eventually collected for Galveston to the $31,000 for the Port Royal disaster, she wrote, "I name these as mere points of interest, without prejudice. . . . the results largely depending upon the locality, the acquaintance, social interests and class of people comprising the sufferers."[70] Barton ensured that Blacks were entitled to the resources at all the distribution centers; she also contacted the principal of the local Black high school to form a separate Red Cross Society. He consulted his "foremost women teachers . . . to form a society with all proper officers, seal, etc., and fit themselves to receive a little money."[71] Donations came from Blacks in communities across the country, including survivors from Port Royal, and $397 was collected. Blacks used the funds to distribute Bibles, clothing, and books but saved most of the money for a home for indigent Blacks.[72] By providing Blacks with their own relief fund rather than relying only on Whites' largesse, Barton ensured that Blacks could determine themselves the best way to use the money.

AFTERMATH

The ward relief stations closed on October 25, 1900, and the Red Cross warehouses closed a few days later. Barton stayed in Texas for two months, but once the worst of Galveston's problems had been met, she and her staff headquartered in Houston. They distributed supplies to people in towns and villages over a thousand-square-mile area that had suffered severe damage. Typical of Barton's policy of restarting local work, she provided strawberry plants to farmers in six storm-swept counties. In those areas, farmers had been accustomed to supplying the earliest strawberries to northern markets, but the hurricane washed away every plant and no money was available to buy more. Barton contacted the farmers' dealers in other states and delivered over a million plants to the waiting growers. The crop was ready for market by the following February.[73]

Disaster songs and poems appeared and provide some idea of the outpouring of support for survivors. "The Texas Cyclone," written by William W. Delany in October 1900 for a New York publisher, was an ode to the helpers: "Now we'll help each poor soul the dark scene to forget, relieving their misery wherever it's met; for the poor and the homeless by the cyclone's dread night we'll send clothing and food down in Texas to-night."[74] A souvenir program for a Baltimore concert to aid the Galveston survivors included the poem "The Ruined City." It ended with: "For in this glorious nation are few who duty shirk, and all whose means permit them, will aid the noble work."[75] Even though geographically remote from Galveston, these functioned to help the community to heal.[76]

Newspapers also attempted to lift their readers' spirits with promising stories of hope. For example, one editorial stated, "The sentiment was Galveston will, Galveston must survive and fulfill her glorious destiny. Galveston shall rise again."[77] Barton's letter to the Texas governor supported this view: "Nowhere have a people shown themselves so ready to meet disaster—brave, resolute, sympathetic, capable and enduring, they are sure to recover. Though fought to the death, they are not conquered; though stricken, they are not slain."[78] Although some people moved away from Galveston and never returned, most were determined to stay and rebuild. After the disaster, the response of administrators at UTMB was positive. The rallying cry for restoration was issued shortly after the storm when one leader stated, "The University of Texas stops for no storm."[79] Indeed, after the hurricane, the University of Texas Board of Regents and state legislators became more generous in appropriations to support the school that had survived such a terrible disaster.

Without a doubt, Galvestonians appreciated relief aid. After the calamity, Barton emphasized how they had all collaborated with the Red Cross, and she left Texas on a wave of public support. The Central Relief Committee unanimously adopted resolutions of thanks and rendered "homage to the woman who is the life and spirit of the Red Cross."[80]

In due time, Galvestonians rebuilt their city, raised the city's grade level above sea level, and built a 17-foot seawall that protected the city from future hurricanes. They also instituted governmental reforms that included a commission form of government that abolished ward representation and secured political control for elites. Progressives approved of this idea for local government, even though it reduced minorities' political strength. Although Blacks had a strong community at the time, segregation hampered their civic activities.[81] They participated in relief and recovery events, but they had to fight for their right to do so. Following the destruction of their hospital, the Black community was aided when the city came through with a new hospital for them in 1902, one that Black physicians and nurses staffed.[82]

CONCLUSION

The size of the 1900 Galveston hurricane in terms of death and destruction was astounding. The initial task was to establish relief committees, sanitation measures, and emergency health care facilities. Indeed, public health concerns for fresh water, food, medical and nursing care, housing, and burying the dead were paramount. Nurses were part of the larger relief efforts of several organizations, and they worked at the disaster site, in hospitals, and with the Red Cross distribution centers. Under difficult conditions, they evaluated survivors who needed immediate hospitalization; provided hands-on medical and nursing care; distributed food, clothing, and disinfectants; provided supplies for shelters; and helped prevent major outbreaks of epidemics.

Aided by a large humanitarian relief effort, city leaders then began rebuilding the city's infrastructures. Galvestonians were the recipients of generous monetary aid. Although the city lost a huge part of its population, the fact that it was reinhabited at all is a key achievement. Historian David G.

McComb asserts that the 1900 storm was Galveston's "finest hour, and demonstrated that rationality and determination can prevail." The people cared for the ill and injured, cleared the streets, disposed of the bodies, rebuilt commercial buildings and homes, and undertook progressive government reforms. Although the city survived, however, it did not prosper afterward.[83]

Other survivors showed despair, shock, and disbelief. One archival source hinted that a wounded woman was left behind at St. Mary's Infirmary. Considering the dire circumstances in which the health care workers were operating, it is not surprising that some potential survivors could have been left behind. To acknowledge such acts openly, however, is no doubt difficult, even guilt-provoking. After all, the health care workers were trained in saving lives, not in abandoning them. This possibly accounts for the fact that only one such situation was written about, and even then, the woman in question was reported to have encouraged her potential rescuers to leave her behind and attend to others who had greater chances of survival. Is it possible that this heroic accounting served, at least in part, to assuage the consciences of the workers who abandoned their desperate attempts to save her? Tragically, in catastrophic human disasters, the dead and injured are not the only victims. Indeed, most health care workers are undoubtedly traumatized survivors themselves, if only in a psychological sense.

Assumptions about social class shaped the Red Cross workers' responses to the disaster, and contemporary societal and cultural tensions over gender also developed. For some, the disaster became a stage for the performance of masculinity, but for others, gendered understandings of the work men and women should do were indistinct. Racial and class antagonisms briefly lifted as people responded to the disaster. And for some, like the Sisters of Charity of the Incarnate Word, the storm became a cherished part of their legacy. One year after the disaster, they opened a new St. Mary's Orphanage, and for years thereafter they paused and remembered all those who perished during the great calamity.[84]

Clara Barton and the Red Cross brought much-needed national help to Galveston. In addition, Barton was instrumental in helping White middle-class women to hold new authority positions in relief activities previously held by men, and she aided Black survivors through the establishment of their independent Red Cross society.[85] Yet discord had arisen, and after her return from Galveston to Washington, DC, Barton faced criticism over her handling of money. This opposition continued in the following years, and she resigned as head of the American Red Cross on May 14, 1904. The following year, the Red Cross reorganized to begin actual nursing and medical services during wartime and disasters.[86]

In closing, health care personnel need to examine disaster sources in all their complexities, including biased accounts that are sometimes self-serving or prejudicial in nature. As we begin to come to terms with recent global disasters, health care workers need to be cognizant of how the persons affected by those events choose to interpret them, and what sociocultural influences they bring with them. Without these perspectives, all people involved in relief work would be handicapped in their efforts to maintain a holistic approach to post-disaster care.

STUDY QUESTIONS

1. Discuss the memoirs, oral histories, and other writings after the 1900 hurricane. How do these writings complicate assumptions about gender? How might the type of disaster influence who or what becomes the target of blame?
2. What are the ethical dilemmas for nurses as they make the transition from emergency room triage, where the sickest person is treated first, to triage during disasters when those less critically ill are often evacuated first?
3. Often after disasters, decisions are made in determining who lives and who dies. Discuss the nursing implications for this situation.

NOTES

1. Associated Press Release from Galveston, Texas, September 9, 1900; and "Monday's Work," *Galveston News*, September 10, 1900, 1.
2. Alice Block to Jennie Robinson, in Casey Edward Greene and Shelly Henley Kelly, eds., *Through a Night of Horrors: Voices From the 1900 Galveston Storm* (College Station, TX: Texas A&M University Press, 2000), 51. This memoir and 32 others, including letters and oral histories, were compiled for the

centennial anniversary of the 1900 storm. Images of the original documents are available at http://www.gthcenter.org/exhibits/storms/1900/Manuscripts.html (accessed July 5, 2006). They are housed in the Rosenberg Library, Galveston and Texas History Center, Galveston, Texas.

3. D. Shiller, "Ike Death Toll Increases as Three Bodies Found," *Houston Chronicle*, September 29, 2008. http://www.chron.com/disp/story.mpl/chronicle/6029478.html (accessed October 12, 2008); and J. Forsyth, "226 Still Missing Following Hurricane Ike: Many May Never Be Found," WOAI AM Radio, October 6, 2008. http://radio.woai.com/cc-common/news/sections/newsarticle.html?feed=&article=4355377 (accessed October 12, 2008).

4. J. Burnett, "In Galveston, Texas, Hospital Weathers Storm." http://www.npr.org/templates/story/story.php?storyId=94680768&ft=1&f=1003; http://www.utmbhealthcare.org/ (accessed October 16, 2008). The response for Galveston was slow. In November 2008, University of Texas System regents announced 3,800 layoffs of nurses, technicians, and other hospital employees at UTMB due to financial losses resulting from the storm.

5. Ellen Beasley, *The Alleys and Back Buildings of Galveston: An Architectural and Social History* (Houston, TX: Rice University Press, 1996); Juan Ockman, ed., *Out of Ground Zero: Case Studies in Urban Reinvention* (Munich and New York; Prestel Publishers, 2002); and Raymond W. Gastil and Zoe Ryan, eds., *Information Exchange: How Cities Renew, Rebuild, and Remember* (New York: Van Alen Institute, 2002).

6. Edward T. Linenthal, *The Unfinished Bombing: Oklahoma City in American Memory* (New York: Oxford University Press, 2001); Mark Pelling, *The Vulnerability of Cities: Natural Disasters and Social Resilience* (London: Earthscan Publications, 2003); and Lawrence J. Vale and Thomas J. Campanella, *The Resilient City: How Modern Cities Recover From Disaster* (New York: Oxford University Press, 2005).

7. Rutherford H. Platt, *Disasters and Democracy: The Politics of Extreme Natural Events* (Washington, DC: Island Press, 1999); Ted Steinberg, *Acts of God: The Unnatural History of Natural Disaster in America* (New York: Oxford University Press, 2000); Steven Biel, ed., *American Disasters* (New York: New York University Press, 2001); Ronald J. Daniels, Donald F. Kettl, and Howard Kunreuther, eds., *On Risk and Disaster* (Philadelphia: University of Pennsylvania Press, 2006); and Thomas A. Birkland, *Lessons of Disaster: Policy Change After Catastrophic Events* (Washington, DC: Georgetown University Press, 2007).

8. Committee on Disasters and the Mass Media, Commission on Sociotechnical Systems, National Research Council, *Disasters and the Mass Media* (Washington, DC: National Academy of Sciences, 1980); Jonathan Benthall,

Disasters, Relief and the Media (London: Tauris, 1993); and Ann Larabee, *Decade of Disaster* (Champaign: University of Illinois Press, 1999).

9. Kevin Rozario (2005). "Making Progress: Disaster Narratives and the Art of Optimism in Modern America," in *The Resilient City*, 27–54.

10. Resources on nursing care for this disaster are scarce. Personal documents such as diaries, letters, and chronicles of nurses' actions are unavailable. A primary source that is accessible is Clara Barton's report to the American National Red Cross, entitled "To the People of the United States." This document, along with survivors' original oral histories, memoirs, and letters, are in the Galveston and Texas History Center of the Rosenberg Library in Galveston, Texas, and they are available online. A methodology in cultural history also is used that involves looking more closely at material culture in the form of songs, poems, and sketches composed just after the disaster. Other primary sources are located at the Sisters of Charity of the Incarnate Word Archives in Houston, Texas. The American National Red Cross Society's papers are located at the National Archives in College Park, Maryland, and were helpful in revealing financial documents and Barton's frustration afterward when discord arose over her financial dealings.

11. R.R. Dynes, *Organized Behavior in Disaster* (Lexington, MA: heath Lexington Books, 1970); E.L. Quarantelli, "Organizational Behavior in Disasters and Implications for Disaster Planning," The Disaster Research Center Report Series 18 (Newark, DE: Disaster Research Center, 1985); and T.E. Drabek, *Human System Responses to Disaster: An Inventory of Sociological Findings* (New York: Springer-Verlag, 1986).

12. Alfred L. Brophy, *Reconstructing the Dreamland: The Tulsa Riot of 1921, Race, Raparations, and Reconciliation* (New York: Oxford University Press, 2002); Vale and Campanella, eds., *The Resilient City*; Rozario, "Making Progress," 33–46; and Patricia Bellis Bixel and Elizabeth Hayes Turner, *Galveston and the 1900 Storm* (Austin: University of Texas Press, 2000).

13. Patricia D'Antonio, "Nurses—and Wives and Mothers: Women and the Latter Day Saints Training School's Class of 1919," *Journal of Women's History* 19, no. 3 (2007): 112–136.

14. Bixel and Turner, *Galveston and the 1900 Storm*; Greene and Kelly, *Through a Night of Horrors*; and David G. McComb, *Galveston, A History* (Austin: University of Texas Press, 1986; repr. 2002).

15. Beasley, *Alleys and Back Buildings*.

16. http://www.utexas.edu/utpress/excerpts/exmarroe.html and http://memory.loc.gov/ammem/aap/timeline2.html (accessed May 27, 2009). According to a National Association for the Advancement of Colored People document,

Texas ranked third in numbers of lynchings, behind Georgia and Mississippi, with 335 from 1889 to 1918; 75 percent of these were Blacks.

17. Bixel and Turner, *Galveston and the 1900 Storm*.

18. After Reconstruction, Southern legislatures passed laws requiring segregation of Whites and Blacks in public transportation and eventually in schools, restaurants, and other public places. In *Brown v Board of Education* in 1954, the U.S. Supreme Court declared segregation in public schools unconstitutional.

19. Anonymous letter, September 8, 1900. 1900 Online Manuscript Exhibit, MSS # 22-0045. http://www.gthcenter.org/exhibits/storms/1900/Manuscripts/Anon_letter/index.html (accessed October 12, 2008).

20. "Galveston Storm, 1900," 1900 Storm file, Villa de Matel Archives, Sisters of Charity of the Incarnate Word, Houston, Texas (hereafter cited as VMA); and J.B. Gleissner, "Reminiscences of September 8, 1900: A Small Tribute to the Heroines Whether They Are Living or Dead," 1938, VMA. In 1900, Catholics in Texas were in the minority in a Protestant-dominated culture, but Galveston had one of the oldest Catholic traditions in the country. It was here that the Sisters of Charity of the Incarnate Word had opened the first Catholic hospital in Texas in 1867, St. Mary's.

21. "Galveston Storm, 1900."

22. http://www.history.noaa.gov/stories_tales/cline2.html (accessed May 23, 2009).

23. Eleanor Hertford to Mr. Gonzales, September 7, 1900. http://www.gthcenter.org/exhibits/storms/1900/Manuscripts/Gonzales/index.html (accessed May 23, 2009).

24. Walter Davis to Mother, September 14, 1900. http://www.gthcenter.org/exhibits/storms/1900/Manuscripts/Davis/1.html (accessed May 23, 2009).

25. Lloyd R.D. Fayling, http://www.gthcenter.org/exhibits/storms/1900/Manuscripts/Fayling/index.html (accessed May 23, 2009).

26. Gleissner, "Reminiscences of September 8, 1900."

27. http://www.gthcenter.org/exhibits/storms/1900/Manuscripts/JHHawley/index.html (accessed May 23, 2009).

28. J.E. Weems, *A Weekend in September* (College Station: Texas A&M University Press, 1957; repr. 1980), 90.

29. HK to Editor: The Editor's Letter-Box, *Trained Nurse and Hospital Review* 25 (November 1900): n.p.

30. A.J. Smith, "The Medical Department and the Galveston Storm," *The University Record* III, no. 1 (1901): 53–69.

31. L. Blackburn, "She Recalls Big Job on Isle Flood," *The Houston Press*, April 13, 1956. This history was written over half a century later. When an oral history of this sort is found, it is important to keep in mind its limitations due to the lengthy passage of time. In this case, an examination of a 1900

nursing journal verified much of the nurse's story. The October 1900 issue of *Trained Nurse and Hospital Review* appealed for nurses to aid each other by describing the tragic deaths of two nurses, one a student and the other a graduate nurse. See "Latest From Galveston," *Trained Nurse and Hospital Review* 25 (October 1900): 292.

32. "Scenes at Galveston," *Houston Daily Post*, September 11, 1900, p. 7.

33. "History of St. Mary's Infirmary, Galveston, Texas," 1900, Catholic Archives of Texas, Austin, Texas.

34. G.A. Kreps, "The Federal Emergency Management System in the United States: Past and Present," *International Journal of Mass Emergencies and Disasters* 8, no. 3 (1990): 281; and C.B. Rubin, ed., *Emergency Management: The American Experience, 1900–2005* (Fairfax, VA: Public Entity Risk Institute, 2007). This situation persisted until World War II.

35. "Monday's Work." See also: http://www.gthcenter.org/exhibits/storms/1900/ Manuscripts/Focke/04-0028_1.html (accessed May 23, 2009).

36. Paul Lester, *The Great Galveston Disaster: Containing a Full and Thrilling Account of the Most Appalling Calamity of Modern Times* (Philadelphia: Globe, 1900), 431–432.

37. Henry Cortes, 1957 memoir, in Greene and Kelly, *Through a Night of Horrors*, 127.

38. http://www.gthcenter.org/exhibits/storms/1900/Manuscripts/Austin/index. html (accessed May 23, 2009).

39. Mary Louise Bristol Hopkins, http://www.gthcenter.org/collections/oralhist/ index.htm#H (accessed May 23, 2009).

40. http://www.gthcenter.org/exhibits/storms/1900/Manuscripts/Rollfing/index. html (accessed May 23, 2009).

41. Mrs. Winifred Black, "Shot for Cutting Dead Woman's Ears," MSS #80-0019, 1900 Storm Online Manuscript Exhibit, Baltimore, Committee in Aid of the Galveston Sufferers Concert Program, http://www.gthcenter.org/ exhibits/storms/1900/Manuscripts/Baltimore/index.html (accessed June 2, 2009). See also Lester, *The Great Galveston Disaster*.

42. Jan Harold Brunvand, *The Big Book of Urban Legends* (New York: Paradox Press, 1994), 152.

43. Clarence Ousley, *Galveston in 1900* (Atlanta, GA: W.C. Chase, 1901).

44. "Monday's Work" and "Organizing Relief," *Galveston News*, September 10, 1900, 1.

45. Charles Law to Wife. http://www.gthcenter.org/exhibits/storms/1900/Manu scripts/Storm_Letter/3.html (accessed May 23, 2009).

46. "Monday's Work"; "Organizing Relief."

47. Sylvia G.L. Dannett, *Profiles of Negro Womanhood*, Volume II of Negro Heritage Library, (Yonkers, NY: Educational Heritage, Inc., 1966); Joyce Ann

Elmore, "Black Nurses, Their Service and Their Struggle" *American Journal of Nursing* 76, no. 3 (March 1976): 435–437; M. Elizabeth Carnegie, *The Path We Tread: Blacks in Nursing Worldwide, 1854–1994* (New York: National League for Nursing Press, 1995); "Surgical Relief," *Galveston Tribune*, September 12, 1900, n.p.; "Suggestions and Advice, *The City Times*, September 29, 3, no. 5 (1900): n.p. Curtis was instrumental in the establishment of Provident Hospital School in Chicago. This hospital, through its medical and nursing schools, played a significant role in educating Black men and women in the health care fields.

48. "Supplies and Medicine," *Galveston Tribune*, September 12, 1900, n.p.
49. "Aid for Storm Victims," *New York Times*, September 12, 1900, 2. See also http://www.galvestonhistory.org/hrc-fact-sheet.htm (accessed November 16, 2006).
50. "Fifth Ward Hospital," *Galveston Daily News*, September 16, 1900, n.p.
51. "2400 Bodies Had Been Recovered," *The Daily Picayune*, New Orleans, September 12, 1900.
52. Katherine Vedder Pauls, February 3, 1970, http://www.gthcenter.org/collections/oralhist/index.htm#P (accessed June 1, 2009).
53. "Third Reading: Our Legacy," Hurricane 1900 folder, VMA.
54. "Hospital Opportunities," *Galveston Daily News*, September 16, 1900, n.p.
55. Hospital records, St. Mary's Infirmary, 1900, VMA.
56. "Red Cross Society Will Afford Practiced Help and Money Will Be Raised," *The New York World*, September 12, 1900, 3.
57. Clara Barton, "To the People of the United States," 1900 Storm Online Manuscript Exhibit, Red Cross Records, MSS # 05-000. http://www.gthcenter.org/exhibits/storms/1900/Manuscripts/RedCross_7/index.html (accessed July 5, 2006). Included is "Report of Mrs. Mussey," pp. 42–43; and "Report of Mrs. Fannie B. Ward," p. 47. See also Caroline Moorehead, *Dunant's Dream: War, Switzerland and the History of the Red Cross* (London: HarperCollins, 1998).
58. Barton, "To the People of the United States;" and Bixel and Turner, *Galveston and the 1900 Storm*.
59. Elizabeth Hayes Turner, *Women, Culture, and Community: Religion and Reform in Galveston, 1880–1920* (New York: Oxford University Press, 1997).
60. Portia B. Kernodle, *The Red Cross Nurse in Action, 1882–1948* (New York: Harper and Brothers, Publisher, 1949).
61. "Report of Mrs. Mussey," 43. In 1900, the Red Cross was responsible for obtaining supplies instead of providing nursing care, although the general perception was otherwise. In 1889 after the Johnstown flood, most of the nursing was handled by a branch of the American Red Cross from Phila-

delphia not associated with Barton. See Kernodle, *The Red Cross Nurse in Action*.

62. "Red Cross Society Account to Star Drug Store," Galveston, Texas, November 8, 1900, and "Texas, Galveston Hurricane." Both documents are located at the National Archives Gift Collection, Records of the American National Red Cross, 1881–1916; Box 58, folder 863, National Archives Building, College Park, Maryland (hereafter cited as NABCP). See also http://www.gthcenter.org/exhibits/storms/1900/Manuscripts/Baltimore/index.html; and http://www.gthcenter.org/exhibits/storms/1900/Manuscripts/Rollfing/index.html (accessed May 23, 2009).

63. Report of Mrs. Fannie Ward, in Barton, "To the People of the United States," p. 46.

64. Ibid.

65. Marian Moser Jones, "Confronting Calamity: The American Red Cross and the Politics of Disaster Relief, 1881–1939," PhD Dissertation, Columbia University, 2008. Proquest Dissertations and Theses, Publication #AAT 3317567, p. 182.

66. "Suggestions and Advice."

67. http://www.gthcenter.org/exhibits/storms/1900/Manuscripts/Rollfing/index.html (accessed May 23, 2009).

68. "Luke No Fool," *The City Times*, September 29, 1900; 3 (5): n.p.

69. Barton, "To the People of the United States," 11.

70. Ibid., 4.

71. Ibid., 11.

72. Ibid., 10–12; and "Full Report, 1900"; "Texas, Galveston Hurricane," NABCP; and Bixel and Turner, *Galveston and the 1900 Storm*.

73. Barton,"To the People of the United States," 20–22; and "Full Report," NABCP.

74. William W. Delaney, "The Texas Cyclone," MSS #99-0005, 1900 Storm Online Manuscript Exhibit, http://www.gthcenter.org/exhibits/storms/1900/Manuscripts/Texas_Cyclone/index.html (accessed June 2, 2009).

75. W. Elbert Dando, "The Ruined City," MSS #80-0019, 1900 Storm Online Manuscript Exhibit.

76. Revell Carr, "We Will Never Forget: Disaster in American Folk Songs From the Nineteenth Century to September 11, 2001," *Voices: The Journal of New York Folklore* 30 (Fall–Winter 2004). http://www.nyfolklore.org/pubs/voic30-3-4/disaster.html (accessed April 3, 2010).

77. "Galveston," *Galveston News*, September 13, 1900, n.p.

78. Barton, "To the People of the United States," 34.

79. Faculty and Staff, *The University of Texas Medical Branch at Galveston: A Seventy-Five Year History by the Faculty and Staff* (Austin: University of Texas Press, 1967), 62.

80. Typed copy of "Resolutions of the Central Relief Committee of Galveston,"
     Box RG 200, National Archives Gift Collection, Records of the American
     National Red Cross, 1881–1916; Box 58, folder 863, NABCP.
81. Robert A. Calvert, Arnoldo De Leon, and Gregg Cantrell, *The History of Texas*, 3rd
     ed. (Wheeling, IL: Harlan Davidson, Inc., 2002), 250; McComb, *Galveston,
     A History*; and D.A. Williams, *Bricks Without Straw: A Comprehensive His-
     tory of African Americans in Texas* (Austin, TX: Eakin Press, 1997).
82. Bixel and Turner, *Galveston and the 1900 Storm*.
83. McComb, *Galveston, A History*, 149.
84. "Third Reading: Our Legacy."
85. Bixel and Turner, *Galveston and the 1900 Storm*.
86. Moorehead, *Dunant's Dream*, and "Full Report," NABCP.

CHAPTER 3

The San Francisco Earthquake and Fire, 1906: "A Lifetime of Experience"

Barbra Mann Wall and Marie E. Kelly

Was it only a week I spent in the camp? I asked my friend . . . after what seemed a lifetime of experience.[1]

In 1906, Lucy Fisher wrote these words in the *American Journal of Nursing* (*AJN*) about her experiences as a nurse after the April 18, 1906, San Francisco earthquake and fire. In 1906, San Francisco ranked as one of the major cities in the United States with a population of a half-million people. Its location over the San Andreas Fault, however, made it prone to earthquakes.[2] While tremors were not new to the city, the 1906 earthquake proved to be devastating. Modern analysis estimates that it registered 8.25 on the Richter scale. The shaking lasted nearly 60 seconds, and people from Oregon to Los Angeles to Nevada felt the tremors. Although the earthquake was destructive, fires, compounded by the lack of water, became raging infernos over the next 3 days. The quake and resulting fire are remembered as causing one of the worst natural disasters in the history of the United States, with a death toll estimated to be 3,000. More than 28,000 buildings burned, half of San Francisco's population was homeless, and 225,000 injuries occurred[3] (see Figure 3.1).

Fisher worked 7 days and nights at a makeshift hospital in Golden Gate Park. Her dramatic experiences and those of other nurses and health care workers who witnessed the terrible events can be pieced together in materials published in the form of letters and written reminiscences. In their accounts, few people expressed concerns about pandemonium, likely because of a rapid military response; rather, many of the stories focused on the excitement of working in a great calamity.[4] These sentiments were

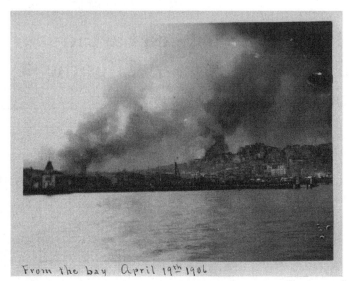

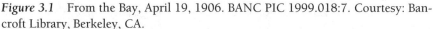

Figure 3.1   From the Bay, April 19, 1906. BANC PIC 1999.018:7. Courtesy: Bancroft Library, Berkeley, CA.

not purposely wished for. However, according to Rebecca Solnit, emotions "graver than happiness but deeply positive" are not uncommon after disasters. Disasters bring out the best in people and provide them with a common purpose.[5] As nurses worked at the front lines of this disaster, their senses sharpened, and they became totally absorbed in their work.

THE RED CROSS AND MILITARY RESPONSE

In 1905, Congress had reincorporated the American Red Cross by a new charter that designated it an official relief organization. Clara Barton had retired, and a Progressive reformer in the person of Mabel Boardman and a central committee of business and government leaders led the organization. This designation gave the agency national standing, but none of the leaders had any field experience.[6] As was customary, local resources were initially mobilized and then collaborated with the Red Cross. The Red Cross nursing recruitment was slow, and the *San Francisco Chronicle* pleaded for nurses from all over the country.[7]

Initially, San Francisco business leaders formed a Committee of Fifty to manage the crisis, with former mayor James Phelan in charge. He also was named head of the finance committee and, as such, had authority over the allocation of relief funds. Because the Red Cross was still in its reorganization phase, it assumed a secondary role. President Theodore Roosevelt, however, without consulting the Committee of Fifty, impulsively declared the Red Cross as the best organization to take over the relief work, and he named Dr. Edward T. Devine, a special Red Cross agent, as its representative in San Francisco. He was to control all relief funds. This caused a furor when the local committee felt insulted over the President's distrust of them, and after Devine's arrival, he, Phelan, and the other business leaders agreed to consolidate their efforts and work as one body. The Red Cross received relief contributions, and the finance committee allocated them. Roosevelt reversed himself as well.[8] The Congress hastily approved $2.5 million for relief, which was supplemented by more than $10 million that Phelan's committee raised in contributions.[9]

Mayor Eugene Schmitz of San Francisco quickly called in the military to meet immediate needs. As the fires gained momentum, they burned over 3 days, with the city's water system destroyed. The military took charge of firefighting, restoring order, distributing tents, serving meals, establishing communication lines, organizing food and clothing distributions, and setting up field hospitals and dispensaries. To care for the homeless, the U.S. Army set up 28 refugee camps in city parks and squares, including Golden Gate Park, the Presidio, Fort Mason, and Harbor View. It also divided the city into seven districts, with Army officers, physicians, and Red Cross representatives in charge. The Army and Red Cross eventually provided earthquake cottages of durable redwood that replaced the tents. Tens of thousands of survivors sought refuge in camps or poured out of the city to surrounding towns[10] (see Figure 3.2).

NURSING AND MEDICAL RESPONSES TO THE DISASTER

The Mechanics' Pavilion: "Given No Alternative"

Various private groups rushed into action. In her account to the *AJN*, nurse Lucy Fisher noted that she was asleep when the first quake rumbled at 5:13 a.m. She awoke and immediately thought she was facing death, which she

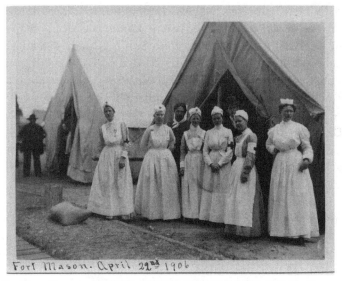

Fort Mason. April 22nd 1906

Figure 3.2   Fort Mason, April 22, 1906, BANC PIC 1999.018:11. Courtesy: Bancroft Library, Berkeley, CA.

looked at calmly though not bravely, because she "was given no alternative." After quickly dressing, she ran to check on a friend and then walked down the streets with another nurse to check the extent of damage. They passed a Nurses' Home, where several people on the front porch told Fisher and her companion that most of the nurses had gone to the Mechanics' Pavilion, which had been opened as a hospital for the injured. The Central Emergency Hospital at the City Hall had been destroyed (Figure 3.3), and the patients and most of the supplies there had been carried over to the nearby Pavilion. At this point, Fisher recalled, "a lump came into my throat at the significance of that message," as she realized that her "duty was so unquestionable that without a word even having passed between us we started toward the Pavilion."[11]

Fisher and other nurses were typically trained in 2- to 3-year nursing programs that stressed an ideology of discipline, self-sacrifice, order, and, as nursing leader Adelaide Nutting called it, "an apprenticeship to duty."[12] Thus, Fisher felt an obligation that compelled her toward the disaster scene. By the time she arrived at the Pavilion, other local nurses, Catholic sisters,

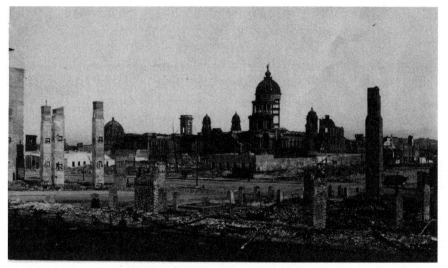

Figure 3.3   San Francisco's 1906 Earthquake: City Hall, April 1900. CHS 2009.123; FN-36064, SF-EQ (1906). Courtesy: California Historical Society, San Francisco, CA.

physicians, and out-of-town doctors attending the California Medical Convention were already working there.

Dr. Rene Bine, a young San Francisco physician, was one of them. He also related his experiences in the hours and days after the disaster. He had commandeered an automobile with his father's pistol in hand. At first, the driver took him to several hospitals for the doctor to check on his patients and then returned him to the Pavilion. Bine and others broke into hardware and drug stores to get medical supplies and ransacked department stores for pillows and mattresses for the injured.[13] One man recalled taking an enthusiastic Salvation Army woman with him. "When we arrived at a drugstore under the St. Nicholas," he wrote, "she jumped out, and, finding the door locked, seized a chair and raising it above her head smashed the glass doors in and helped herself to hot water bags, bandages, and everything which would be useful in an emergency hospital."[14] Apparently, these volunteers deemed lives more important than possessions, and they felt justified in taking the supplies.

Dr. Margaret Mahoney was another volunteer at the Pavilion. After the quake, she quickly dressed and ran toward a collapsed building to try to free any survivors, but it was to no avail because there were none. Fearing that there might be other injured people who needed her help, she then checked on her patients at two different hospitals and subsequently went to the Pavilion to offer her services. On her way, she wondered at how few casualties were on the streets, as many seemed to have escaped unharmed. As she entered the Pavilion, however, she witnessed a dead body carried out in a wicker basket coffin and more than 300 injured persons inside. Still, Mahoney noted, "Within all was perfect order; the wounds of the injured bandaged; coffee being served, every attention given."[15]

At first, Fisher and her companion were not permitted into the Pavilion until they said they were nurses. Instantly, that word allowed them entrance. They faced a scene of mattresses strewn on the floor, nearly all occupied by patients. An improvised surgery was well equipped and already in operation with operating room tables, dressings, instruments, and hot and cold sterilized water from the destroyed emergency hospital. Patients constantly were being admitted and tended not only by physicians and nurses but also by ministers, priests, and Catholic sisters, among others. But to Fisher, it was not "perfect order." Rather, there was much confusion as everyone hurried about trying to help the sufferers. Fisher and her friend were told to "pitch in," which they quickly did. Since the surgery area was well staffed, Fisher was particularly concerned about the critical cases that might be overlooked in the confusion, and she went around the room with extra blankets, hot water bags, and coffee for people in immediate danger. In the process, she observed for those "with feeble pulses and blue lips."[16]

Fisher and her friend worked in the main part of the building, pinning pillowcases to their waists to carry dressings. In addition to dressing changes, they gave hypodermic injections for stimulation and anesthesia. Because of the confusion and the danger of duplication of drugs, the nurses pinned tags onto patients with the name and quantity of the drug, and the time it was administered. People were constantly rearranging the mattresses, making it considerably difficult to keep up with patients' locations. Once, Fisher went to get a sterilized basin for a dressing change only to find that her patient had been moved. In addition, the enthusiasm of so many wanting to help led to a duplication of effort. Humorous incidents did occur, "incidents in a drama that we were all a part of and were to us what the fool is to the tragedies of Shakespeare," wrote Fisher, "a moment's respite and relaxation for overwrought emotions." However, these short periods did not overcome the tragedy of the situation. Nurses patched up survivors with cuts from glass and helped patients with broken bones and burns. Fisher talked with a woman who was badly burned and had lost all three of her children. Three weeks later, as Fisher did follow-up visits for the Red Cross, she came upon this woman again, who had found one of her daughters but not the other two.[17] Nurses also cared for patients who eventually died of shock. Typical of a patient death was a woman who was admitted to a hospital at 1 p.m. on April 18 suffering from shock. She received two doses of strychnine and one of nitroglycerine by hypodermic injection but died at 5:15 that day.[18]

The patients and personnel at the Pavilion experienced several aftershocks, but the most devastating incident occurred when the fires reached the Pavilion itself. Health care personnel whispered this news to each other and quickly moved 354 patients to the rear entrance, where they were placed in ambulances and other vehicles and taken to hospitals at the Presidio or Golden Gate Park. Months later, as Fisher recalled, some people with "wild imaginations" had hinted that patients had been "chloroformed" while others had been shot. While these reports later were proven false, Fisher worried about them. To her *AJN* readers, she noted that the physician in charge remained in the building until all the patients and equipment had been removed.[19] Dr. Mahoney also wrote that all were evacuated within an hour.[20]

What was especially difficult for nurses was determining where they were most needed. All they could do was to go to each hospital and inquire within, which took a considerable amount of time. Fisher and two other nurses eventually went to the California Woman's Hospital, and they rode in a machine that was new to them and therefore anxiety provoking: the automobile. As Fisher exclaimed, "Paul Revere's ride might justly be compared to ours but nothing less sensational." Although she had lived through the earthquake and fire, she thought she surely would be killed in the speeding car. However, the "hell wagons," as they often were called, became "chariots of mercy" as they were the salvation of many. Indeed, the *San Francisco Chronicle* referred to automobiles as "the most heroic messenger service"[21] (see Figure 3.4).

Fisher was not needed at the California Woman's Hospital, so she went to the hospital at the thousand-acre Golden Gate Park. She recalled,

> From the hour of the earthquake . . . quests for lost relatives and friends began. At the Pavilion faces were eagerly scanned by distracted people

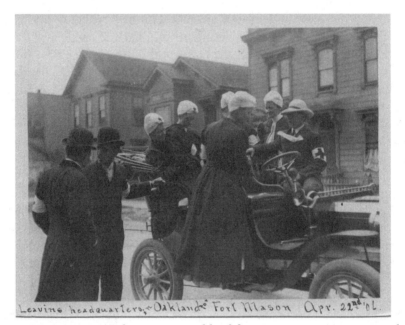

Leaving headquarters; Oakland, Fort Mason   Apr. 22nd '06

Figure 3.4   Leaving Headquarters in Oakland for Fort Mason via an automobile, April 22, 1906. BANC PIC 1999, 018:9. Courtesy: Bancroft Library, Berkeley, CA.

seeking their lost ones. In the hospitals and camps these searches continued during the days that followed and have not yet ceased. . . . "The cry of Rachael weeping for her children and refused to be comforted because they were not," was the picture at the Pavilion and at the Park Hospital and in the camps that made so many of us who looked upon it feel that words of comfort would be almost a mockery, and that all we could do was to offer a silent sympathy.[22]

At Golden Gate Park, nurses lived in a different kind of world where, in Fisher's words, "Old things had passed away, and all things had become new and terrible, and if . . . that continuity of life is dependent upon adaptability to environment, we possessed that qualification in a high degree."[23] They donned long white smocks they had brought with them and worked in the field where patients arrived throughout the night. The nurses had to plan for continually changing conditions. They readied beds on mattresses on the ground, relieved pain with morphine injections, and gave strychnine hypodermically for stimulation. At first, Fisher tried to obtain orders from one of the physicians before giving the injections, but it took so long to find him that he eventually told her to use her own judgment, which she promptly did. In all the excitement, she found that she developed additional strength to meet the unusually heavy demands, and her senses "became unusually keen."[24]

Throughout the first 3 days and nights, the boom of dynamite sounded as firemen, frustrated by broken water mains, used explosives to create firebreaks in a desperate measure to check the progress of the fire.[25] This proved to be futile. Fisher could see the crimson sky in the distance, and her eyes burned from the falling ashes. She and the other nurses cared for firemen who had been injured and other patients who suffered from the "fire dust." The third night she made rounds with some medical students who helped her carry a lantern and supplies, such as "boracic acid" solution and cotton, which she used for cleansing patients' eyes. By the fourth day, the winds had died down and the firestorms had ended. Throughout, Fisher had been too excited to sleep, and by the end of the week, she realized she had dozed but 10 hours.[26]

Even though the nurses did not work for the Red Cross, they wore arm bands with Red Cross labels and placed these symbols on ambulances and automobiles to facilitate passing through the lines of sentries. Fisher likened the situation at the Golden Gate Park to a "battlefield," with the Red Cross symbols on arms, the wounded lying on the ground, and the many soldiers who guarded the camp. By April 20, there were estimates of 100,000 refugees in the park and 254 people treated at the hospital. Physicians, nurses, medical students, and untrained helpers provided the work. Fisher constructed a distance between herself and some women who were "unprofessional nurses," in her view. While many were no doubt sincere in their motives, Fisher saw them as a hindrance rather than a help. She also noted the blurring of boundaries of social class. She witnessed doctors who did carpentry work, supervised the commissary department, and put up tents. Others who had not known the likes of hard labor cooked over smoky stoves and served large numbers of workers with food. Indeed, groups that had never socialized with each other before felt solidarity as they met immediate survival needs. After working for a week, an exhausted Fisher eventually went to a friend's home in Oakland.[27]

The Presidio Refugee Camp: "Like Civil War Times"

After the Mechanics' Pavilion burned, many of the injured were taken to the Presidio, which included a 300-bed general hospital and smaller post hospital. Anna Blake was not a nurse but a patient at the general hospital. She had been at the Clara Barton Hospital with a painful ear condition and was transferred to the Presidio during the first week of the earthquake. She wrote several letters to her mother and grandmother about her situation. Much of the letters contain personal information, such as requests for her eyeglasses. Other parts reveal the fears and suffering she experienced during the earthquake and fire and the relationship she had with her nurses.[28]

Blake's letters illustrated the pathos occurring around her. While she was being transported to the Presidio, she remembered the awful silence, punctured only by intermittent booms of dynamite. The ambulance in which she was riding had to travel through crowded streets in intense heat with flames over 2 miles long and a mile high that followed them.[29] At the end of April, she wrote to her mother that it "seems like Civil War times" because soldiers were in the room day and night. A nurse named Mrs. Cunningham cared for her at first at the Presidio but was transferred later, much to Blake's sorrow. One of her doctors also left for another hospital, and she found his replacement to be "snippy."[30] She was placed in Ward G at first, which she labeled a "mousetrap": The wall was cracked, the windows unhinged, and plaster loose from the ceiling. Eventually, Blake transferred to Ward C where things improved.

On April 25, she wrote to her mother, "We all have our lives and no broken limbs and fortunately my sickest days are over, so don't worry. If I only had Miss Cunningham."[31] She also confided to her mother about her fear of vaccination, to which she had to subject herself. Indeed, patients had little control over what was happening to them. Five minutes passed, and then she continued her letter: "The deed is done, and I suppose I must accept that with the rest. I positively refused to have it on my arm like the rest so I have it on my leg. Carried my point for once."[32] Thus, amid the powerlessness Blake felt as a patient, by this act, she restored some control over her situation.

On May 25, Blake penned a letter to her grandmother and provided details of the dire conditions in the camp:

> The first week here was like a week in Libby Prison. Over a hundred of us were crowded together in one room of the barracks. There were rich women

and poor women, white, yellow and black, from all quarters of the city. . . . There was no heat, scant food and little water. We were allowed no communication with the outside and sentries guarded the place day and night, no one being allowed to enter but priests and nuns and wearers of the Red Cross. Then conditions began to improve.

Later, when a fire broke out at the Presidio, she heard soldiers crying, "Shoot anyone caught looting" and "Get the patients out." They feared a riot, but soon the wind changed, which kept her ward from burning. That fire, however, frightened her more than the big one in the city. She, too, heard tragic stories from fellow patients who had lost children and other family members. Indeed, "the bravest women were those who had been the richest and had lost the most."[33]

Dr. Bine, who had worked at the Mechanics' Pavilion initially, went to the Presidio, where more than 10,000, at his estimation, slept outside, including Dr. Mahoney and her family (see Figure 3.5). Tugs brought in food from Oakland and other areas. He then oversaw the Harbor View refugee camp, which held 2,800 people. Camp payrolls noted that nurses worked 7 days a week, 10- to 12-hour shifts, and were paid $60 a month. Bine, on the other hand, worked 14-hour days for $150 a month. On Monday, April 30, he wrote that sanitary conditions in the camp were improving. The camps were well organized, with latrines, garbage disposal systems, washing facilities, and running water. Bine was able to distribute hot cocoa to the camp refugees, and even though he was drenched by rains, he wrote, "I never felt better in my life. We sleep on the ground & it is better than the country and lots of fun. We have a good supply of rations & are in OK shape all around."[34]

Despite sanitation measures, this camp and others were at risk of typhoid fever epidemics, and the Department of Health reported 289 cases in San Francisco between April and August. A special health commission formed with representatives of the medical profession, U.S. Army, public health and marine services, and city and state boards of health. The commission initiated inspections and disinfecting crews, set up isolation hospitals and water and food control measures, obtained laboratory supplies from Hahnemann Hospital and the University of California College of Agriculture, and arranged for the removal of 509 dead animals.[35]

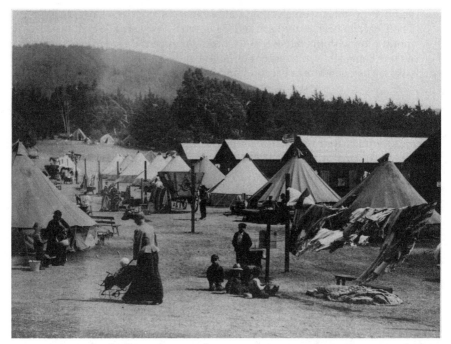

Figure 3.5   A windy day at the Presidio, San Francisco Refugee Camp, April 1906.
FN-26267. Source: California Historical Society, San Francisco, CA.

Oakland: "Working in the Thick of the Suffering"

The largest number of refugees went to Oakland, just across the bay from San Francisco. William Randolph Hearst, the newspaper icon and editor of the *Examiner*, sent a special relief team from Los Angeles, which included doctors, nurses, and journalists. One nurse was Nellie May Brown. She and other members of the relief team arrived the day after the quake and immediately went out to the Presidio, where thousands of refugees had assembled. They were not allowed to land, however, and came back to Oakland, where they established a hospital. Brown wrote several letters and postcards to her mother, detailing her anxieties, her concern for her brother Ralph, and reassurances of her own safety. The letters also are revealing for the sentiments she felt about her work. Upon her arrival, she said, "Words cannot describe the horror of the scene—people are leaving everything & are crowding the ferries and every other transport which will carry them out of it. The whole city will eventually be swept away completely." At the camp in Oakland, two to three doctors and newspapermen worked with each group of 10 nurses. Unlike Lucy Fisher, Brown was able to sleep, but she still confided to her mother that they should "bear up . . . and try to help others."[36]

By the next day, Brown was well rested and "working in the thick of the suffering—at last experiencing the horrors of the field hospital." She was in the first squad sent out to one of the nearby forts. Because of the threats of disease, they were all vaccinated. She, too, was having the "experience of a lifetime."[37] In addition to working in Oakland, on April 22, Brown and other nurses went into the city to relieve nurses in different hospitals. They experienced the fright of aftershocks, and a pall fell over the entire relief party when one of the physicians fell down some stairs and his revolver discharged, killing him instantly.[38]

Other Responses: "We Render Many Services Not In a Nurse's Line"

Other nurses from across the country volunteered. Sister Mary Veronica Ryan, the superintendent of Mercy Hospital Training School in Chicago, was instrumental in sending 30 Mercy nurses to assist survivors in San Francisco.[39] Then, in June 1906, the *AJN* published a report of a variety of nurses' experiences during the disaster. Genevieve Cook, editor of the *Nurses' Journal of the Pacific Coast*, had volunteered for duty at the Presidio General Hospital but was asked instead to do private duty for one of the officers whose wife was seriously ill. Another nurse who worked for the Red Cross Society had to walk to the Presidio camp with her family, but beforehand, she spent the first night in one of the central parks. She immediately put her nursing skills to work caring for newborns and sick babies with measles and pneumonia, and she calmed the refugees and sent the bedridden to other facilities. She wrote that "we render many services not in a nurse's line." Eventually she opened a clinic.[40]

Elizabeth Ashe, a graduate from Presbyterian Hospital Training School in New York, established a camp for convalescents in a neighboring county. She put her plan before the various authorities (no other data are given about the plan), who accepted her proposal. She wanted to pay the nurses small salaries to have one for every 25 or 30 patients, and while some nurses, such as those working with Dr. Bine, did receive payment, the relief committee denied Ashe's request. She also sent a nurse to Telegraph Hill, one of the few areas left unscathed by the fire, to care for refugees there. "It would be a splendid thing to have a nurse in each camp, but that seems to be out of the question," she wrote.[41]

Children's Hospital of San Francisco: "Grateful That I Am a Trained Nurse"

At the time of the disaster, the Directress of Nursing at Children's Hospital of San Francisco (CHSF) was Katherine Brown.[42] Her tenacity in the face of personal hardship, her spirit of adventure as a nursing leader, and her prior nursing experience were all called into play on that fateful April day in San Francisco. A native of Philadelphia, Brown received her nurse's training at the Protestant Episcopal Hospital School of Nursing in that city. Like the education of Fisher and others at the turn of the 20th century, Brown's schooling required stamina and determination. These students routinely worked 70–90 hours a week caring for patients during the day in the hospital, then attended lectures and studied in the evening. After completing her training, Brown worked as the only graduate nurse in charge of a 50-bed hospital and the education of 15 student nurses. Working often 16-hour days during the height of a typhoid epidemic, Brown contracted a near-fatal case of typhoid fever.[43]

Following her convalescence, Brown was not content to relinquish the independence that her nursing career had allowed. In a bold move, she traveled west via the transcontinental railroad. Brown had accepted the position in Salt Lake City, Utah, as Directress of St. Mark's Hospital. The hospital had been established to serve hundreds of workers from the surrounding railroad and mining camps.[44] Prevalent illnesses included lead poisoning, appendicitis, and typhoid fever, and traumatic injuries from accidents were common. Besieged by the hospital's financial instability and gross overcrowding, however, she resigned after a year and accepted the position at CHSF.[45]

All of her prior experiences prepared her for her tenure as Directress at CHSF during the earthquake and fire. The hospital consisted of a building for pediatric cases aged infant to 15 years, a maternity building, a woman's building for gynecology cases, and a pediatric orthopedic building. There was also a separate nurses' residence. Brown was a proponent of the strict discipline and character development of the Nightingale Training School model. These values and the experience she had gained in caring for trauma patients in Utah would serve her well in leading the CHSF nurses in the aftermath of San Francisco disaster.

In a letter to her cousin dated May 15, 1906, Brown wrote that her first sensation when awakened by the earthquake was of "the house . . . shaking as though in the grasp of a great giant."[46] Her professionalism and dedication to her patients is captured in the letter to her family when she retold how she rallied her subordinate nurses minutes after the disaster struck:

> The nurses had rushed out of their rooms and were coming pell mell down the stairs . . . when I opened my door someone called, "Oh Miss Brown, what shall we do?" I answered rather fiercely, "Do? Put something on and come over and see what has happened to our patients!"[47]

In true character, Brown went right to work, organizing the nurses, whom she commended for their "splendid cooperation and lack of hysteria." The CHSF nurses must have been relieved to find that all of their patients had survived the quake, except a "one week malnutrition baby who was thrown to the floor by the swaying of the building and only lived for a few hours."[48]

After she and the nurses tended to the other patients, Brown directed her nurses to begin cleaning up the damage caused by the quake and to prepare for other patients from downtown hospitals that were already in flames. The CHSF was relatively unscathed because of its location outside of the downtown area. By noon, the hospital was filled with earthquake survivors. As in the other areas of the city, there was no running water. The nurses worked under extreme conditions without a sewage system, lights, or heat for the next 6 weeks. Orderlies dug trenches where the nurses carried out the refuse from the wards. A cook stove outdoors served as the kitchen.[49] Brown related feeling a sense of personal fulfillment in the letter to her family in April 1906: "I want to say that never in my life have I been as grateful that I am a trained nurse, a superintendent of a training school, and in San Francisco, as I am this minute."[50]

DISCUSSION: FOCUSED AND ENERGIZED

Newspapers praised nurses for their self-sacrifice. Indeed, in each nursing text, the women described themselves heading toward the disaster area when most residents were trying to escape or, in Katherine Brown's case, preparing immediately to care for the injured in her hospital. What compelled them to do so? Surely they felt a sense of responsibility to care for those in need—to provide the skilled services for which their years of training had prepared them. But for many, it was more than merely their occupational roles that drew them toward the disaster scene, more even than their sense of altruism. It was also a personal force that some were perhaps slow to acknowledge but that is commonly found in intensive care units, emergency rooms, and other sites where life and death are held in the balance. It is a force fed by adrenalin and sustained by feelings of intensity and excitement—feelings that challenge people to apply themselves fully and to give their all to the tasks at hand.

Fisher's own prejudice that men were not naturally fit for nursing was dispelled when she observed three in particular who showed as much gentleness, self-sacrifice, intelligent sympathy, and fine skills as any female nurse.[51] She closed her article in the *AJN* by paying tribute to the many people who undertook the responsibility of caring for the patients who were brought to the Golden Gate camp throughout that first week:

> I know that within my own soul there developed a deeper and greater reverence for human nature in the aggregate as I realized the real divinity of manhood shining forth in deeds of glad self-sacrifice which were manifested in a tireless devotion to the injured; in the performance of tasks that ordinarily might be classed as menial but were done with such an unselfish spirit that the work became glorified.[52]

Nurses provided both physical and psychological first aid, and they helped with evacuations (see Figure 3.6). Their work combined knowledge, skill, bravery, empathy, being present for their patients, and sometimes merely offering a "silent sympathy," which some men did as well as any woman. On April 25, 1906, reflecting on what she had observed in San Francisco after the earthquake, one woman stated, "I really believe that in the heat of the excitement the women were more collected than the men."[53]

LINGERING QUESTIONS

While people crossed many social boundaries after the disaster, there were some problems. Certainly, Anna Blake, the patient at the Presidio hospital, experienced pain and suffering along with thousands of other survivors. In addition, the Red Cross was the object of complaints of withholding relief at key times. Whereas Dr. Mahoney had praised the government's role in caring for survivors at the Presidio, she described "the saddest chapter in the history of our disaster" when the Red Cross and other organized charity workers arrived. Refugees resented them. "These trained workers," wrote Mahoney, "joined with the local relief committee. Being in the habit of dealing with paupers they undertook to pauperize a self-respecting community." Pauperism involved independent people shifting into dependent roles, and it was a major concern of the day.[54]

It is unknown whether or not nurses were involved; nevertheless, to Mahoney, these charity workers hoarded supplies, insulted the people, and tried to drive them from the bread lines. Even though money was plentiful

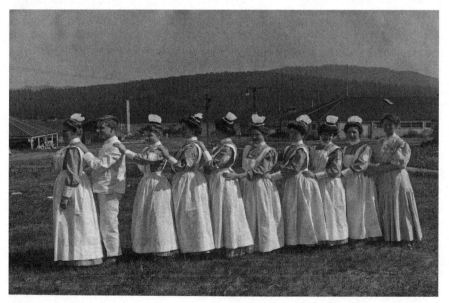

Figure 3.6   Nurses of the City and County Hospital, 1907. FN-26267, Courtesy: California Historical Society, San Francisco, CA.

and new clothing was on hand, they distributed second-hand materials and required people to stand in line all day and answer humiliating questions to get them. One secretary of a local charity told Mahoney, "Put them on their mettle. Make it hard for them." As Mahoney said, "Who were the people to be so treated[?] Human beings who had been through a most dreadful calamity." She was insulted that the relief agencies accused people of staying in the tents because they liked that kind of life and did not want to pay any rent, when thousands had no other shelter to use, or when the Red Cross suggested opening a pawnshop so that people could sell the few articles of value they had saved from the fire, even though there were millions of dollars in the relief fund. Mahoney scathingly concluded that "our crowning sorrow was the relief distribution. . . . May all other stricken communities be spared the combination of Red Cross, trained charity workers and a relief committee composed of wealthy men."[55] Although the Red Cross had raised record amounts of funds, people were left living in temporary structures and impoverished.[56]

A gaping hole in this disaster report includes the voices of Black nurses. Philip L. Fradkin surmised that the Black community may have lacked the means to document personal experiences, or archivists and librarians simply did not seek their stories. We do know that Namahyoke Curtis, who had worked as a nurse in Galveston in 1900, worked in San Francisco as well through a commission from William Howard Taft, then Secretary of War. This well-respected woman worked day and night until her own health became impaired. In addition, Blacks in Los Angeles were enthusiastic in tending to Black refugees coming to their city. They organized societies for the refugees' benefit, raised $500 for relief to be used for clothing and other provisions, met trains, and personally cared for the refugees.[57]

One problem for native San Franciscans was the care of Chinese survivors. Chinese immigrants and children of immigrants had been in San Francisco since the gold rush days, and in the 1850s, they began to congregate in the area between Nob Hill and the financial district. More than 35,000 lived in the area known as Chinatown in 1906, and the number of deaths after the earthquake is unknown. One newspaper described them as "swarming in the vacant lots and parks." When Ashe wrote that she wanted a nurse in each camp, was she thinking about the Chinese survivors as well? Her account raises more questions than answers in this respect. The city impressed many of the surviving Chinese into street cleaning work.

City leaders also planned to relocate Chinatown, which had been almost entirely destroyed, much to the dismay of the Chinese themselves. The newspaper speculated that one reason President Roosevelt initially charged the neutral Red Cross with relief work was because of rumors that San Franciscans were treating Chinese badly, which they denied.[58]

Within six days, a committee was formed to decide where to move the Chinese survivors, without asking them. The decision was to relocate them to a distant, bleak peninsula, but the Chinese resisted. Chinese residents in New York had raised $2,500, with more expected, in relief for Chinatown. The Chinese consul praised President Roosevelt for taking it upon himself to see that everyone benefited from the relief. By mid-April, the Chinese delegation in Washington, DC, announced that the Dowager Empress herself, speaking from the Forbidden City in China, demanded that her people stay in their original area. Threatened by the Chinese government with the loss of lucrative trade, the city leaders relented.[59]

CONCLUSION

Ted Steinberg argued that civic leaders engaged in "seismic denial" after the 1906 earthquake; they blamed most of the damage on the fire rather than the earthquake itself in order to build a vision of the disaster that would be consistent with growth and development of the city. In that way, any risks that could occur from earthquakes have been forgotten, especially regarding policies to reinforce vulnerable buildings.[60] While lessons often go unlearned after disasters, one positive occurrence after the 1906 earthquake and fire was a change in how nurses organized to respond. The May 1906 issue of the *AJN* reported that the Red Cross Society, "even in its imperfect organization has been a power and a blessing. Will the nurses of this country learn a lesson from this greatest national calamity?"[61] Subsequently, the December 1907 issue began a regular department on Red Cross work. Because of their experience in the 1906 disaster, the San Francisco County Nurses' Association joined the state's Red Cross branch as a body, bringing a total of 188 nurses enrolled in the state. As an example, Katherine Brown from CHSF joined the California branch of the Red Cross in 1907.[62] Thereafter, the American Nurses Association and the Red Cross worked together to develop new nursing standards for volunteers, and the National Committee on Red Cross Nursing was created, with Jane Delano as the first chairwoman.[63]

While concrete outcomes such as the above are important, it also helps to analyze nurses' and other caretakers' experiences during and after the earthquake and fire. They performed meaningful work that was deeply rewarding to them. Their discipline and coolness enabled them to respond quickly to emergencies and help bring about control over a chaotic situation. By reading their stories, we find that they turned the disaster into an opportunity, and they were proud of their work. Their experiences during the 1906 earthquake and fire can provide significant insights into the meaning of nursing, stimulate new avenues of research, and help us develop new interpretations of that important area of study, disaster nursing.

STUDY QUESTIONS

1. What comprised nurses' work during the disaster? Physicians' work? What specific roles did physicians carry out that nurses did not? Was there any blurring of roles?
2. The chapter describes emergency workers breaking into buildings for supplies. Discuss the ethical dimensions of "looting" in times of crisis. Relate that to images after recent disasters, such as the 2010 earthquakes in Haiti and Chile.
3. Rumors abounded about patients being left to die as nurses and other workers fled the Mechanics' Pavilion. Most of the rumors were false. Discuss the ethical problems a nurse might face in such a crisis. Consider the obligation to care versus the need to survive and responsibilities to families versus responsibilities to patients.
4. What does abandonment mean to you?

NOTES

1. Lucy B. Fisher, "A Nurse's Earthquake Story," *American Journal of Nursing* 7, no. 2 (November 1906): 84–98. Quotation is on p. 98.
2. The Spanish had established San Francisco in 1776, and it was a small town until gold was discovered in 1848. It then became a supply station for the gold miners and eventually a boom town. A classic history of the West

is Ray Allen Billington's *Westward Expansion: A History of the American Frontier* (New York: Macmillan Publishing Co., 1982). See also Patricia Nelson Limerick, Clyde A. Milner II, and Charles E. Rankin, eds., *Trails: Toward a New Western History* (Lawrence, KN: University Press of Kansas, 1991); Walter Nugent, *Into the West: The Story of Its People* (New York: Random House Vintage Books, 1999); Valerie J. Matsumoto and Blake Allmendinger, eds., *Over the Edge: Remapping the American West* (Berkeley: University of California Press, 1999).

3. "Earthquake and Fire," and other articles on the earthquake in *The Call-Chronicle-Examiner*, April 19, 1906, 1. Newspaper editors collaborated to publish one paper on April 19. See also http://www.zpub.com/sf/history/1906earth.html (accessed August 15, 2009). For extended analyses of the earthquake, see Philip L. Fradkin, *The Great Earthquake and Firestorms of 1906: How San Francisco Nearly Destroyed Itself* (Berkeley, CA: University of California Press, 2005); Dennis Smith, *San Francisco is Burning: The Untold Story of the 1906 Earthquake and Fires* (New York: Penguin Group, 2005); Simon Winchester, *A Crack in the Edge of the World: America and the Great California Earthquake of 1906* (New York: HarperCollins Publishers, 2005); Rand Richards, *Historic San Francisco, a Concise History and Guide* (San Francisco: Heritage House Publishers, 2007).

4. Kevin Rozario, "Making Progress: Disaster Narratives and the Art of Optimism in Modern America," in *The Resilient City: How Modern Cities Recover From Disaster*, eds. Lawrence J. Vale and Thomas J. Campenella (New York: Oxford University Press, 2005), 44.

5. Rebecca Solnit, *A Paradise Built in Hell: The Extraordinary Communities That Arise in Disaster* (New York: Viking Press, 2009), 5.

6. Marian Moser Jones, "Confronting Calamity: The American Red Cross and the Politics of Disaster Relief, 1881–1939," PhD diss., Columbia University, 2008. Proquest Dissertations and Theses, Publication #AAT 3317567, 182; Charles Hurd, *The Compact History of the American Red Cross* (New York: Hawthorn Books, Ind., 1959); Caroline Moorehead, *Dunant's Dream: War, Switzerland and the History of the Red Cross* (London: HarperCollins, 1998).

7. "Urgent Call for Nurses," *San Francisco Chronicle*, April 22, 1; "Nurses and Supplies Needed," *San Francisco Chronicle*, April 23, 2; Portia B. Kernodle, *The Red Cross Nurse in Action, 1882–1948* (New York: Harper and Brothers Publishers, 1949), 43. In the May 1906 issue of the *American Journal of Nursing*, the editors commented on the work of developing the Red Cross, with specific rules for the enrollment of volunteer and paid nurses, but no official nursing department yet existed in the Red Cross agency.

8. Series of telegrams by William W. Morrow, President of the California Red Cross, in William W. Morrow, "The Earthquake of April 18, 1906, and the Great Fire in San Francisco on that and Succeeding Days—Personal Experience, Inauguration of Red Cross and Relief Work," San Francisco Public Library. See also "President Asked to Rescind Proclamation Reflecting on San Francisco," *San Francisco Chronicle*, April 23, 3.
9. "Department Reports of the San Francisco Relief and Red Cross Funds (A Corporation)," March 19, 1907, San Francisco Public Library History Center (hereafter cites as SFPLHC); Letter from James D. Phelan to William H. Taft, November 28, 1906, The 1906 San Francisco Earthquake and Fire Digital Collection, Bancroft Library (hereafter cited as BL).
10. Report from George Torney, Chief Sanitary Officer, U.S. Army Hospital, Presidio of San Francisco, April 20, 1906. http://archives.gov/exhibits/sf-earthquake-and-fire/aftermath.html; Timeline of the San Francisco Earthquake, April 18–23, http://www.sfmuseum.net/hist10/06timeline.html (accessed July 15, 2009). See also Eugenie L. Birch, "Learning From Past Disasters," in Eugenie L. Birch and Susan M. Wachter, *Rebuilding Urban Places After Disaster: Lessons From Hurricane Katrina* (Philadelphia: University of Pennsylvania Press, 2006), 132–148.
11. Fisher, "A Nurse's Earthquake Story." First quotation is on p. 84; second is on p. 86.
12. M. Adelaide Nutting, "Apprenticeship to Duty," in *A Sound Economic Basis for Schools of Nursing and Other Addresses* (1926, repr. New York: Garland Publishing Company, 1984), 350. See also Susan Reverby, *Ordered to Care: The Dilemma of American Nursing, 1850–1945* (New York: Cambridge University Press, 1987); Tom Olson and Eileen Walsh, *Handling the Sick: The Women of St. Luke's and the Nature of Nursing 1892–1937* (Columbus: Ohio State University Press, 2004).
13. Typed copy of Rene Bine to Folks, n.d., MS 3640, folder 6, California Historical Society, San Francisco, CA (hereafter cited as CHS).
14. "Personal Recollections During the Eventful Days of April, 1906," B.L. http://www.oac.cdlib.org/view?docId=hb4p3007dw&brand=oac4&doc.view=entire_text (accessed July 31, 2009).
15. Margaret Mahoney, "The Earthquake, The Fire, The Relief," July 28, 1906, SFPLHC, 4; "Heartbreaking Scenes at the Pavilion," *San Francisco Chronicle*, April 19, 4.
16. Fisher, "A Nurse's Earthquake Story," 88.
17. Ibid., 89.
18. Report from George Torney, Chief Sanitary Officer, U.S. Army Hospital, Presidio of San Francisco, April 20, 1906. http://archives.gov/exhibits/sf-earthquake-and-fire/aftermath.html (accessed July 31, 2009).

19. Fisher, "A Nurse's Earthquake Story," 90.

20. Mahoney, "The Earthquake."

21. Fisher, "A Nurse's Earthquake Story," 94. These were Lucy's words, but Fradkin credits the *Chronicle* with using the term "chariots of mercy." Fradkin, *The Great Earthquake*, 102. See also "Keep Out of the Way of the Automobiles," *San Francisco Chronicle*, April 22, 1906, 2.

22. Fisher, "A Nurse's Earthquake Story," 93.

23. Ibid, 94.

24. Ibid, 95.

25. "Blow Buildings Up to Check Flames," *The Call-Chronicle-Examiner*, April 19, 1906, 1.

26. Fisher, "A Nurse's Earthquake Story," 95.

27. Ibid., 98. See also "Vast Army Now in the Park," *San Francisco Chronicle*, April 21, 5.

28. Blake was the daughter of a San Francisco attorney and the great niece of a California Supreme Court judge and former mayor of San Francisco.

29. Anna Blake to Grandma, 1906, http://www.oac.cdlib.org/ark:/13030/hb7489p15c/?brand=oac4 (accessed July 31, 2009).

30. Anna Blake to Mother, 1906, http://www.oac.cdlib.org/ark:/13030/hb7t1nb645/?brand=oac4; Anna Blake to Mamma, April 26, 1906. The 1906 San Francisco Earthquake and Fire Digital Collection, BL (accessed July 31, 2009).

31. Anna Blake to Mamma, April 25, 1906, in ibid. and at http://www.oac.cdlib.org/view?docId=hb0p30047m&brand=oac4&doc.view=entire_text (accessed July 31, 2009).

32. Anna Blake to Mamma, April 26, 1906, ibid. The 1906 San Francisco Earthquake and Fire Digital Collection, BL.

33. Anna Blake to Grandma, May 25, 1906, in ibid and at http://www.oac.cdlib.org/ark:/13030/hb1f59n7x9/?brand=oac4 (accessed July 31, 2009).

34. Rene Bine to Folks, Monday, April 30, 1906, MS 3540, folders 5 and 6, CHS.

35. "Resume of Work of Sanitation Performed by the San Francisco Board of Health, From April 18, 1906, to Date," *California State Journal of Medicine* 4, no. 9 (September 1906): 242–246.

36. Nellie May Brown to Mother, April 19, 1906. Bancroft (BANC) MSS 99/173 cz#1, MS 75C1, in files labeled Fresno and Oakland, California, 1906 April 19–22, BL. Also located at http://www.oac.cdlib.org/ark:/13030/hb258004mn/?brand=oac4, the 1906 San Francisco Earthquake and Fire Digital Collection, BL (accessed August 15, 2009).

37. Nellie May Brown to Mother, April 20, 1906, in ibid.

38. Nellie May Brown to Mother, April 22, 1906, in ibid.

39. Joy Cough, RSM, *In Service to Chicago: The History of Mercy Hospital* (Chicago: Mercy Hospital and Medical Center, 1979).

40. "Editorial Comment—The San Francisco Disaster," *American Journal of Nursing* 6, no. 9 (June 1906): 581–592. Quotations are on p. 583. Another daunting task for nursing leaders in the city was finding hospital experiences for nursing students. Among the hospitals destroyed were the Waldeck, St. Mary's, St. Winifred's, St. Francis', Clara Barton, Pacific, McNutt, Mary Patton, and Hahnemann. Nursing leaders hoped that the training schools in the neighboring cities would take the students, but they were having great difficulty reaching them.

41. Ibid.

42. The Children's Hospital of San Francisco is the forerunner of the University of California San Francisco Children's Hospital.

43. Katherine Brown, Professional Autobiography, n.d. Barbara Bates Center for the Study of the History of Nursing, University of Pennsylvania, Philadelphia, PA. (hereafter cited as BBCHN).

44. http://www.stmarkshospital.com (accessed October 10, 2009).

45. Brown, Professional Autobiography.

46. Katherine Brown to Cousin, May 15, 1906, BBCHN.

47. Ibid.

48. Ibid.

49. Ibid.

50. Katherine Brown to Family, April, 1906, BBCHN. Brown continued to demonstrate remarkable courage and fortitude in her nursing career. During World War I, as a Red Cross nurse and in the service of the Army Nurse Corps, she served as chief nurse of Base Hospital #34 in Nantes, France. See Brown, Professional Autobiography, BBCHN.

51. Fisher, "A Nurse's Earthquake Experience," 97.

52. Ibid., 96.

53. "Praise Bravery of the Women," *San Francisco Chronicle*, April 25, 1906, 6.

54. Mahoney, "The Earthquake," 8.

55. Ibid., 6–8.

56. Jones, "Confronting Calamity."

57. "Los Angeles: Negroes Caring for Their Race," *Los Angeles Herald*, April 23, 1906, n.p.; Fradkin, *The Great Earthquake*; Sylvia G.L. Dannett, *Profiles of Negro Womanhood*, Volume II of Negro Heritage Library, (Yonkers, NY: Educational Heritage, Inc., 1966); Joyce Ann Elmore, "Black Nurses, Their Service and Their Struggle," *American Journal of Nursing* 76, no. 3 (March 1976): 435–437; and M. Elizabeth Carnegie, *The Path We Tread: Blacks in Nursing Worldwide, 1854–1994* (New York: National League for Nursing Press, 1995). Curtis had also volunteered during the Spanish American War, and for her wartime work, she received a government pension.

58. "Care of Chinese Hard Problem," *San Francisco Chronicle*, April 23; "President Asked to Rescind."
59. Winchester, *A Crack in the Edge of the World*; Fradkin, *The Great Earthquake*; "Chinese Will Aid Afflicted," *San Francisco Chronicle*, April 25, 2.
60. Ted Steinberg, "Smoke and Mirrors: The San Francisco Earthquake and Seismic Denial," in *American Disasters*, ed. Steven Biel (New York: New York University Press, 2001), 103.
61. "Editorial Comment," *American Journal of Nursing* 6, no. 8 (May 1906): 503.
62. Letter from the American Reed Cross to Katherine Brown, July 23, 1907, BBCHN.
63. Kernodle, *The Red Cross Nurse in Action*; Hurd, *Compact History*. The Red Cross Nursing Service under the direction of Jane Delano oversaw deployment of thousands of nurses overseas during World War I and their induction into the Army Nurse Corps.

CHAPTER 4

The Monongah Mine Disaster, December 1907: "A Roar Like a Thousand Niagaras"

John C. Kirchgessner

What at first seemed like distant thunder in a few seconds was transformed into a roar like a thousand Niagaras. Like the eruption of a volcano the blazing gas reached the surface and vomited tongues of red flame and clouds of dust through the two slopes.[1]

The above quotation in the Pittsburgh newspaper announced the mine explosion that had occurred on December 6, 1907, in Monongah, West Virginia. It was the deadliest mine disaster in American history, with the lives of at least 361 men and boys lost. The explosion was thought to have been caused by the ignition of methane gas.[2] The Fairmont Coal Company owned and operated Monongah Mines 6 and 8, founded in 1899 and 1905, respectively. Ironically, the day after the explosion, another newspaper noted that the mines were inspected daily and were among Fairmont Coal Company's safest, most modern, and best equipped mines. Indeed, they were believed to be among the best mines in the world. "Whatever criticisms have been made about the safety of the West Virginia mines cannot apply to those at Monongah."[3]

Monongah is situated on the West Fork River, approximately 6 miles above the city of Fairmont and 25 miles below Clarksburg. Many precautions were put in place to help decrease the likelihood of a disaster. However, a disaster did happen, and it had far-reaching implications for decades to come. In spring 2010, the United States and the world experienced the aftermath of two coal mine disasters: one in China's Wangjialing mine and the other in the Upper Big Branch mine in Moncoal, West Virginia. At a time when mine safety and the victims of mine disasters are on the minds

of many, we are reminded that American coal miners for over a century
have dealt with the harsh conditions of their workplace and the ever present danger inherent in their occupation. It is too early to determine unequivocally what precipitated the Upper Big Branch disaster on April 5,
2010. However, it appears that many of the same causes that led to the
Monongah mine disaster in December 1907, namely, coal dust, methane
gas, equipment, and human error, also contributed to the Upper Big Branch
mine disaster. The Monongah disaster serves as an excellent case study
when analyzing the care provided during mining disasters. At the same
time, it illustrates the influence of native and immigrant cultures found in
West Virginia and a "culture of danger" inherent in mining. Significantly,
even though class and ethnic differences often created tensions and led to
conflicts, sometimes violent ones, those factors were overshadowed in the
response to the Monongah disaster.

The Appalachian mountain range extends from Maine to Tennessee. Labor migrations from around the world transformed the region traditionally
known as Appalachia, which includes the states of West Virginia, Virginia,
Kentucky, and Tennessee. Although the region has many commonalties
related to culture, topography, and resources, each state and region has its
own individual and unique qualities. West Virginia is known for its mountainous and often remote terrain. Topographically, the state can be divided
into two regions: (a) the Appalachian Mountains, in the eastern third of the
state, and (b) the hills, valleys, and hollows of the Allegheny Plateau in the
western two-thirds of the state. It is the topography that is significant in
the population development of the inhabitants of West Virginia, as well as
the development of industry. The entire region is rich in natural resources,
including timber, minerals, coal, and natural gas. The best known of the
region's many resources is bituminous coal.

PETER AND STANISLAUS URBAN

On December 6, 1907, brothers Peter and Stanislaus Urban trudged
through the cold early morning drizzle to begin their workday in the miles
of underground tunnels found in Monongah Mine 8. The Urban brothers
represented the diversity of miners found in the coal fields of northern
West Virginia at the turn of the twentieth century. They were born of Polish decent, and Peter had emigrated from Romania only 5 months before,

in July 1907.[4] Like many immigrant coal miners before him, he spoke little English when he came through Ellis Island, and he had no training in the mining of coal before taking the job his brother found him in the mine. As with thousands of other immigrants throughout the nation, Peter came to America with his wife and three of his children (two daughters remained in Poland) hoping for a life of political and economic freedom.[5]

The mining town of Monongah had its own distinct blend of cultures. It was populated mostly by immigrants from Italy, Poland, and Austria–Hungary, with a smaller number of Turks, Greeks, and Blacks. The newly arrived immigrants joined the first- and second-generation Irish, Welsh, Scottish, English, and German miners whose fathers and grandfathers immigrated to West Virginia when the mining industry began in the last half of the nineteenth century.[6] Generally, each group of immigrants lived and socialized with members of their respective nationalities, but they often worked together in the mines. As an immigrant employee of the Fairmont Coal Company, Peter Urban was conscripted to work inside the mines. Urban, like many of the Italian, Polish, and eastern European immigrants who settled in northern West Virginia, was willing to challenge the cultural, class, and vocational barriers facing him in order to live and work in his new country.[7]

As the Urban brothers reached the opening of Monongah Mine 8 on that cold December morning, they were joined by other miners who were scheduled to work the day shift. They had a full 12 hours to spend inside the mine, but they considered themselves fortunate to have the work. Just 2 months before, in October 1907, the U.S. stock market had crashed, initially causing a panic on Wall Street; the effects of the crash continued to be felt in the mining communities of West Virginia that December. By 1907, coal had become the sole source of fuel for American railroad and shipping industries but, perhaps more importantly, it had become the only source of energy to produce electricity, iron, and steel, all used to build many of the major American cities.[8] As construction diminished in the economic slump, a decrease in the demand for coal led the Fairmont Coal Company to slow down production in the Monongah Mines.

The day before the disaster, December 5, was St. Nicholas's Day, a holiday celebrated by many of the region's Roman Catholic immigrants, and the mines had been closed. Before the brothers and their fellow miners could enter the mine on December 6, the mines' fire boss had to determine that the mines were safe for entry; thus, the men and boys scheduled for work that morning had to wait until the "all clear" sign was given by the night shift fire boss, 21-year-old Lester Emmitt Trader. Then, the mine foreman opened the gates to the mines.

Trader, young and relatively inexperienced, was responsible for assessing the mines for dangerous conditions during his 12-hour shift the night of December 5. While walking through the mines' passages, tunnels, and roads, he checked for the accumulation of methane gas, coal dust, and any structural changes. All could contribute directly to explosions and/or roof falls, and the miners knew that these were the most common dangers they faced daily while underground. In addition, Trader sprinkled water throughout the main passages to help keep the coal dust down. However, unlike other mines in the region, the Monongah mines did not water down the individual rooms that were off the main passageways. Thus, Trader did not sprinkle the rooms in which miners used explosives to extract the coal and load the coal cars.[9]

Mines 6 and 8 were connected underground and contained a total of 475 working rooms that created a large underground network.[10] As historian and former U.S. Assistant Secretary for Mine Safety and Health Davitt McAteer, noted, Trader continued on his rounds and noted in his fire boss's book that there were trace amounts of methane gas in certain locations throughout the mines, areas that were believed to be the only ones in which methane collected.[11] At the end of his shift, he placed the book with his findings in the fire boss's shed but never reported them directly to the mine foreman, as was the custom. Trader was also unaware that methane gas had been discovered in two locations in Mine 6 on December 4, the last day the mine was in operation.[12]

THE EXPLOSION

After the gates to the mine opened around 6:00 a.m., Peter and Stanislaus went to their designated mine room and began digging coal in Mine 8. By midmorning, the mines were in full operation, and coal was being hauled out by the carload. About 10:30 a.m., 14 cars were being pulled out and up the incline to the mine's tipple by a wire rope; all was going well until a coupling pin on one of the cars snapped.[13] At that moment, all 14 cars, each of which weighed 3 tons, plunged 1,500 feet back into Mine 6.[14] They tore out rails and electrical wiring and ripped out the wooden props and partitions that formed the stabilizing skeletal structure of the mine. The cars also took with them the check boards found at each mine's portal. These check boards were the sole source of identifying which miners had entered the mine that morning. Later, many of the identifying tags used by each miner were found among the debris strewn both inside and outside the mine, while others were never found.

As the cars tore through the mouth of the mine, they ripped many of the curtains that were used to keep methane gas and coal dust from circulating throughout the mines in the event of an accident. They also destroyed the mine's huge ventilating fan—the main source used to move clean, oxygen-rich outside air into the mine. Consequently, coal dust and methane circulated at dangerously high levels and created an atmosphere ripe for disaster.[15] Moments after the crash, the horrific explosion occurred deep in Mine 6. It also resulted in subsequent cave-ins that hampered the rescue work that ensued over the next hours and days. The opening to Mine 8 was completely obliterated, and Mine 6's entry was entangled with debris. The explosive force was so great that a second ventilation fan housed in Mine 8, 30 feet tall and weighing several tons, was "lifted like a toy and wafted across the river."[16] The explosion literally spewed tons and tons of equipment, coal, and timber out of the mines. It was reported that flames shot more than 60 feet into the sky. Many surrounding company buildings were destroyed as well. Those living in Monongah immediately knew what had happened. Even more impressive, however, was that those living up to 8 miles away in Fairmont also knew, as their houses shook, windows broke, and streets buckled.[17] In the ensuing minutes and hours, several smaller localized explosions and fires also occurred, each consuming life-giving oxygen.

The human loss inside the mines was even more devastating, and the exact number of lives lost would never be known. Many of those who were working near the openings of the mines were tragically obliterated, as they were spewed out of the mines with the debris. Inside, many men and boys died immediately as a result of traumatic injuries that included decapitation, amputation, burns, crushing, and blunt force trauma.[18] There were those, however, who exhibited no physical injuries at all. These were the miners who were working deep in the mine and in rooms off the main passageways. Rescuers found many of these miners simply remaining where they had last sat down to rest, with no trauma to their bodies at all. They became the victims of another deadly element of the disaster—poisonous gas.

"After damp" and "black damp" are the most common gases produced after a mine explosion. Made up of carbonic acid and nitrogen, and carbon dioxide and nitrogen, respectively, these gases are devoid of one essential element, oxygen. Two other deadly gaseous mixes are "choke damp" and "white damp"; both are also devoid of oxygen.[19] Those who survived an explosion and their rescuers had to contend with an atmosphere of these deadly gasses that could result not only in physical complaints but also rapid death by asphyxiation. The miners were well aware of these dangerous gases and used heavy, specially designed canvas curtains to block off areas and prevent their infiltration. Much of the infrastructure, however, including trap doors and curtains, were ripped apart in the explosions of Mines 6 and 8 and, as noted earlier, the main source of fresh air and oxygen to the mines, the ventilation fans, were destroyed in the initial explosions.

Peter Urban survived the disaster, and in January 1908 he described it at the Marion Coroners Inquisition, including what he and his brother experienced, and his state of mind inside the mine shortly after the initial explosions:

> All I know [is] we went to work that morning and we had no cars; so we started to dig coal and then we went in 8; then at the time while we were eating there was a noise, or report; then I told my brother we better run—something had happened. He says: 'Oh, what happened? I don't think anything happened,' and took a pick and goes to the face and started work. Then we started to run; then I don't remember nothing [sic]. I don't know where I came or what became of me . . . I was so frightened I don't remember anything . . . When I came to—had my mind together—I recognized I was at home.[20]

After the citizens of Monongah recovered from the initial jolt, they rushed outside and toward the mines. Chaos and panic soon developed as miners' families congregated around the mine openings, and the first rescue workers attempted to enter the mines. Wives, mothers, and children of miners, many non-English speaking or limited in their command of the language, were beside themselves trying to find out whether or not their loved ones were safe. The *Illustrated Monthly West Virginian* reported in January 1908, "The scenes at the mines during the work of rescue were pitiful in the extreme. For several days frantic women grouped about the opening of the mines and their shrieks of agony were enough to move the hardest heart to pity. Grief-stricken mothers, wives, sweethearts, and sisters waited and watched and wept. Some prayed, some sung [sic], and some, in their very ecstasy of sorrow were hysterical and laughed."[21] By December 9, the crowds became overwhelming, and the *Pittsburgh Dispatch* reported that people from all areas of West Virginia, Maryland, and Pennsylvania had come to the mine. Some were relatives of the victims, while others came out of morbid curiosity. A train from Baltimore also ran an excursion to Monongah, bringing hundreds of people.[22]

THE RESCUE

Rescue work began immediately, with the first party entering Mine 6 approximately 25 minutes after the initial explosions. As McAteer noted, there were no organized rescue teams to respond to mine disasters in 1907. Although such systems existed in Europe at the time, the state of West Virginia and the nation did not have any plans in place. Thus, each rescue effort was "an ad hoc affair," very much dependent upon volunteers.[23] Volunteers came easily, however, as it was part of the unwritten Miners' Code that no one was left behind, and everything that could be done was carried out to rescue fellow miners. As historian Paul Rakes noted, the code was "an informal but sacred code [that] produced a common understanding among workers that, in a disaster, the miners on the surface would work ceaselessly until recovering the last body." Rakes further noted that this was a cultural mandate, not a law of political or industrial nature that required miners to further risk their lives for fellow miners.[24]

The Miners' Code existed among deep-seated class and ethnic conflicts that were embedded in the diversity of cultures in Appalachian mines. The *New York Times* reported that the rescue efforts were coordinated by American-born miners. Although cultural tensions sometimes occurred between Americans and foreign-born miners, they all cooperated with the rescue organizers.[25]

This cooperation helps to illustrate a phenomenon that developed in West Virginian mining communities, namely, mining carried with it a significant risk for fatalities that resulted in an almost passive acceptance of deaths and injuries. Rakes noted that "between 1890 and 1907, at least 26,434 deaths occurred in the nation's coal mines."[26] An acceptance of death and injury and the overall sense of fatalism among miners reflected the self-image and the public's perception of miners at the turn of the twentieth century. It was clearly a masculine enterprise pursued by stoic men who accepted the fate of their vocational decisions.[27] This "culture of danger" that surrounded mining and the often overly dramatized lack of conscience of the coal barons were not the only factors that contributed heavily to mining fatalities. During the Industrial Age, technology became a significant contributing factor in the number of mining deaths. As mines modernized mechanically and mining activities extended deeper and deeper into the earth, the deeper mines were known to have greater amounts of methane gas. In addition, greater use of machinery often resulted in large amounts of coal dust—all of which potentially created a volatile underground atmosphere that could result in disaster at any given time.

This hazardous environment significantly affected the first rescue crew at Mine 8, who returned to the surface around noon on December 6. Any further rescue attempts had to wait until fans were put in place—it was essential that ventilation and oxygen be restored to the mines before other men were sent to rescue. Over the next several hours, through the means of telephone and telegraph, the region, state, and nation became aware of the magnitude of the event at Monongah. Local, state, and federal relief in the form of personnel, supplies, and funds poured into a community desperately in need.[28] The region's and nation's newspapers, the New York Times among them, continued to report the rescue and cleanup efforts over the coming days and weeks.

A second rescue crew was sent into Mine 8 around 4:00 p.m. after moaning was heard by a rescuer coming from a ventilation shaft, also known as a "toad hole." The rescuer was lowered into the hole, followed by others. The party found Stanislaus and Peter Urban; Stanislaus was mortally wounded as a result of falling when the brothers attempted to escape the explosions. Peter was found protecting his brother, his eyes glassy and sobbing. As the rescuers attempted to move the Urbans to safety and care, Stanislaus died.[29] Peter was brought to the surface and would become the only person known to have been rescued from the disaster. Dr. F.W. Hill, one of the physicians at the scene, described Peter Urban's initial condition: "At the time, he was taken out only sufficiently to find if he was conscious and to send him home. . . . His pulse was very weak and he was not rational. He was in a condition of shock. There did not seem to be any evidence of external injury or violence."[30] By dusk of December 6, the rescuers returned to the mouth of the mine and confirmed that there was little hope of finding other survivors. The men and women who had congregated at the mine knelt down in the falling snow and prayed, offering a miners' benediction.[31]

CARE OF SURVIVORS, RESCUERS, AND FAMILIES

Among the volunteers to report to the mines within the first hours after the disaster were 12 physicians from Fairmont who were accompanied by nurses. Shortly after arriving at Mine 6, the doctors and nurses established an emergency hospital in the local blacksmith shop to care for the people whom they anticipated would be brought out of the mine over the next several hours and days. They also planned for the streetcar and railroad companies to transport survivors, once stabilized at the emergency hospital, to hospitals in Fairmont.[32] Within the first 24 hours, however, it became apparent that the nurses' and physicians' services were not required for any survivors, because there were none. Rather, they were needed for the rescuers who battled fatigue and deadly gases. On December 7, *The Fairmont West Virginian's* headline read: "Death List Appalling: Mine Horror Increases in Awfulness as it Becomes Apparent that Over 400 Have Perished." A second emergency hospital was established to care for the rescuers overcome by "after damp" and "black damp" gases.[33] Rescuers were taken from mines weak and sometimes unconscious but, as noted by the *Pittsburgh Dispatch*, "after being out of the mine a few hours they have fully recovered."[34]

There were reports that some men did survive and were taken to the West Virginia Miners Hospital 3 in Fairmont for further care or comfort. Two in fact were outside the mine when the explosion occurred. Rescuers took Patrick McDonald and W.C. Bice to the hospital on a special train from Monongah. McDonald, a motor man in Mine 6, was hurled over 100 feet; he was found unconscious with severe burns over his face and chest. Bice was transported to the Miners Hospital with crushing injuries to his chest and abdomen. His injuries were so extensive that he died a few hours after admission.[35] Both cases illustrate the type of injuries the physicians and nurses treated on a daily basis at the Fairmont Miners Hospital 3. As a state-funded facility that opened in 1901, the hospital offered acute care services free of charge to miners, railroad workers, and lumber men.

Mine injuries, such as those of McDonald, were the greatest challenge to the nurses and physicians at Miners Hospital 3. Traumatic injuries, including burns, crushed limbs, broken backs, lacerations, and fractured skulls, were all too common. While surgical methods to repair and stabilize skull and spinal injuries were known at the time, few patients survived. Nursing at Miners Hospital 3 was, at the very least, rigorous and demanding. Many patients who were admitted required amputations, care of fractures, suturing of wounds, and treatment for burns. Few survived amputations, spinal trauma, or head trauma, and patients with major trauma, including massive crushing injuries to the lower limbs, often required intensive postoperative nursing care. Severe hemorrhaging and the resultant shock from many of the injuries were the immediate complications that the physicians and nurses had to manage. Some patients were merely cleaned and comforted until they died.[36]

Many patients who initially survived the traumatic injury later suffered and died from postoperative infections. Burns in particular were problematic with resultant secondary infections, and they often had poor outcomes. Nurses and physicians used compounds containing phenol, alcohol, and arsenic to treat infections. They also used mercury compounds, considered some of the most effective germicides of the time, as disinfectants; however, these had side effects, and hospital personnel were warned of these in references regarding mercury's use. Nurses also used arsenic for skin infections.[37]

COLLABORATIVE EFFORTS AFTER THE DISASTER

Morticians were busy after the December 6 explosion. At the peak of the rescue effort, dead bodies were recovered at such a rapid rate that the local morticians could not keep up with caring for the bodies. Their personnel were in great demand, and coffins were in short supply. Five railroad carloads of coffins arrived in Monongah the day after the explosion, but they were not enough; 100 of the coffins came from Zanesville, Ohio.[38] A temporary morgue was set up in a new bank building so that the bodies could be prepared before their families came to identify them. A tent was also set up as an Italian morgue near Our Lady of the Most Holy Rosary of the Vale of Pompeii, the local Italian Catholic church. After the morticians completed their work, the bodies were buried as rapidly as possible. At one point, funerals were conducted continually in local churches; priests had to be brought in to assist with the numerous Italian and Polish Catholic funerals. On the Monday following the disaster, a total of 40 funerals were conducted in Monongah.[39] Workers at the local cemeteries had to rapidly dig graves to accommodate all of the dead, and a new cemetery was established and soon filled. As one journalist wrote, the grieving survivors stood over "the cold rows of open graves in the sodden, half-frozen, rain-drenched and snow-flecked West Virginia soil," the dreary weather only compounding their grief.[40]

Almost immediately, Fairmont Coal Company and the town of Monongah began making arrangements to care for the families. As McAteer noted, "The initial support efforts were spontaneous: those with something to contribute did so."[41] Each member of the town realized the gravity of the situation.[42] Within the first days, several relief committees organized both in Monongah and Fairmont. The mayor of Monongah called upon the people of the region and state to help in any way they could. His plea eventually reached many Americans beyond West Virginia, such that relief in the form of supplies, personnel, and money came from all over the nation. Until 1907, the American Red Cross only provided aid after natural disasters. The magnitude of this disaster, however, made the Red Cross's leaders realize that they needed to set a precedent and respond to human-made disasters as well.[43] The organization collected $3,700 in donations and sent a social worker to Monongah to help the relief committee and the survivors.[44]

AFTERMATH

The search and rescue effort went on for days and weeks, and slowly the mines gave up their dead. What remained to be answered, however, was just how many men and boys were in the mine at the time of the explosion. Record keeping was generally poor. It was a known practice for boys to assist their fathers in the mines, but they typically were not counted among those employed.[45] Thus, there could have well been more than the approximately 380 men usually working the day shift. The *Fairmont Times* reported that there were 425 men who went to work in the mines that morning. On December 8, the *New York Times* noted, "It is now believed that the number of dead will not reach 400 . . . it was discovered that many miners believed to have been entombed had escaped because they had not gone to work Friday after Thursday's holiday. It is said that 406 men were in the mine when the explosion occurred."[46] The exact count was further confounded by the destruction of the check boards that remained the most reliable way to know who was in the mine on any given shift.[47]

Most of the recovery effort was completed before December 17, when the *Fairmont West Virginian* reported that the "excitement was over," as well as the search for the bodies in Mine 6, and little was expected to be done in Mine 8. Only a few bodies had been found over the couple of days before this report, and the condition of Mine 8 did not lend itself to easily recovering any more. Mine 8 had sustained far worse damage than Mine 6, and many of its rooms were reported to have cave-ins of over 200 feet long. It was decided that should there be bodies under such destruction, they would be beyond recognition.[48] On December 24, the *Fairmont Free Press* announced that 342 bodies had been recovered. While most had been identified, some were beyond recognition. Throughout the next 2 months, bodies were discovered occasionally as cleanup and reconstruction continued; the final and official number of those recovered was 361.[49]

Two hundred fifty women were widowed, and 1,000 children were left fatherless; some children became orphans, and many survivors were in Europe. For those in West Virginia, winter was knocking on the door, and many families were dependent upon the weekly pay the miners brought home; few had cash reserves, and in a matter of minutes their economic livelihood had been snuffed out. The Fairmont Coal Company established commissaries for the widows and children and provided supplies needed for the rescue parties.

The Monongah Mines Relief Committee was established as the central relief organization to assist in providing support to families. The committee determined that each widow would receive $300 and each surviving child $100 for a total of $175,000 and an additional $25,000 for aged dependents and unborn infants.[50] W.M.O. Dawson, governor of West Virginia at the time, recognized that the state could not afford to provide all of the aid and put out an appeal for donations to the Relief Committee on December 14. This resulted in donations from citizens throughout the United States, which included other miners, senators, unions, and industrialists.[51] Donations also came from France and Germany. The Fairmont Coal Company provided each widow with an additional $150 and $75 to each child younger than 16 years old.[52]

As word of the event spread throughout the nation and the world, the citizens of Monongah and the surrounding mining towns questioned how and why the disaster occurred. Almost immediately, investigations were organized to find the cause of the disaster. Among the organizations that assisted in the investigation were the West Virginia Department of Mines, the Fairmont Coal Company, the Ohio Department of Mines, the Pennsylvania Department of Mines, and the U.S. Department of Commerce. In addition, French and Belgian mining experts contributed to the effort.[53] According to McAteer, two causal theories emerged. The first blamed the runaway coal cars that ignited methane and coal dust after crashing back into Mine 6. The second theory centered on the improper use of explosives within Mine 8, which caused methane gas or coal dust to ignite, thus setting off a series of explosions throughout both mines.[54] The coroner of Marion County, West Virginia, also established a jury in January 1908 to further investigate the explosion.[55] Throughout the investigations, the Fairmont Coal Company "made every effort to absolve itself of any responsibility. The coroner's jury, composed of men of power and influence who were associates of the company's owners, eventually exonerated the company of any wrongdoing."[56]

CONCLUSIONS

As nurse historian Barbra Mann Wall noted, contextual factors, including time, place, and economics, help to shape how people interpret and make sense of disasters.[57] In many ways, Monongah was "the perfect disaster" in that it had a number of contributing factors that came together on December 6, 1907. These factors included human error, mechanical error, lack of policy, and the right season. If perhaps the same factors had come together on a summer day, the event may not have been so cataclysmic. The U.S. Department of Labor Mine Safety and Health Administration noted:

> The greatest explosion hazard in coal mines comes from methane gas. All coal seams contain some methane and when the barometer falls during colder weather, more of that methane migrates into the mine air than normal. Pockets of methane may accumulate in areas of the mine in which gas checks are infrequent. When an ignition source is present in that area, there exists the potential for a deadly explosion. Colder weather can also dry out the air inside a coal mine. During summer, warm air coming into the mine brings moisture that condenses on mine surfaces and traps the coal dust.[58]

The drying effect of colder air makes coal dust more likely to get suspended in the mine atmosphere, which can also contribute to an explosion, and likely it did on December 6, 1907.

The Monongah disaster became embedded in the conscience of many Americans and affected even those living in the native lands of the immigrant miners. It was a "wake up call" and had a profound impact on future policy devised to help prevent further disasters. For example, the Monongah disaster prompted the Pennsylvania State Mining Commission to take action to protect miners from machinery. After 1907, the federal government became formally involved in mine safety, and the U.S. Bureau of Mines was established in 1910. In addition, after 1907, the establishment and enforcement of child labor laws became more aggressive because of the loss of so many young boys at Monongah. By 1912, mines had to provide rescuers with equipment to prevent their being overcome by "after damp" and "black damp" gases.

The Monongah citizens' response to the disaster also illustrates the transnational nature of early twentieth century West Virginia. By 1907, the state had moved from a predominantly agrarian-mountaineering culture composed of native-born Americans to a culture in touch with the world economy through manufacturing industries. Many nationalities comprised the workforce.[59] In addition to the Polish Urban brothers, miners included American-born, Italian, Slavic, Greek, Lithuanian, Irish, Hungarian, Scottish, and Latvian men and boys. Many blacks also mined in West Virginia.[60] This transition influenced every thread of West Virginia's cultural fabric, its economy, religion, language, and customs. In the next decades, conflicts continued over unionization and the exploitation of coal miners. In the face of disaster, however, the region's citizens responded as one, embodying the resilience of the mountaineers and miners as they carried out their grim tasks and the Miners' Code.

STUDY QUESTIONS

1. What factors contribute to prompt responses to disasters from local, state, and federal governments?
2. Speculate about how race and ethnicity of the miners might have affected the response.

3. What were the nursing priorities for victims injurede in mining disasters? Differentiate immediate needs from those several days later. What might a survivor of methane gas exposure require? Speculate about complications that survivors might experience after being trapped under debris and wreckage for some time.
4. In lieu of continued mining disasters from methane gas explosions, what suggestions do you have to decrease risks for miners?

NOTES

1. John P. Cowan, "Roar Like A Thousand Niagaras Tells of Death Underground," *Pittsburgh Dispatch*, December 7, 1907, 1.
2. Ibid., and Davitt McAteer, *Monongah: The Tragic Story of the Worst Industrial Accident in US History* (Morgantown: West Virginia University Press, 2007). McAteer was former Assistant Secretary of Labor for Mine Safety and Health.
3. *The Fairmont-West Virginian*, December 7, 1907.
4. West Virginia Press Services, "Andrew Urban's Father Was Sole Survivor of 1907 Monongah Mine Disaster," *The Times-West Virginian*, August 1, 1991.
5. Thomas J. Koon, "Only Known Monongah Mine Disaster Survivor Came Here From Poland," *The Times-West Virginian*, October 3, 1999.
6. McAteer, *Monongah*, 76.
7. Michael E. Watson, "Sadly in Need of Organization: Labor Relations in the Fairmont Field, 1890 to 1918," in *Culture, Class, and Politics in Modern Appalachia*, eds. Jennifer Egolf, Ken Fones-Wolf and Louis C. Martin (Morgantown, WV: West Virginia University Press, 2009), 142–149.
8. McAteer, *Monongah*, 8.
9. Ibid., 18
10. Ibid., 63
11. Ibid., 20; and Mark Reutter, "The Historical Context: Coal Mining and Accidents in Northern West Virginia." http://www.makingsteel.com/Coaland Accidents.html (accessed May 27, 2009), 2. Reutter notes, "Northern West Virginia coal . . . gives off large quantities of methane (natural gas) while mined. While not poisonous, methane is flammable, and when mixed with as little as five percent air, becomes highly explosive. . . . During the process of extracting coal, part of the coal seam is reduced to a fine dust, which can be just as explosive as methane mixed with air. If coal dust is allowed to accumulate, the smallest spark from a match or a moving machine part in the mine may blow enough of the dust into the air to form an explosive

cloud. Unless blocked by seals or other means, the cloud can almost instantaneously penetrate every passageway until the whole mine is devastated by explosions."

12. McAteer, *Monongah*, 20.
13. Coal mine tipples were "originally the place where the mine cars were tipped and emptied of their coal, and still used in that sense, although now more generally applied to the surface structures of a mine, including the preparation plant and loading tracks." http://www.irs.gov/businesses/small/article/0,,id=139342,00.html#t (accessed January 5, 2010); "Coupling Pin Snaps, Causing Disaster," *Pittsburgh Dispatch*, December 7, 1907, 1.
14. McAteer, *Monongah*, 5.
15. Ibid., 116.
16. Ibid., 1.
17. Lacy Dillon, *They Died in Darkness* (Parsons, WV: McClain Printing Company, 1976), 73.
18. Eugene Wolfe, "December 6, 1907: No Christmas at Monongah," *Golden Seal Reprints*, Winter 1993, 33.
19. McAteer, *Monongah*, 132–133.
20. West Virginia Mine Investigating Committee: Report of Hearings, *Transcript of Testimony: Taken at an Inquisition Held at Fairmont, Marion County, W. Va.*, January 6–15, 1908, 265.
21. "Events in West Virginia: The Monongah Catastrophe, Most Appalling Disaster in the History of Coal Mining," *The Illustrated Monthly West Virginian*, January 1908, 1.
22. *Pittsburgh Dispatch*, December 9, 1907, 1.
23. McAteer, *Monongah*, 127.
24. Paul Rakes, "A Combat Scenario: Early Coal Mining and the Culture of Danger," in *Culture, Class and Politics in Modern Appalachia*, eds. Jennifer Egolf, Ken Fones-Wolf, and Louis C. Martin (Morgantown: West Virginia University Press, 2009), 69.
25. "350 men Entombed in Mine Explosion," *The New York Times*, December 7, 1907, 1.
26. Rakes, "A Combat Scenario," 58.
27. Ibid., 69.
28. "Monongah Sends Out Appeal for Aid Which Being Generously Responded To," *The Fairmont West Virginian*, December 9, 1907, 1. On Sunday, December 8, W.H. Moore, the mayor of Monongah, sent out an appeal for aid to the citizens of West Virginia, in it he stated: "To the People of West Virginia : . . . Many of our best men are under the hills. In this great calamity we appeal to the people of the State for substantial support. We deeply

appreciate your sympathy, but this will not satisfy the hungry or clothe the orphans and widows. We appeal to the Mayors, Ministers, Boards of Trade, Business Men, Leagues, Ladies Aid Societies. . . . This is no time for sentiment. Our homeless need substantial aid. . . ."

29. McAteer, *Monongah*, 135; Koon, "Only Known Monongah Mine Disaster Survivor."

30. West Virginia Mine Investigating Committee: Report of Hearings, 239.

31. "400 Killed by Terrific West Virginia Mine Explosion," *Pittsburgh Dispatch*, December 7, 1907, 6.

32. "Explosion Causes Great Loss of Life at Monongah," *The Fairmont Times*, December 6, 1907, 1.

33. "Death List Appalling," *The Fairmont West Virginian*, December 7, 1907, 1.

34. "Destruction Greater as Men Work Farther Into Wrecked Mines," *Pittsburgh Dispatch*, December 9, 1907, 3.

35. "Death List Appalling."

36. John C. Kirchgessner, "The Miners' Hospitals of West Virginia: Nurses and Healthcare Come to the Coal Fields, 1900–1920," *Nursing History Review* 8 (2000): 159–164.

37. Ibid. See also Clara Weeks Shaw, *A Text-Book of Nursing* (New York: D. Appleton and Company, 1903), 104, 143, 145.

38. Eugene Wolfe, "December 6, 1907: No Christmas at Monongah," 35; "100 Coffins Shipped," *Pittsburgh Dispatch*, December 7, 1907, 1.

39. McAteer, *Monongah*, 153.

40. Eugene Wolfe, "December 6, 1907: No Christmas at Monongah," 36.

41. McAteer, *Monongah*, 171.

42. Ibid.

43. Ibid., 175.

44. Marion Moser Jones, "Confronting Calamity: The American Red Cross and the politics of disaster relief, 1881–1939," PhD diss., Columbia University, 2008. Proquest Dissertations and Theses, Publication #AAT 331756, 328. Jones noted that when Red Cross leaders decided to "embrace industrial accident prevention and relief as part of its relief mission, it landed in the middle of a shifting and politically charged relationship between employer and employee at a critical juncture in American labor relations." Thus, their future actions to alleviate the human suffering caused by industrial accidents "often neutralized the conflicts between labor and management. This result, while seeming to benefit both parties, ultimately favored the interests of the conflict-wary employers."

45. McAteer, *Monongah*, 220.

46. "Fire Stops Rescue at Monongah," *The New York Times*, December 8, 1907, 3.

47. McAteer, *Monongah*, 219.

48. "Excitement Is All Over at Monongah: Search for Bodies Is Nearly Done," *The Fairmont West Virginian*, December 17, 1907.
49. Lacy Dillon, *They Died in Darkness,* 33.
50. "Monongah Mines Relief Committee," *The Fairmont West Virginian*, December 14, 1907.
51. Ibid.
52. McAteer, *Monongah*, 191.
53. McAteer, *Monongah,* 162.
54. Ibid.
55. Ibid., 160.
56. Shirley Stuart Burns, "Monongah: The Tragic Story of the Worst Industrial Accident in U.S. History," Southern Historical Association. http://www.thefreelibrary.com/Monongah:+The+Tragic+Story+of+the+Worst+Industrial+Accident+in+US . . . -a0218657012, (accessed March 30, 2010).
57. Barbra Mann Wall, "Healing After Disasters in Early Twentieth-Century Texas," *Advances in Nursing Science,* 31, no. 3 (July–September, 2008): 211–224.
58. "Colder Weather Brings More Danger to Underground Coal Mining." http://www.msha.gov/MEDIA/PRESS/1996/NR961011.HTM (accessed September 20, 2009).
59. "Introduction: Networks Large and Small," in *Transnational West Virginia: Ethnic Communities and Economic Change, 1840–1940*, eds. Ken Fones-Wolf and Ronald L. Lewis (Morgantown: West Virginia University Press, 2002), ix–xiv.
60. McAteer, *Monongah*.

Nurses' Response Across Geographic Boundaries in the Halifax Disaster, December 6, 1917: Border Crossings

Deborah A. Sampson

I am sending. . . a corps of our best State surgeons and nurses in the belief that they may be of service to you in this hour of need.[1]

Massachusetts Governor Samuel W. McCall sent these words to Halifax, Nova Scotia, leaders immediately upon hearing of the December 6, 1917, harbor explosion that devastated the city. Halifax was the most important World War I North American seaport. As New England nurses participated in humanitarian intervention, disaster responses, and international cooperation, they crossed geographic boundaries to provide care amid chaos. Significantly, this episode illustrates the interrelatedness of American and Canadian nursing history and culture, particularly in terms of the role of nurses in Canada–United States relations. In doing so, it demonstrates early twentieth-century Nova Scotia/New England women's migration patterns as well as the disaster-related patient care knowledge of nurses in early twentieth-century New England.

During World War I, the Halifax, Nova Scotia, harbor was one of the largest and busiest Atlantic shipping ports. It was a crossroad for transportation needs in North America and the nexus for wartime shipping for both Canada and the United States.[2] Ships carrying soldiers, munitions, and supplies across the Atlantic to Europe originated from the Halifax harbor. Returning ships with war-wounded soldiers stopped at the Halifax docks to disembark cargo and people or before sailing with their cargo to other North American ports. Halifax, strategically located at the largest ice-free

North American harbor, and its people, shipyards, and rail system, were vital to North American commerce and war efforts.[3]

On a beautiful, clear, and unusually warm early winter morning, December 6, 1917, two wartime-related ships collided in the busy and crowded Halifax harbor as a result of miscommunication between the harbor pilot and the ship captain. Of the almost 50,000 residents and several thousand soldiers stationed in Halifax, approximately 2,000 people were killed, 10,000 injured, and many thousands left homeless. The maimed and injured survivors required immediate care. Disaster relief of unthinkable proportions was critically needed.[4] The city's survivors and nurses and the residents of other Canadian towns near Halifax responded immediately, but the magnitude of the hardship could not be alleviated with regional resources. Within hours, the Boston, Massachusetts mayor and other leaders of the city received news of the disaster and sent the first of many relief trains loaded with supplies and relief workers, chiefly surgeons and nurses, which arrived in Halifax 2 days later. The state of Massachusetts and the New England region continued to send supplies and relief personnel, including nurses—relief that was so appreciated by the people of Halifax that annually the city of Halifax still sends a Christmas tree to Boston Common in remembrance. Few in Massachusetts, let alone the United States, know about the important history of this disaster, which affected North American wartime transportation and nearly destroyed a thriving city, let alone the significance of the Christmas tree. No one in Halifax has forgotten.

Public and academic historians, primarily in Canada, have analyzed the disaster itself: the work of physicians, social workers, and lady volunteers; the reconstruction of the public infrastructures; and the long-term effects of the disaster on residents of Nova Scotia.[5] Samuel Prince's scholarly analysis of the Halifax explosion, the immediate response, and the lasting effects on the city and its people is considered to be the foundational work upon which all other disaster analysis and planning have since developed.[6] However, little historical analysis has examined the role, contributions, and dynamics of an important group of women involved with the disaster—the nurses who cared for the injured.[7] As often happens, the role of physicians and political leaders is well known, but the activities of the largest group of professional relief workers—the nurses —remain invisible. Perhaps most importantly, this research helps inform current debates and scholarship about international relief endeavors after natural and human-made disasters and the role of integrating health care professionals and other relief workers into a geographically specific and culturally distinct milieu. It also improves understanding of activities of vital, yet often overlooked, disaster relief providers, the nurses, who are so often on the front lines of disaster care.

PEOPLE AND PLACES

This is a story, in part, of the interrelatedness of geography, people, place, and shared identities based on race, culture, and historical roots. The Canadian Maritime provinces of Nova Scotia and New Brunswick are contiguous parts of the North American region that also comprises the New England states of Maine, New Hampshire, Vermont, Massachusetts, Connecticut, and Rhode Island. These geographic regions share the continuous geography of the North Atlantic Ocean, coastline mountain ranges, and large river systems, as well as a complex ethnic heritage and history (see Figure 5.1).

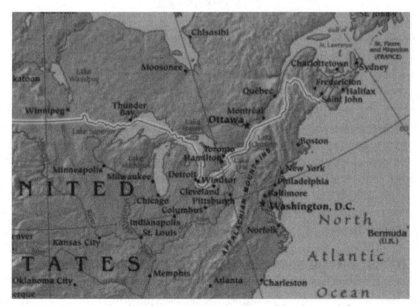

Figure 5.1   New England and Nova Scotia (in the public domain).[8]

From earliest known times, the indigenous peoples who lived in the region often roamed throughout the large areas of coastal and inland regions without regard, of course, to national "boundaries." The earliest European settlers throughout this region were of western European English- and French-speaking heritage. Family migrations, trade, and knowledge flowed from one area to another from the 1600s to the present in spite of the national border established in the late eighteenth and early nineteenth centuries.[9]

Established in 1749 as a British port, Halifax was a major strategic center for British power during the American Revolution in the late 1700s, and British loyalists in the Boston area and other New England seacoast towns fled to Halifax beginning in 1774.[10] Halifax remained a major British military position during the War of 1812. Prior to the U.S. Civil War in the 1860s, because of the frequency of Boston and New England seacoast ship transportation, Halifax was also a major destination for Black slaves escaping slavery in the United States with the help of abolitionists from Canada and the United States.[11]

THE DISASTER

One of the ships involved in the 1917 Halifax explosion was the Mont Blanc, a French ship loaded with highly volatile munitions. The other, the Imo, was an aging cargo ship used to transport relief supplies from North America to Belgians suffering wartime deprivations. After colliding with the Imo, the Mont Blanc caught fire and exploded. It was vaporized 10 minutes later, resulting in a mass disaster that has been one of the defining moments in Canadian history. The explosion, still the largest nonnuclear human-made explosion in history, sent a 2,000-foot black smoke plume skyward and caused a pressure wave that obliterated buildings within a mile of the harbor. Many schools, churches, businesses, and homes, including the military hospital filled with soldiers recuperating from World War I battle wounds, collapsed or were seriously damaged, and buildings 10 miles away sustained heavy damage.[12] The Black settlement, Africville, on the back side of a harbor jetty, was flattened, never again to be rebuilt.[13] Almost all windows shattered throughout the city, with the millions of flying glass shards injuring hundreds. A post–explosion-related 50-foot tsunami poured water over the devastated area and washed virtually everyone and everything in its path back into the harbor, including Miq Mac natives and their winterized wigwam settlement in a small waterfront cove.[14] Fires from overturned wood and coal stoves in damaged buildings ravaged the remains of the city, which was soon covered with oily residue from the smoke plume. Whole neighborhoods disappeared, and the main commerce area of the busy harbor, the harbor side rail yard, the docks, and the downtown business district were unrecognizable. Main railway and waterfront transportation terminals were in shambles. With telegraph cables down, communication to the outside world was limited. Food, water, beds, and adequate shelter were scarce, whereas sanitation facilities, electrical power, and fuel for heating and cooking were suddenly unavailable.[15] The basic needs of everyone in the city were threatened amid the rubble.

To make matters worse, many of Halifax's citizens thought the explosion was a German wartime attack, and untrue but credible rumors circulated among the frantic and shocked population that German submarines were in the harbor and threatened more destruction. The situation was indeed bleak, yet the disaster would become worse when, in less than 24 hours, a major blizzard blanketed the city with snow, blackened slush, and ice.

THE INITIAL RESPONSE

When the first shock of the explosion was over, people immediately started helping the wounded. The uninjured tried to free those trapped in the rubble, and every wheeled vehicle, including trucks, cars, horse-drawn wagons, and handcarts, was used to transport the survivors to hospitals through streets piled with wreckage and bodies. Many survivors were dazed or dying, many were in tattered rags that had been clothing, some were naked after the blast stripped away any trace of clothes, and most were bleeding and in pain. Others who were physically unharmed were so emotionally stunned that they wandered in a stupor until found by friends, family, or kind strangers and directed to places of succor and safety.

Patients arrived at the remaining hospitals and other hastily organized emergency care facilities with horrific trauma. Flying glass, some pieces still embedded in victims, had slashed the faces of people who had stood at windows watching the Mont Blanc burn, and those still gazing when the explosion shattered windows had glass shards embedded in eyes, faces, necks, and other body parts. The sound wave concussion ruptured eardrums, leaving some survivors deaf, and propelled others through the air, often resulting in massive multiple-system trauma, including internal injuries, traumatic brain injury, and fractures. Numerous crush injuries occurred as well when people were caught in falling rubble or were lifted off their feet and slammed to the ground. People close to the explosion who survived and others caught in damaged buildings that caught fire suffered serious burns.[16]

As Halifax buildings lay in ruins, the sun still shone over the city, although people near the harbor were covered with black soot, and wooden buildings caught on fire from overturned coal and wood stoves. This necessitated a response from local military and civic leaders in Halifax, who formed a relief oversight group under the direction of Canada's Lieutenant Colonel McKelvey Bell. They wasted no time in trying to assess the situation and identify structurally sound hospitals and other buildings to use as relief stations. Several hospitals were intact enough to be used for the wounded, whereas schools and other large public and private buildings were organized as makeshift hospitals, relief stations, emergency lodging, and boarding homes for relief workers.[17]

Canadian towns near Halifax immediately sent relief in the form of clothes, food, and medical supplies, and women's groups mobilized quickly. Available nurses in Halifax initially provided the urgent aid, including those from the five hospitals with schools of nursing in the immediate Halifax region: Victoria General Hospital; Grace Maternity Hospital; Children's Hospital; the Halifax Infirmary (later part of Victoria General); and the Nova Scotia Psychiatric Hospital, located across the harbor in Dartmouth where student nurses helped support the immediate relief efforts.[18] The Victoria Order of Nurses (VON), the Canadian equivalent of visiting and public health nurses' associations, sent nurses from Toronto, Montreal, and Ottawa, and they subsequently organized and staffed the critically needed dressing stations throughout the city.[19]

As citizens and soldiers using commandeered vehicles brought bodies and injured alike to the hospitals, nurses, physicians, and other staff sorted those who could be saved from those judged too traumatically injured to survive. Thus, nurses attended to conscious victims first, doing what was absolutely necessary, such as washing and bandaging wounds, hurriedly assisting physicians with emergency surgical procedures, and creating some sort of order.[20] Barbara Orr, who was 14 years old at the time of the explosion and the only survivor of her immediate family, recalled being transported by soldiers in a fish delivery wagon to the newly completed and relatively undamaged Camp Hill Military Hospital, where she was left in a corridor near the entrance among other injured patients covered in black grime. Only when she called out did an orderly recognize that she, perhaps the only one among a hallway of motionless bodies, was still alive.[21]

The scene in the hospitals was inconceivable, as whole families and cartloads of injured amassed there. Each hospital had only a hundred or fewer beds but now housed more than 1,000 emotionally and physically traumatized people suffering from burns, lacerations, eye injuries, fear, pain, and shock. Food, water, bedding, bandages, medicines, and equipment were becoming scarcer, whereas sanitation facilities, power, heat, lighting, and sterilizing mechanisms were nonexistent. Window openings, devoid of glass, were covered by blankets or hastily installed rubble tacked up to the frames. Every inch of floor space was taken up by injured and bleeding people, many moaning, crying, or calling for help. Before outside help arrived, available Halifax physicians and nurses were inundated with frantic families looking for loved ones amid the dead, dying, and injured. Unhurt and less seriously injured survivors found ways to leave Halifax on trains they found at undamaged rail lines at the edge of the city. Although some of these survivors went to other Canadian cities and towns, where they were cared for by kin or willing strangers, others traveled to Boston, where they were welcomed by anxious family members and friends.[22] In the first 24 hours, however, thousands of people who needed care for injuries remained in Halifax. It was into this landscape of turmoil and trauma that the outside relief nurses stepped.

THE BOSTON RESPONSE

In Governor McCall's initial telegram to Halifax (which would not be received because of damage to the communication system), when he volunteered Boston physicians and nurses, he stated, "I need hardly say to you that we have the strongest affection for the people of your city, and that we are anxious to do everything possible for their assistance at this time. We are ready to answer any call that they may make upon us."[23] Word of the disaster spread throughout Boston, and the city responded with shock, disbelief, worry, concern, and an outpouring of help.

In the late nineteenth century until the Great Depression of the 1930s, economic depression in Nova Scotia and neighboring New Brunswick was a stimulus for out-migration from these Canadian Maritime provinces to the more economically vibrant New England region. Travel back and forth between Halifax was particularly convenient because several trains and steamships left Boston daily bound for Halifax and other Maritime cities.[24] Young Maritime women often left Canada to pursue independence, education, jobs, and economic opportunity in the large cities of coastal New England, with metropolitan Boston a particular draw for these women. Not only did educational and economic opportunity abound, but also many families and friends from home were in the Boston area. This allowed increased networking for introductions and decreased loneliness through social support during difficult times. Frequently, sister would follow sister, or young women would immigrate and live with other family members already established in Boston.

At the time of the Halifax disaster, population migrations between Canada and the United States were relatively unimpeded by legal or physical border barriers until the 1930s, when the United States implemented stronger entry requirements, border controls, and visa laws.[25] Until then, Boston was an "Eldorado for Maritime girls" and, for young women of the early twentieth century, "going to Boston was a rite of passage into adulthood."[26] Economic forces generated job opportunities for women that simply did not exist in the Maritimes, even in cities like Halifax, and trained nursing was of particular interest. Nursing provided an attractive opportunity as a secure occupation for "respectable" Caucasian English-speaking middle-class Maritime women. Not only were women of this economic, racial, and ethnic class favored by Boston-area nursing schools of the time, but nursing wages were also quite good. In 1917, for example, new graduate nurses in Boston could earn from $50 to $100 per month and also receive room and board; not an inconsiderable sum when the average family income was $925 per year.[27] Boston Chapter Red Cross nurses not only received good wages but also had additional instruction in patient care during disasters.[28]

Although Canadian nursing schools developed in tandem with those in the United States, albeit at a slower rate, New England nursing schools offered less competition for more spots for Maritime women. As Susan Reverby noted, English-speaking Canadian women comprised the largest non-U.S. minority in American training schools prior to 1930.[29] Half of Boston-area training school slots and graduate nursing positions in the city were filled by Canadian women, most of whom were from the Maritimes.[30] Moreover, Boston-area nursing schools and nursing agencies, such as the Waltham, Massachusetts Training Home for District Nurses, actively advertised and recruited women from the Halifax area.[31] In 1910, only Canadian-born women in domestic service and garment trades outnumbered those in nursing in Boston.[32] Maritime women, then, could pursue independence, travel, and the adventure of living in a major metropolitan area by becoming nurses in New England, and many did.

In the wake of the several disasters in the Boston area, including the Great Boston Fire of 1890 and other fires in nearby Salem and Chelsea that destroyed both cities, the Massachusetts Public Safety Committee had organized a well-funded disaster response program that included members of the state military guard trained in disaster relief and a cadre of nurse volunteers, primarily from Boston and the surrounding area. In addition, the American Red Cross had chapters in many major cities, including Boston, with organized units of physicians and nurses who were ready to respond to wartime or disaster needs.[33] Thus, Massachusetts was poised to have readily organized and available resources to send over the well-traveled and direct rail lines not only to war allies but also to historical and actual Canadian cousins 800 miles away who were in need.

Within 12 hours of receiving word of the Halifax explosion, the Massachusetts Public Safety Committee and other Boston leaders formed the Massachusetts Halifax Relief Commission. By noon of the day following the explosion, the commission dispatched a train with 12 physicians, 10 nurses, 4 railroad managers, and 6 members of the Boston press along with a carload of supplies, the first of many relief trains sent to Halifax (see Table 5.1).

Within hours, the train encountered a snowstorm that escalated into the type of Nor'easter that produces white-out conditions, gale force winds, and massive snowfalls.[34] The train stopped frequently so that impassable snow drifts could be shoveled off the tracks. It finally arrived on December 8 despite the blizzard.[35] Another train transported the Boston Red Cross Hospital Unit, headed by Samuel Wolcott of the Red Cross and Dr. W.E. Ladd of the Boston City Hospital. The unit had 22 physicians and 73 nurses (67 women and six males) along with 14 civilian workers. At the same time, Dr. E.A. Codman, a Boston ophthalmologist affiliated with the Massachusetts Eye and Ear Hospital, arrived by train with 10 physicians and 4 nurses whom he had educated in eye diseases and surgical care, along with nine civilians.

Table 5.1   An Inventory of Supplies on the Massachusetts Halifax Relief Commission Train, December 6, 1917

564 fracture pillows
1,000 pillows
1,368 muslin bandages
53 splints
330 gauze compresses, 9 × 9 in.
4,000 gauze compresses, 4 × 4 in.
432 flannel bandages
1,196 bandages, 3 in.
2,694 gauze bandages
2,700 gauze compresses
1,200 gauze sponges
1,000 four-tail bandages
1,720 gauze rolls
204 flannel bandages
890 slings
8 standard oil heaters
4 boxes lanterns, glass
21 pairs cotton blankets
36 heavy gray Army blankets
6 litters
3 bedpans
4 urinals

Red Cross supplies
498 sweaters
226 flannel pajamas
333 convalescent gowns
8,300 gauze compresses, 4 in.
9, 354 bandages, 1 in.
1 crate gauze sponges
378 triangular bandages
1 box miscellaneous

Medical supplies
50 tubes morphine sulphate, 1/8 grain, hypodermic
5 tubes atropine, 1/150 grain
100 salt solution tablets
1,000 aspirin tablets
500 calomel, 1/10-grain tablets
500 cascara, 3-grain tablets
9 lb ether 1/4-lb cans
6 lb ether 1/2-lb cans
10 gal alcohol
1/2 gal tincture of iodine

Continued

Table 5.1   (*Continued*)

100 corrosive tablets
1 pint carbolic acid, 95% solution
1 quart boric acid, 4% solution

Additional supplies purchased in St. John, New Brunswick
10 gal alcohol
1 gal tincture iodine
5 lb cotton
5 lb boric ointment
30 lb Vaseline
8 oz tincture digitalis
500 caps camphor in oil
1 gal aromatic spirits of ammonia
1 gross assorted catgut tubes
11 skeins No. 1 white twisted silk
8 oz 4% cocaine
4 oz 1% atropine
1 pint olive oil
12 pairs dressing scissors
12 pairs dressing forceps
1 dozen 4-oz tins
1 1/2 dozen glass stoppered bottles (empty)
2 dozen rolls adhesive 7 × 36 in.
4 dozen rolls adhesive 2 × 60 in.
4 pints brandy
1 gross safety pins

Boston was not the only place in New England that sent help. The Providence, Rhode Island, hospital sent 52 physicians and 52 nurses, and the Rhode Island Red Cross sent a train with 60 physicians and 60 nurses. Major G.M. Elliot of the Maine Guard arrived with 12 physicians and 13 nurses. The Red Cross in New York City and Washington also sent relief, although in smaller numbers and with few nurses.[36]

After the first relief trains arrived, some of the physicians and nurses found their way to whatever facilities they could, since little time had been available for Haligonian[37] leaders or the military officers in charge of the disaster to organize a worker triage system. Some of the nurses dispersed throughout the city to relieve Canadian nurses in the hospitals. Others, such as those with Codman and Ladd, set up emergency care in makeshift hospitals at the YMCA, college buildings, churches, the Salvation Army, or the hastily organized relief and dressing stations. Specialized units such as Codman's remained together throughout their stay in Halifax. This was especially important because the

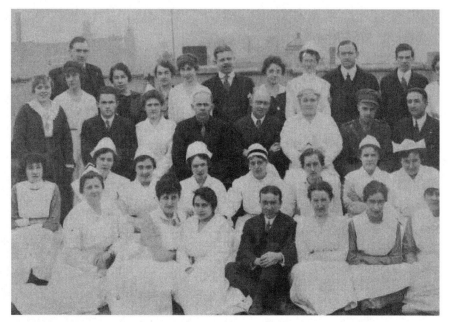

Figure 5.2   Dr. E.A. Codman and part of his staff, Halifax M.C.A. Emergency
Hospital, December 6, 1917. Courtesy: Janet F. Kitz/Private Collection.

nurses were trained in assisting during eye surgery and postoperative care.
Hundreds of patients with serious eye injuries were tended in the first few
days after the arrival of the Codman team.[38] (see Figure 5.2).

The out-of-town relief nurses, including those of the VON, were
housed primarily in private homes throughout the city or slept in makeshift places in the hospitals and dressing stations where they worked. A
few of the most fortunate, such as those on the first Massachusetts Relief
Commission train, were housed in the luxury of the Nova Scotia governor's
home in a relatively undamaged and elegant section of Halifax.[39] Although
some nurses had quarters in luxury homes and may not have suffered, others living in relief stations; improvised shelters; and, in the case of Haligonian nurses, their own damaged homes, certainly suffered in the cold and
dark until services for heat, light, and order could be restored. Whatever
the luxury of the accommodations, given the overwhelming situation of
damaged buildings, lack of resources, and a deluge of traumatized people,
the nursing staff, whether relief or resident, undoubtedly had little time to
enjoy what comfort that may have been provided.

"ACT PROMPTLY AND EFFICIENTLY IN EMERGENCIES"[40]: CARING FOR THE SURVIVORS

After they arrived, the relief nurses replaced their Halifax counterparts, many of whom had worked nonstop for days. The nurses continued what the Halifax nurses had started: prioritizing immediate activities, triaging patients according to need and probable viability, bandaging wounds and stanching bleeding, assessing and diagnosing types and severity of injuries, assisting in surgery and providing anesthesia, cleaning soot-covered patients, and medicating patients in pain. They also instituted environmental sanitation methods, directed hospital staff and lay volunteers, helped families find loved ones among the injured and dead, and worked with authorities to identify and catalogue the victims.[41]

All nurses would have been prepared, to some degree, to "act promptly and efficiently in emergencies," as announced in the Training School for Nurses of the Massachusetts General Hospital brochure.[42] Indeed, training school curricula and textbooks in the early 1900s included content on providing emergency treatment for trauma patients, such as splinting and casting fractures and using available materials for emergency bandaging and immobilization. Books also taught laceration management and types of suturing, burn classification and management, and identification and prevention of hemorrhage and infection. Management of head injury, foreign body removal, care of orthopedic injuries and paralysis, mechanisms of tissue repair, administration of anesthesia, management of precipitous births when no physician was available, and care of premature infants were also expected of nurses.[43] The nurses' training also included classroom lectures by physicians on the care of patients with acute psychiatric conditions, and training in principles and practices of environmental hygiene, sanitation for sewage disposal, sanitary water filtration, and food preparation and safe storage.[44]

The nurses learned to classify burns as first, second, or third degree and would have cared for burns in a manner typical of the time: breaking blisters and trimming the tissues; removing burned tissue; administering pain relief with morphine or opium; and applying oily dressings such as those saturated with "carron oil" (linseed oil and lime water), petroleum jelly, or even plain boric acid followed by a paraffin mesh dressing.[45] The nurses were taught that shock was a life-threatening sequelae of bleeding, unapparent internal injuries, and burns. Textbooks instructed nurses on ways to prevent shock by having the injured lay with feet elevated above the head. A critical focus of nursing care in the pre-antibiotic era was the prevention of infection. Thus, trained nurses, and particularly the Red Cross and Massachusetts Public Safety Committee disaster response nurses, would have had lessons in skills necessary for managing the immediate Halifax situation and patient needs.

The nurses' abilities to work efficiently in such dreadful conditions were apparent. W.B. Moore of Kentville, Nova Scotia, and one of the Canadian physicians who provided disaster relief, commented on the heroism, stamina, courage, and calmness of the nurses working after the explosion: "The trained nurses . . . showed their professional superiority . . . [and] . . . coolness, combined with acuteness of perception and rapidity of action as to constitute a veritable godsend to the afflicted, and the hardworking surgeons." He also commented on the nurses' "qualities of initiative, brains, and efficiency, under such circumstances as would test a man."[46] Indeed, the nurses in the Halifax disaster blurred gendered boundaries by exhibiting traits, behaviors, and qualities usually attributed to men—intelligence, agency, and competence in spite of horrific conditions.

The nurses also expanded their own practice during the disaster as they undertook activities that would be reserved for physicians in less desperate times. Given that physicians had to perform major surgery, nurses made medical decisions about patients' conditions, such as who would be routed to surgery ahead of others, whose injuries were immediate, and who could wait. Moore stated as much when he noted in his memoir report that he often left in the middle of attending a patient to go to someone more severely injured; the medical care of the first patient was left to nurses.[47] The nurses were also responsible for determining who would receive pain-relieving morphine and how much to give without physician advice. Moreover, pregnant women gave birth in unprecedented numbers within the first few days of the explosion; birth attendance and care of high-risk infants were the responsibility of nurses and family members.[48]

As the urgent aftermath passed and order was restored, the American nurses joined with their Canadian colleagues to care for convalescing patients, but only for a short time.[49] Most of the New England relief units stayed in Halifax for a month, and few remained beyond the February following the explosion. However, other reconstruction and social service disaster relief from New England, particularly Massachusetts, continued for more than a year as Halifax struggled with rebuilding.

DISCUSSION

The linkage between Halifax and the New England states was more than a tie related to the imperatives of commerce and war. It is difficult to over-estimate the cultural, familial, and economic ties of Maritime Canada and the New England states of Massachusetts, Rhode Island, Maine, and New Hampshire. These geographic regions had very old and intertwined cultural and geographic histories of place. First and foremost, until the American Revolution, no actual national boundary existed between the areas. People, whether of Native American background or European ancestry, passed freely from one region to the other. Maritime Canada and New England were the same "place," since both were British colonial territories with no international boundary for several hundred years after European settlement. Until the 1930s, few restrictions stood in the way of immigration or border crossing between eastern Canada and the New England states. Unlike immigrants during the waves of European and Asian migrations occurring in the late 1800s and early 1900s, Canadians from the Maritime provinces were not required to register when crossing the U.S. border or vice versa. Thus, in 1917, Maritime Canadians, particularly those of English-speaking British, Scottish, or Irish Protestant heritage, were simply not viewed as "the other" by New Englanders.

Halifax and Maritime Canada also shared with New England a heritage of refuge—of opportunity, collaboration, and cooperation. At the outset of the American Revolution, for example, British Loyalist leaders in colonial New England areas, particularly Boston, escaped the rebellion by relocating to Halifax, a coastal city used by the British as war headquarters. Later, during the era of American slavery, New England and Canadian abolitionists collaborated to help runaway slaves reach the safety of slavery-free Canada. Then, throughout the industrial era of the 1800s, the New England coastal cities of Boston and Lynn, Massachusetts, and Providence, Rhode Island, had attracted laborers from farms and fishing villages in Nova Scotia who found the factory work to be more lucrative, steady, and less dangerous than farming the rocky soil of Cape Breton or fishing the capricious Atlantic Ocean. Nor was it unusual for Nova Scotians to seek education in the United States, particularly in the Boston-area schools.

Many Canadian young women came to the New England states in the late 1800s and early 1900s to find work as teachers, nurses, household help, shop girls, and factory workers. Indeed, in the early 1900s a significant percentage of student nurses in the prestigious Massachusetts hospitals, such as the Massachusetts General Hospital, Boston City Hospital, and Providence (Rhode Island) Hospital, were English-speaking Canadian women of Scottish and British heritage. In Waltham, Massachusetts, an affluent suburb of Boston, the prestigious Waltham Nurses Agency was established for the purpose of placing trained nurses of Canadian Maritime heritage in upper- class home nursing situations throughout the Boston area. Even today, Haligonians speak of "going down to Boston" as if they were taking a trip to the mall. The New England states welcomed Maritime Canadians, who spoke the same language, shared many of the same cultural values and ethnicity, and enhanced the economic progress of New England industrialization.

Thus, Nova Scotia Canadians were a prominent presence in New England at the time of the Halifax explosion. Many of the nurses in the New England contingencies who responded to the Halifax disaster were either of Canadian Maritime origins or had family and friends from Halifax or Nova Scotia. For example, of the 10 nurses on the Halifax Relief Commission train, 6 were graduates of Massachusetts General Hospital and 2, the McInness sisters, were from Nova Scotia.[50] They had a strong identity based on an historical, ethnic, and emotional connection to the eastern Canadian cities' residents. Some nurses, such as those attached to the Red Cross units and the Massachusetts Commission, were already prepared to respond to the disaster. Others were employees of physicians such as Codman, and they had special skills to help disaster patients. Moreover, the exigencies of World War I, patriotic fervor, and feelings of being allies with Canada against German aggression lent an underlying perspective of unity for New Englanders when Halifax was severely damaged. These issues played a significant part in the willingness of the nurses to venture off to an unknown situation. Other nurses and volunteers on response trains either cared dearly about Halifax and Nova Scotians or had an overwhelming need for adventure. Nurses with needed skills and deep cultural roots in Canada had what was necessary to volunteer without hesitation for the disaster response.

CONCLUSION

The presence and activities of nurses were critical aspects of the disaster relief after the explosion that destroyed much of Halifax, Nova Scotia, in 1917. Nurses from Halifax, other parts of Canada, and the New England states worked together in hospitals, dressing stations, and damaged homes. They demonstrated qualities of initiative, character, calmness, acumen, intellect, and professionalism that society usually regarded as male prerogatives. Halifax nurses also had to contend with emotions of fear, sadness, worry about loved ones, and sorrow related to the destruction of their homes as undoubtedly did some of the nurses arriving on relief trains who may have been Halifax natives. In addition, as was true in other disasters, the nurses cared for survivors in ways that transcended the standards of nursing practice of the time. Their care demonstrated shifting knowledge and practice boundaries even as geographic boundaries blurred.

STUDY QUESTIONS

1. Nurses responding to disasters often leave home to venture into unfamiliar places and provide care for strangers amid horrific conditions and in unfamiliar environments and cultures. This occurred for nurses from the United States who responded to the Halifax explosion. In what way did race, class, and culture play a part in this disaster compared to others described in this book?
2. Discuss the implications of weather and wartime on the care nurses provided during the Halifax disaster.
3. In what way might transnational migration of the nursing workforce influence a disaster response across other national boundaries?
4. Often, nurses in disasters perform tasks and make decisions at other times that are reserved for physicians, thereby crossing professional boundaries. Discuss why this occurs and how time, place, and situation in other patient care circumstances might shape how and when nurses cross professional practice boundaries.

NOTES

1. Telegram dated December 6, 1917, located in Public Archives of Nova Scotia (hereinafter identified as PANS), Halifax, NS, Series C, General Correspondence folder titled "Massachusetts-Halifax Relief Committee 1917–1918,

Halifax Relief Commission," accession numbers MG 36 I Series C Folder 113.2.

2. Many extensive descriptions and analyses of the explosion have been published documenting the events. Among them are: John Griffith Armstrong, *The Halifax Explosion and the Royal Canadian Navy: Inquiry and Intrigue* (Vancouver, BC: The University of British Columbia Press, 2002); Michael J. Bird, *The Town That Died: A Chronicle of the Halifax Disaster* (Halifax, NS: Nimbus Publishing Ltd., 1995); David B. Flemming, *Explosion in Halifax Harbor: The Illustrated Account of a Disaster That Shook the World* (Halifax, NS: Formac Publishing Company, Ltd., 2004); Joyce Glasner, "On the Front Lines of the Disaster," *The Beaver* (December 2007/January 2008): 18–24; Janet F. Kitz, *Shattered City: The Halifax Explosion and the Road to Recovery* (Halifax, NS: Nimbus Publishing Ltd., 2004); Laura M. McDonald, *Curse of the Narrows* (Halifax, NS: Formac Publishing Company Ltd., 2005); Joan M. Payzant, "The Dartmouth Side of the Explosion," in *Ground Zero: A Reassessment of the 1917 Halifax Explosion in Halifax Harbor*, eds. Alan Ruffman and Colin D. Howell (Halifax, NS: Nimbus Publishing Ltd., 1994), 35–44.; David Sutherland, "Halifax Harbor, December 6, 1917: Setting the Scene," in *Ground Zero: A Reassessment of the 1917 Halifax Explosion in Halifax Harbor*, eds. Alan Ruffman and Colin D. Howell (Halifax, NS: Nimbus Publishing Ltd., 1994), 3–8; Jay White, "Exploding Myths: The Halifax Harbor Explosion in Historical Context," in *Ground Zero: A Reassessment of the 1917 Halifax Explosion in Halifax Harbor*, eds. Alan Ruffman and Colin D. Howell (Halifax, NS: Nimbus Publishing Ltd., 1994), 251–274.

3. Ibid.

4. Data concerning the numbers of Halifax population dead, injured, and missing vary somewhat between data sources. Few firm numbers existed about the actual population that included visitors, sailors, and non-Caucasian residents. Any person unfortunate enough to have been near the explosion point, simply vanished. Body parts were found at some distance from the explosion. Because Halifax was a wartime shipping city and travel occurred without need for documentation between other parts of Canada, the U.K., or the U.S. for that matter, some victims may not be accounted for. The Halifax civilian and military leaders in charge of the explosion worked diligently at the time of the explosion and for years after to identify all the dead, but some bodies remained unidentified; those missing were presumed dead; and as with other disasters, categorization of those lost and injured is an estimate. I have attempted to use all report data to arrive at a "best guess." Armstrong, *The Halifax Explosion*; Bird, *The Town That Died*; Michelle Herbert Boyd, *Enriched by Catastrophe: Social Work and*

Social Conflict After the Halifax Explosion (Black Point, NS: Fernwood Publishing Company Ltd., 2007); William J. Buxton, "Private Wealth and Public Health: Rockefeller Philanthropy and the Massachusetts-Halifax Relief Commission/Health Commission," in *Ground Zero*, 183–194; Russell R. Dynes and E. L. Quarantelli, "The Place of the Explosion in the History of Disaster Research: The Work of Samuel H. Prince," in *Ground Zero*, 55–68; Glasner, "On the Front Lines of the Disaster"; PANS, Halifax, Nova Scotia, Paper titled "Synopsis" #89.6 in folder titled "History of Halifax Relief Commission—notes compiled by W. E. Tibbs," accession number MG 36 Series C#89; PANS, Halifax, Nova Scotia, 1918 Report (unpublished) from David Fraser Harris, MD. In folder titled "Medical History of the Disaster by Dr. David Fraser Harris" (copy of report also in author's possession), accession number MG 36I C-118-119 (hereafter identified as Harris, "Medical History of the Disaster by Dr. David Fraser Harris"); Kitz, *Shattered City*; Archibald MacMechan, "The Halifax Disaster," in *The Halifax Explosion: December 6, 1917*, ed. Graham Metson (Toronto, ON: McGraw-Hill Ryerson, 1978), 11–75; McDonald, *Curse of the Narrows*; T. Jock Murray, "Medical Aspects of the Disaster: The Missing Report of Dr. David Fraser Harris," in *Ground Zero*, 229–244; Samuel H. Prince, "Catastrophe and Social Change, Based Upon a Sociological Study of the Halifax Disaster," in *Political Science* (New York: Columbia University, 1920); Abraham C. Ratshesky, "Report of the Halifax Relief Expedition, December 6 to 15, 1917," in *The Halifax Explosion: December 6, 1917*, ed. Graham Metson (Toronto, ON: McGraw-Hill Ryerson, 1978), 136–146; Henry Roper, "Archibald MacMechan and the Writing of the 'Halifax Disaster,'" in *Ground Zero*, 3–8; White, "Exploding Myths."

5. See Neena Abraham, "Medical Memories of the 1917 Explosion," in *Ground Zero*, 245–250; Boyd, *Enriched by Catastrophe*; Buxton, "Private Wealth and Public Health"; W. J. Connolly, "The Halifax (Nova Scotia) Explosion of 1917: An Epilogue," *Journal of the Royal Society of Medicine* 80 (1987): 774–775; Richard B. Goldbloom, "Halifax and the Precipitate Birth of Pediatric Surgery," *Pediatrics* 77 (1986): 764; Kitz, *Shattered City*; Janet F. Kitz, *Survivors: Children of the Halifax Explosion* (Halifax, NS: Nimbus Publishing, Ltd., 1992–2000); Chryssa N. McAlister, T. Jock Murray, Hesham Lakosha, and Charles E. Maxner, "The Halifax Disaster (1917): Eye Injuries and Their Care," *British Journal of Ophthalmology* 91 (2007): 832–835; Chryssa N. McAlister, T. Jock Murray, and Charles E. Maxner, "The Halifax Explosion of 1917: The Oculist Experience," *Canadian Journal of Ophthalmology* 43 (2008): 27–32; Suzanne Morton, "'Never Handmaidens': The Victorian Order of Nurses and the Massachusetts-Halifax Health Commission" in *Ground Zero*, 195–206; Michael L. Nance, "The Halifax

Disaster of 1917 and the Birth of North American Pediatric Surgery," *The Journal of Pediatric Surgery* 36 (2001): 406–408; Linda J. Quiney, "Filling the Gaps: Canadian Voluntary Nurses, the 1917 Halifax Explosion, and the Influenza Epidemic of 1918," *Canadian Bulletin of Medical History* 19 (2002): 351–373; "The Halifax Disaster," *Canadian Bulletin of Medical History* 8 (1918/1986): 59–62.

6. Dynes and Quarantelli, "The Place of the Explosion in the History of Disaster Research"; Prince, "Catastrophe and Social Change."

7. Morton, "'Never Handmaidens.'" Although several authors have identified that nurses were part of the relief effort, only a few have discussed in what way these activities occurred. For example, Morton analyzes the tensions between authorities and Victoria Order of Nurses (VON) nurses.

8. Library of Congress Geography and Map Division. 2007. Washington, DC; Central Intelligence Agency. DOI: g3300 ct002230, http://hdl.loc.gov/loc.gmd/g3300.ct002230. No Claim to Original U.S. Govt. Works.

9. Betsy Beattie, *Obligation and Opportunity: Single Maritime Women in Boston, 1870–1930* (Montreal, QC: McGill–Queen's University Press, 2000); Howard Zinn, *A People's History of the United States, 1492–Present* (New York, NY: Harper Perennial, 1995).

10. Armstrong, *The Halifax Explosion*; McDonald, *Curse of the Narrows*.

11. Ratshesky, "Report of the Halifax Relief Expedition."

12. Armstrong, *The Halifax Explosion*; McDonald, *Curse of the Narrows*; Sutherland, "Halifax Harbor, December 6, 1917"; White, "Exploding Myths."

13. Glasner, "On the Front Lines of the Disaster."

14. Personal conversation with Gary Shutlak, Archivist, PANS and Allan Marble, Professor (emeritus) Dalhousie University, November 20, 2006, Halifax, Nova Scotia; Armstrong, *The Halifax Explosion*; Jennifer Burke, "Turtle Grove: Dartmouth's Lost Mi'kmac Community," in *Ground Zero,* 45–54; David A. Greenberg, T.S. Murty, and Alan Ruffman, "A Numerical Model for the Halifax Harbor Tsunami Due to the 1917 Explosion," *Marine Geodesy* 16 (1993): 153–167.

15. Bird, *The Town That Died*; Dynes and Quarantelli, "The Place of the Explosion in the History of Disaster Research"; Harris, "Medical History of the Disaster by Dr. David Fraser Harris"; MacMechan, "The Halifax Disaster."

16. Harris, "Medical History of the Disaster by Dr. David Fraser Harris"; Kitz, *Survivors: Children of the Halifax Explosion*; for examples of supporting documents, see PANS, Halifax, Nova Scotia, Series C, General Correspondence folder titled "Red Cross Civilian Relief Report 1917," "History of Explosion and Relief Committee," accession numbers MG 36 I Series C 36–104.

17. Harris, "Medical History of the Disaster by Dr. David Fraser Harris." Halifax Ladies College, the YMCA and Knights of Columbus building were some of the facilities used as hospitals.

18. Harris, "Medical History of the Disaster by Dr. David Fraser Harris"; Marble, conversation; Kathryn M. McPherson, "Nurses and Nursing in Early Twentieth Century Halifax" (master's thesis, Dalhousie University, 1982).

19. Victorian Order of Nurses for Canada, *V.O.N. 50th Anniversary, 1897–1947* (Montreal, QC: Southam Press, 1947).

20. Harris, "Medical History of the Disaster by Dr. David Fraser Harris"; Kitz, *Survivors: Children of the Halifax Explosion*; James G. Mahar and Rowena Mahar, *Too Many to Mourn: One Family's Tragedy in the Halifax Explosion* (Halifax, NS: Nimbus Publishing Ltd., 1998).

21. Kitz, *Survivors: Children of the Halifax Explosion*.

22. PANS, Halifax, Nova Scotia, Series C, General Correspondence folder titled "Massachusetts-Halifax Relief Committee 1917–1918, Halifax Relief Commission," accession numbers MG 36 I Series C Folder 113. The Massachusetts-Halifax Relief Commission offices in Boston functioned as a clearinghouse for Boston residents to receive information about the safety, well-being, and needs of Halifax family and friends. See multiple correspondence discussing Boston relatives' concerns for Halifax and Halifax residents who left after the explosion and are in Boston with relatives.

23. The actual telegram is located in PANS, Halifax, Nova Scotia, Series C, General Correspondence folder titled "Massachusetts-Halifax Relief Committee 1917–1918, Halifax Relief Commission," accession numbers MG 36 I Series C Folder 113.2.

24. Beattie, *Obligation and Opportunity*; Blair Beed, *1917 Halifax Explosion and American Response* (Halifax, NS: Dtours Visitors and Convention Center, 2002); Kitz, *Shattered City*; McDonald, *Curse of the Narrows*.

25. Beattie, *Obligation and Opportunity*; Susan M. Reverby, *Ordered to Care: The Dilemma of American Nursing, 1850–1945* (New York, NY: Press Syndicate of the University of Cambridge, 1987).

26. Beattie, *Obligation and Opportunity*, 108.

27. David Friday, *Profits, Wages and Prices* (Rahway, NJ: Harcourt Brace Howe, 1920); Massachusetts Board of Registration for Nurses, *Eighth Annual Report for the Year Ending Dec. 31, 1917* (Boston, MA: Wright & Potter Printing Company State Printers, 1918); The Training School for Nurses of the Massachusetts General Hospital, *Announcement for 1917*.

28. The Training School for Nurses of the Massachusetts General Hospital, *Announcement for 1917*.

29. Reverby, *Ordered to Care*.

30. Beattie, *Obligation and Opportunity*; Reverby, *Ordered to Care*.

31. Ibid.; and Victorian Order of Nurses for Canada, *V.O.N. 50th Anniversary, 1897–1947*. This training school was owned by Dr. Alfred Worcester, Professor of Hygiene at Harvard University.

32. Beattie, *Obligation and Opportunity*, 131–143.

33. Ratshesky, "Report of the Halifax Relief Expedition"; American Red Cross, "Halifax Disaster Provided Year's Biggest Emergency Task for Red Cross Department of Civilian Relief," *Red Cross Bulletin*, December 17, 1917, Washington, DC, 1–2.

34. Copies of meteorology reports from Thursday, December 6, 1917 through Wednesday, December 12, 1917, obtained from the private collection of Gary Shutlak, Archivist, PANS, Halifax, NS; Envelope marked "Jackdaw" titled "Halifax.09:06. December 6, 1917. "A photo documentation of the Halifax Explosion" with data from D. L. Hutchinson, Director of the St. John (NB) observatory and F. B. Ronnan, Halifax Station. The sun was shining on December 6, 1917 and the temperature was 39 degrees. By the afternoon the next day, the temperature dropped to 32 degrees and winds of 34 mph with blizzard conditions arrived in Halifax. Sunday, temperatures rose to 50 degrees and the snow turned to rain, becoming ice when temperatures dropped to 15 degrees at night, making roads impassable. Winds continued through Monday with the "worst blizzard in years" documented in meteorology reports (below) and knee deep drifts. Total snow fall recorded was 23 inches.

35. PANS, Halifax, Nova Scotia, Series C, General Correspondence folder titled "Massachusetts-Halifax Relief Committee 1917–1918, Halifax Relief Commission," accession numbers MG 36 I Series C; Ratshesky, "Report of the Halifax Relief Expedition."

36. Ibid.

37. People from Halifax, Nova Scotia, are referred to as "Haligonians."

38. For discussions of the numbers, types, and treatment of eye injuries, see Abraham, "Medical Memories of the 1917 Explosion"; Boyd, *Enriched by Catastrophe*; Harris, "Medical History of the Disaster by Dr. David Fraser Harris"; Kitz, *Shattered City*; McAlister et al., "The Halifax Disaster (1917): Eye Injuries and Their Care"; McAlister, Murray, and Maxner, "The Halifax Explosion of 1917: The Oculist Experience"; McDonald, *Curse of the Narrows*; Murray, "Medical Aspects of the Disaster"; Ratshesky, "Report of the Halifax Relief Expedition."

39. Ratshesky, "Report of the Halifax Relief Expedition."

40. Training School for Nurses of the Massachusetts General Hospital, *Announcement for 1917*, 24.

41. Harris, "Medical History of the Disaster by Dr. David Fraser Harris."

42. Training School for Nurses of the Massachusetts General Hospital, *Announcement for 1917*, 24.

43. Charlotte A. Aikens, *Primary Studies for Nurses: A Text-Book for First Year Pupil Nurses* (Philadelphia, PA: W.B. Saunders Company, 1915); Beverly Boutilier, "Helpers or Heroines? The National Council of Women, Nursing and 'Woman's Work' in Late Victorian Canada," in *Caring and Curing: Historical Perspectives on Women and Healing in Canada*, eds. Diane Elizabeth Dodd and D. Gorham (Ottawa, ON: University of Ottawa Press, 1994), 17–47; Joan Carter, *Tears, Trials and Triumphs: A History of the Victoria General Hospital School of Nursing, 1891–1995* (Tantallon, NS: Glen Margaret Publishing, Ltd., 2005); Joseph Brown Cooke, *A Nurse's Handbook of Obstetrics* (Philadelphia, PA: J.B. Lippincott Company, 1915); Lavinia L. Dock, *Text-Book of Materia Medica for Nurses* (New York, NY: G.P. Putnam's Sons, 1916); Glasner, "On the Front Lines of the Disaster"; Goldbloom, "Halifax and the Precipitate Birth of Pediatric Surgery"; Jean N. Groft, "Everything Depends on Good Nursing," *Canadian Nurse* 102 (2006): 19–22; Harris, "Medical History of the Disaster by Dr. David Fraser Harris"; Kitz, *Survivors: Children of the Halifax Explosion*; Massachusetts Board of Registration for Nurses, *Eighth Annual Report for the Year Ending Dec. 31, 1917* (Boston, MA: Wright & Potter Printing Company State Printers, 1918); McPherson, "Nurses and Nursing in Early Twentieth Century Halifax"; Morton, " 'Never Handmaidens' "; Quiney, "Filling the Gaps"; Emily A. M. Stoney, and Lucy Cornelia Catlin, *Practical Points in Nursing for Nurses in Private Practice* (Philadelphia, PA: W.B. Saunders Company, 1916).

44. Ibid.

45. Archibald L. McDonald, *Essentials of Surgery: A Textbook of Surgery for Student and Graduate Nurses and For Those Interested in Caring For the Sick* (Philadelphia, PA: J.B. Lippincott Company, 1919); Amy Elizabeth Pope and Thirza A. Pope, *A Quiz Book of Nursing for Teachers and Students* (New York, NY: G.P. Putnam's Sons, 1915). Treatments and nursing care defined in textbooks of the period rarely changed in substantive ways between 1915 and 1920; therefore a textbook published in 1919 would contain care essentially the same as nurses provided in 1917. Barbara Brodie, personal communication, October 20, 2009.

46. Metson, *The Halifax Explosion*, 110–111.

47. Ibid.

48. Cooke, *A Nurse's Handbook of Obstetrics*; and Victorian Order of Nurses for Canada, *V.O.N. 50th Anniversary, 1897–1947*.

49. Harris, "Medical History of the Disaster by Dr. David Fraser Harris"; PANS, Halifax, Nova Scotia, Series C, General Correspondence folder titled "Massachusetts-Halifax Relief Committee 1917–1918, Halifax Relief Commission," accession numbers MG 36 I Series C Folder 113, item 113.99a; Ratshesky, "Report of the Halifax Relief Expedition." A smallpox outbreak occurred in Halifax within weeks after the explosion but was limited to 50–100 cases. Leaders and physicians credited nurses, particularly the VON nurses providing home care, with preventing a full-blown epidemic in the city.

50. Ratshesky, "Report of the Halifax Relief Expedition"; Massachusetts General Hospital Nurses Alumna Association Office, Massachusetts General Hospital, Founders Building, Room 302, "Report to the Training School Advisory Committee, February 14, 1918," unmarked file folder located in lateral file cabinet drawer file; Massachusetts General Hospital Nurses Alumna Association Office, Massachusetts General Hospital, Founders Building, Room 302, "Massachusetts General Hospital School of Nursing, Boston, Mass. A List of Graduates Published 1940," file folder marked "prior to 1915" located in lateral file cabinet drawer file.

CHAPTER 6

The Boston Instructive District Nurses Association and the 1918 Influenza Epidemic: "Intelligent Cooperation"

Arlene W. Keeling

Influenza Situation Here Serious . . . Could Immediately Place Two Hundred Nurses—Can You Provide Them.[1]

On September 23, 1918, James Jackson, the manager of the New England division of the Red Cross, telegraphed these words to the Red Cross headquarters in Washington, DC, asking for nurses. A deadly form of influenza had erupted among the military recruits at Camp Devens, just outside Boston, Massachusetts, almost a month earlier and since then had spread to the civilian population. People were succumbing to the flu at exponential rates; sick and dying patients were pouring into the city's hospitals, where wards were soon overflowing and hundreds of extra cots lined the hallways. In some cases, whole families were ill and convalescent patients could not be discharged because there was no one well enough at home to care for them.[2] The city desperately needed nurses.

Indeed, nurses rather than physicians were needed on the front lines of the flu battle. In 1918, excellent nursing care was the primary treatment for influenza. There was minimal understanding of the disease; there were no antiviral medications to inhibit its progression and no antibiotics to treat the complicating pneumonia that often followed. Instead, bed rest, ice packs, sponge baths, and nutritious fluids were the standard treatments, along with such remedies as aspirin, mustard plasters, Vicks VapoRub, Listerine, and cough syrups. All treatments were best given by a skilled nurse—one who could make astute and critical observations of the patient's condition and intervene accordingly. The problem was that there were not enough trained nurses available to deliver skilled nursing care. In 1918, because of the deployment of large numbers of graduate nurses to military camps at home and abroad to assist in the war effort, the United States was experiencing a severe shortage of professional nurses on the home front. Further aggravating the situation, because of racial discrimination, neither the Army nor Navy Nurse Corps was employing Black nurses. Thus, when the epidemic reached Boston in the late summer, professional nurses were already stretched thin. Because hospitals were soon filled, many very sick people had to remain at home. There, the few public health and district nurses who had not been assigned to the military cause were left to serve on the front lines of the epidemic.

The influenza epidemic in Boston provides a case study that focuses on the public health and visiting nurses' contributions in the first city on the East Coast to be hit by flu. It is an account of a community response to an emergency situation in which the Boston Instructive District Nurses Association (IDNA) nurses played one part. Public health officials, physicians, military, and hospital nurses were all involved on the front lines of the epidemic, and their stories have been told by numerous others.[3]

In Boston, the IDNA's work among thousands of poverty-stricken young immigrants in neighborhoods throughout the city was critical to the community's response to the epidemic.[4] Led by director Mary Beard, an experienced and well-respected leader in the field of public health nursing, the IDNA nurses not only provided direct care but also coordinated the care given by other nurses and volunteers. In addition, the IDNA nurses supervised hundreds of nurses' aides, including "recent graduates of First Aid and Home Nursing Classes with 72 hours of hospital experience."[5] Numerous groups, including Red Cross volunteers, schoolteachers, church auxiliaries, diet kitchens, Catholic sisters, and social service agencies, provided essential support.[6]

SPANISH FLU

The 1918 flu (now known to be H1N1) was a virus like none other. It was called *Spanish flu* because Spain was neutral in World War I and, unlike other countries concerned about their national defense, Spain willingly admitted that it had a major public health problem. The highly contagious and deadly flu came on suddenly and with a vengeance; in fact, the patient could usually recall the exact time of its onset. Military physicians characterized its arrival as "explosive," observing that "no other disease spreads so fast."[7] The symptoms became all too familiar: sneezing, coughing, headache, bone and joint aches, chills, and fever of 102°–104° within a few hours. Extreme prostration followed, and patients "strained to breathe through lungs that rapidly filled with a thin, bloody fluid." In some cases, blood seeped from the nose and mouth.[8] Bronchopneumonia often complicated the situation, in which case mortality was 60%–70%.[9] Death sometimes occurred within 12 to 24 hours, sometimes after a week or more.[10]

What was unique was that this novel flu, instead of affecting mostly the very old and the very young, was deadliest for healthy young adults between the ages of 20 and 40. Among those particularly affected were strong, able-bodied military recruits; young civilian men; and pregnant women. The disease therefore wreaked havoc on young families, particularly in immigrant ghettos, where the virus spread like wildfire. When the parents were ill, families were without means of providing care; when parents died, children were left orphaned.

In 1918, the flu struck in three waves. The first wave came in the spring of 1918 and was a mild version, causing more illness than deaths and occurring sporadically throughout the world. The second wave, occurring primarily in September and October, was lethal. The virus had mutated and was both highly contagious and extremely virulent. It circled the globe, following trade routes and shipping lines. In the United States, the second wave struck in late summer in Boston and within a matter of days spread south along the eastern seaboard, to New York; Philadelphia; Baltimore; and Washington, DC. It then traveled with astonishing speed south and westward across the country along transportation lines, accompanying its hosts on trains and ships. By October 19, the flu had reached epidemic proportions as far away as San Francisco.[11]

THE BOSTON EXPERIENCE

In 1918, Boston, Massachusetts, was a sprawling industrial city and a center of manufacturing and shipping with a population of almost 750,000. Since the mid-1800s, Boston's population had swelled with Irish, Italian, and Jewish immigrants, who provided a steady source of cheap labor for the textile factories and mills. The city also housed military bases where, that summer, thousands of young recruits were stationed prior to deployment overseas.

The terrible outbreak of influenza started at Commonwealth Pier, where sailors quartered there succumbed in droves and were rapidly transferred to the local Chelsea Naval Hospital. The flu then spread to nearby Camp Devens in central Massachusetts, devastating the young recruits there.[12] Military hospitals were soon overflowing, and makeshift hospitals were needed. On September 10, the *Boston Globe* reported that an open-air tented hospital had been erected at Corey Hill in Brookline and had received 200 sailors from Commonwealth Pier and East Boston.[13]

Authorities in Boston had no idea what they were dealing with, being one of the first cities hit by the flu. On September 13, the health department reported its first civilian case. By September 17, newspaper headlines declared that 47 patients had died and 2,273 people had been stricken; indeed, the flu was "epidemic in much of greater Boston."[14] Within the next 24 hours, health authorities recorded 41 more deaths. Fear spread with the flu, prompting the Boston health commissioner to issue a warning against public hysteria. The next week, Massachusetts Lieutenant Governor Calvin Coolidge formed the Emergency Public Health Committee to coordinate statewide efforts to curb the spread of the epidemic and assign resources. The committee's first action was to telegraph the American Red Cross requesting help. Nurses were the top priority. Because health authorities had issued no quarantine or isolation mandates until later, many casualties had already occurred. Consequently, the Boston nurses were fighting an uphill battle from the beginning.[15]

THE NATIONAL RESPONSE

The day after Jackson's telegram, September 24, the American Red Cross National Committee on Influenza assembled in Washington to discuss the epidemic. During that meeting the group drafted a decentralized plan to address the national emergency.[16] The plan was clearly outlined from the start; it left the major response to local authorities and individual local Red Cross Chapters and coordinated that response with the United States Public Health Service (USPHS). Working through 3,684 local chapters in 14 regional divisions, the National Red Cross would assume charge of supplying nursing personnel and would pay the nurses' salaries. The national committee would also furnish emergency hospital supplies when local authorities were unable to do so. The USPHS would "gather facts about the spread of this disease and the adequacy of existing resources" and would determine when and where to send additional nursing personnel and supplies. It would also decide when "nursing personnel and supplies had served their emergent purpose and might be transferred." The USPHS would also mobilize physicians and from time to time ask the Red Cross to distribute official statements about the prevention and care of the disease. Meanwhile, all "general publicity" would be issued by the chair of the Red Cross National Committee on Influenza.[17] In short, the USPHS would manage the medical response and distribute posters and pamphlets educating the public about the illness. The Red Cross National Committee would communicate with its local organizations and direct the nursing response.[18]

Directions to specific localities were equally clear. Each local Red Cross chapter was instructed to immediately organize a Chapter Committee on Influenza to work in close cooperation with their local public health officials and to survey available nursing personnel and hospital supplies within its jurisdiction.[19] Immediately following the meeting, the director of the Red Cross Bureau of Nursing Services, Clara D. Noyes, telegraphed all Red Cross divisions with a directive: "Suggest you organize Home Defense nurses . . . to meet present epidemic . . . Provide nurses with masks."[20]

THE BOSTON IDNA RESPONDS

In Boston, the IDNA Nurses (classified as "Home Defense" nurses a year earlier) did not need to be told to organize for the epidemic: They had been seeing patients with influenza since early September. In fact, the association's newly opened headquarters on Massachusetts Avenue had been made the "administrative center for all home nursing care" related to the flu.[21] Moreover, IDNA superintendent Mary Beard had been serving on the governor's Emergency Public Health Committee and therefore was well aware of the fact that the flu was rampant in the city. In her report to a special meeting of the IDNA Board of Managers on September 25, Beard noted: "The influenza situation overshadows everything . . . the need for nurses is tremendous."[22] According to Beard, as nurses entered homes throughout the city, they found "whole families stricken . . . In one case the father was found in bed, dead; in another room, the mother lay, with two children, all very ill; and in still another, the baby, dying with pneumonia."[23] The epidemic was worse than anything the IDNA nurses had experienced in the 32 years of the association's work.

UNDERLYING STRUCTURE SUPPORTS EPIDEMIC WORK

The Boston IDNA had its origins in 1886, when it was established to provide home nursing care to the city's sick poor.[24] By 1910, the IDNA's work included maternal–infant cases, the inspection of children in nurseries and kindergartens, the management of three milk stations, and the inspection of factory workers. It also involved nursing policyholders of the Metropolitan Life Insurance Company and attending patients with contagious diseases. In all instances, the IDNA's mission was twofold: "curative care [under the direction of dispensary physicians] and preventive education."[25] In 1912, Mary Beard, a 1903 graduate of the New York Hospital training school, had been appointed the IDNA's director. As president of the National Organization of Public Health Nursing and chair of the subcommittee on public health nursing on the Council of National Defense, and internationally known for her work on the Rockefeller Foundation, Beard was well credentialed for the position and had the experience necessary to supervise visiting nurses. She was also familiar with the educational requirements for public health nursing and immediately set about restructuring the organization and opening a training school for public health nurses in collaboration with Simmons College. By 1918, the more efficient and professional IDNA not only had a main office and nine branches, serving "practically the whole of Boston," it also had pupil nurses who could be employed to expand the association's services.[26]

During the epidemic, Superintendent Beard directed much of the nursing response. With her connections to other public health nursing leaders throughout the country and her involvement with the governor's Emergency Public Health Committee, she was in the perfect position to do so. Under Beard's direction, the IDNA coordinated the care of "nurses of all kinds," including 15 from the Board of Health (who had volunteered under the IDNA), as well as 7 tuberculosis nurses, 13 school nurses, 20 baby hygiene nurses, and the Simmons public health nursing students. For the duration of the epidemic, the IDNA nurses also supervised hundreds of attendants, aides, and untrained volunteers, who "poured in the Central House all day long and well into the night offering to help in any way they could."[27]

Throughout the month of September, the IDNA nurses saw 4,664 new patients—more than three times the number they had seen in August.[28] Among these were 64 pregnant women with pneumonia or flu, 13 of whom died and 11 of whom miscarried. Not only the poor needed nurses, but the middle- and upper- class families also sought help, mostly requesting the private duty nurses they had come to expect. According to one IDNA report:

> All day long and up to 11:00 at night the four telephones poured out their pitiful stories. Whole families desperately ill with no one to do the commonest things for them; patients meeting the crisis of pneumonia with no nursing care at all; distracted relatives begging us to give that which did not exist anywhere to be given—nurses to stay till the patients were better.[29]

Because "nurses could not be had in sufficient numbers . . . the fullest utilization of their services" was to be made, and the New England division of the Red Cross declared that "an automobile and driver" be put at each nurse's disposal.[30] It was a mandate that would blur boundaries of class and gender as elite White ladies who comprised the IDNA's Board of Managers worked with the local Red Cross and the Home Guard Motor Corps to transport nurses throughout the city, sometimes volunteering to drive their own automobiles. It was, after all, both patriotic and fashionable to "do one's bit" to help the country during the war. The plan worked: Not only did it save the nurses' time, the automobile transportation allowed the nurses to carry soup, blankets, pneumonia jackets, and other necessary supplies.

NURSING SHORTAGES AND INCREASING SICKNESS

By the end of September the flu situation had gotten increasingly serious. It was now spreading not only through Boston but also throughout the state. So, on September 26, State Commissioner of Health Eugene Kelly once again telegraphed to Washington:

Influenza pneumonia situation . . . throughout Massachusetts very serious. Deaths increasing at alarming rate . . . Many doctors and nurses ill . . . Federal assistance necessary . . . Five hundred doctors and one thousand nurses needed at once.[31]

The reply from Washington was terse: "Can send all the doctors you want but not one nurse."[32]

Meanwhile, although the National Red Cross had few nurses to send to Boston, several localities responded to the city's desperate appeal for help. Among these, Lieutenant Governor McCallum Grant of Nova Scotia sent nurses and doctors in appreciation of Boston's response to the Halifax explosion a year prior (see Chapter 5), and the city of Baltimore sent a "special hospital train, fully equipped with 40 beds" to East Braintree Station near Quincy.[33] On their arrival in Boston, nurses were met at the train station by local Red Cross workers and "escorted to the State House" for their assignments. Most nurses would serve in Boston's emergency tent hospitals and military camps. The majority of civilian nursing would be left to the already- overloaded IDNA nurses and the public health nurses who had volunteered to help them.

On October 6, when the epidemic was rampant in Boston, IDNA Director Beard reported that the district nurses were caring for "3,074 patients ill with influenza or pneumonia." The care that the nurses provided was basic. They put patients to bed, covered them with blankets, and opened windows for fresh air. Following medical orders, or relying on their own nursing expertise and making do with what they had on hand, the nurses bathed patients; changed bed linens; and administered such treatments as ice packs and aspirin to reduce fever, Listerine gargles for sore throats, and mustard plasters and cough syrups to alleviate lung congestion.[34] They also provided nourishment, giving patients "gruels, cereals, milk toast, eggs, milk, etc." in small quantities.[35]

Key to the nurses' routine was the use of gauze masks. These were ordered by the National Red Cross, to be worn "constantly in congested homes, [when] . . . doing anything for the patient."[36] It was a mandate created with the hope of protecting nurses and others from "the bacteria which were floating in the air around each patient" so that they would not contract the disease. The demand for masks was enormous. In Boston, Red Cross volunteers worked seven days a week to produce 83,606 gauze masks during the last week of September and the first weeks of October[37] (see Figure 6.1).

The IDNA nurses not only used the masks themselves but also taught family members how to do so. They also taught family members how to care for flu victims, emphasizing the need for complete bed rest, warm blankets, fresh air, and nourishing fluids. To do so they used home demonstrations and educational circulars in which they encouraged "intelligent coopera-tion" on the part of patients and families.[38] Typical directions included the burning of "all bits of gauze or rags" used to collect nasal discharge; the use of face masks on adult patients; hand washing with "plenty of soap . . . and warm water when possible"; the administration of "a quarter of a glass of water every hour"; and propping the patient up with "two, three, or four pillows . . . whenever breathing is the least bit difficult."[39]

The work was arduous; the telephone at the IDNA headquarters rang incessantly, and nurses and volunteers worked late into the evenings. By the end of October, the nurses had completed 39,690 home visits—more than twice the number they had made in October 1917.[40]

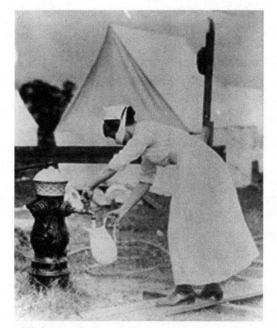

Figure 6.1   Nursing at a tent hospital, 1918, Courtesy National Archives and Records Administration.

THE AFTERMATH

By November, Boston was reeling with "the social wreckage" left in the wake of the epidemic. Often, families were left fatherless; in other cases, when both parents died, children were left orphans. The strain on the IDNA was also bad. 66% of the staff and some of the students had been ill "at one time or another" during the eight weeks of the epidemic.[41] Indeed, every department of the service had been "stressed to the utmost"[42] (see Figure 6.2).

For the IDNA nurses, the follow-up work was twofold: They not only continued to follow up those who had lingering effects of the illness, but they also returned to their maternity and "other preventive work."[43] The flu's sequelae were serious and included "ear troubles" in children, pneumonia, and debilitating muscle weakness and hair loss in adults. In her December report to the Board of Managers, Beard noted that the "follow-up work with the influenza patients . . . had revealed many kinds

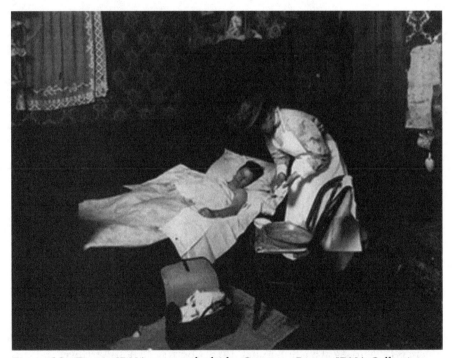

Figure 6.2   Boston IDNA nurse at bedside. Courtesy: Boston IDNA Collection, Howard Gotlieb Archives, Boston University.

of physical ailments left by the epidemic and that large numbers of the patients had been connected with dispensaries and hospitals for "after treatment."[44]

Getting the city back to normal would take the efforts of many. The IDNA nurses turned to affluent citizens for monetary support and to social workers for their skills in placing orphaned children and helping families find work, food, and medicines. Summarizing the work in the association's 1918 annual report, Mary Beard observed: "Our plan of organization has proved itself capable of tremendous expansion in an emergency. . . . [In addition] the universal need for nurses during the epidemic . . . brought a great volume of understanding of our work."[45] Part of that understanding resulted in an increase in donations to the IDNA. Responding to an *emergency bulletin* outlining what the IDNA nurses had accomplished during the epidemic and explaining the need for donations to support their work, 232 citizens contributed money to the association for the first time, and 362 "regular contributors" gave additional sums.[46]

CONCLUSION

As was true after other disasters, the response to the flu emergency was influenced by time and place. The epidemic occurred without warning in Boston in the summer of 1918—in the setting of mobilization of troops and nurses to the battlefront in Europe. Troop movements set up conditions for the spread of disease among formerly healthy young men, while the deployment of nurses led to a serious nursing shortage at home. Boston authorities were slow to mandate isolation or quarantine measures, yet the context was not all negative. As far as preplanning was concerned, a year earlier, public health nurses had been designated as Home Defense nurses charged with the responsibility for responding to emergencies within U.S. borders. As they worked in the chaotic situation of the Boston setting, they played a critical role in the public health response.

Many groups collaborated in the response, and nurses crossed state and national boundaries to help. Volunteers manned diet kitchens to feed whole families, others drove motor cars to ferry nurses across town, and Red Cross volunteers made thousands of face masks. As Boston hospitals rapidly became overwhelmed with patients, community agencies bore the brunt of the responsibility for caring for the sick. Key to this effort was the work of the IDNA, formed some 32 years earlier to care for the sick poor.

Led by Mary Beard, an influential and well- connected public health nursing leader, the IDNA nurses, secure in their training and skill, provided care for patients in their homes in nine districts throughout the city. The nurses were supported by the local chapter of the Red Cross, a network of social agencies, women's volunteer organizations, and churches. Indeed, the spirit of volunteerism that pervaded the community and the "intelligent cooperation"[47] with nurses' instructions on the part of families were essential to the IDNA nurses' attempts to fight the grim disease. Afterwards, nurses, physicians, and social workers continued to see patients with long-term complications. It would take months to return the city to "normal."

STUDY QUESTIONS:

1. What is meant by "intelligent cooperation" in the response to the epidemic?
2. Why was it so important that visiting and public health nurses take an active part in caring for the sick during the epidemic?
3. Discuss the importance of the word *instructive* in the title of the nurses' organization.
4. How did the context in which the epidemic occurred affect the city's response?

NOTES

1. James Jackson, telegram to American Red Cross headquarters, Washington, DC, 5:29 p.m., September 23, 1918. National Archives and Record Administration (NARA), CP box 689, 803.11.
2. Amalie Kass, "Infectious Diseases at the Boston City Hospital: The First 60 Years," *Clinical Infectious Diseases* 117, 2 (August 1993): 276–282.
3. For further reading on the general topic of the flu epidemic in Boston, see Carol Byerly, *Fever of War: The Influenza Epidemic in the U.S. Army During World War I* (New York: New York University Press, 2005). Also see: Alfred W. Crosby, *America's Forgotten Pandemic: The Influenza of 1918,* 2nd ed. (New York: Cambridge University Press, 2003).
4. Social agencies included organizations like the Salvation Army, the Bureau of Communicable Diseases, the Bureau of Child Welfare, the Red Cross, Maternity Centers, the Association for the Aid of Crippled Children, Milk

Stations, Diet Kitchens, and Social Service Departments of local hospitals. "What the Boston Metropolitan Chapter of the Red Cross Accomplished During the Epidemic" (November 18, 1918). NARA, CP box 689, 803.11 Epidemics, Flu, Massachusetts, 2. See also Arlene Keeling, "Midway Between the Pharmacist and the Physician," in *Nursing and the Privilege of Prescription* (Columbus: Ohio State University Press, 2007): 1–27.
5. "What the Boston Metropolitan Chapter of the Red Cross Accomplished," 1–2. Quote is on p. 1.
6. "Vigorous Action to Stamp Out Grippe," *The Boston Globe*, September 18, 1918.
7. Byerly, *Fever of War*, 90.
8. Katrina Rodies, "That Great Call: The Pandemic of 1918," *Nursing and Health Care Perspectives* 19(5): 204–205. Quote is on p. 204.
9. J. Keegan, "The Prevailing Pandemic of Influenza," *The Journal of the American Medical Association,* 71, 13 (1918): 1051–1059. Quote is on p. 1052.
10. Arlene Keeling, "'The Ghetto Was a Hotbed of Influenza and Pneumonia': District Nursing During the Influenza Epidemic," 1918–1919, in *Everyday Nursing Life, Past and Present*, ed. Sylvelyn Hahner-Romback (Stuttgart, Germany: Franz Steiner Verlag, August 2009), 63–80. See also Arlene Keeling, "When the City Is a Great Field Hospital: The Influenza Pandemic of 1918 and the New York City Nursing Response," *Journal of Clinical Nursing* 18 (September 2009): 2732–2738.
11. *Americas' Forgotten Pandemic*, 92–94.
12. http://www.celebrateboston.com/disasters/greatinfluenza.htm (accessed May 18, 2006).
13. "Brookline gets 200 Sick Sailors: Spanish "Grippe" Victims Sent to Corey Hill," *The Boston Daily Globe*, September 10, 1918.
14. "Grippe Making Great Headway," *The Boston Daily Globe*, September 17, 1918, 1.
15. Howard Markel et al. have shown that, although the contagiousness of the disease was deadly, especially in crowded conditions, Boston leaders did not initiate any quarantine or isolation orders to close schools, places of amusement, and other public gatherings until approximately September 25. These interventions reduced person-to-person contact, but they were delayed, with excess deaths occurring before specific actions were taken. By contrast, New York authorities responded quickly after the first cases were reported and before excess deaths occurred; therefore, the city had the lowest death rate in the East coast. See Howard Markel et al., "Nonpharmaceutical Interventions Implemented by US Cities During the 1918–1919 Influenza Pandemic," *Journal of the American Medical Association* 298, 6 (August 8, 2007): 644–654. The authors noted that Pittsburgh and Philadelphia health authorities also responded late and had poor outcomes.

16. Marian Moser Jones, "'The Greatest Mother' and the Great Pandemic" (Unpublished manuscript, April 10, 2009). Paper presented at the National Influenza History Seminar, The University of Michigan, May 14–15 (in press, *Public Health Reports, Supplement*).

17. J. Fieser (January 15, 1941). Report to Mr. Atkinson, January 15, 1941, re: Influenza Epidemic of 1918. NARA, CP Records of the Red Cross, box 557, 500.2 Influenza.

18. Ibid.

19. Ibid.

20. Clara Noyes, "Memo to All Division Directors," (September 25, 1918) NARA, CP box 689, 803.11.

21. Minutes of the IDNA Board of Managers Meeting (October 23, 1918): 1. IDNA Collection, Howard Gotlieb (HG) Archives, Boston. See also Medical Advisory Committee. Red Cross Nurses, Docket, July 23, 1917: 1–3, HG Archives, Boston University (BU), N34, box 11, folder 5. See also IDNA Annual Report, 1918. HG N34, box 13, folder 11, p. 32.

22. Minutes of the IDNA Board of Managers Meeting (September 25, 1918): 2. HG Archives, BU, N34, box 11.

23. IDNA, *Emergency Bulletin*, 1918. HG Archives, BU. N34, box 11.

24. Carrie Howse, "'The Reflections of England's Light': The Instructive District Nursing Association of Boston, 1884–1914," *Nursing History Review* 17 (2009): 47–79.

25. Ibid., 67.

26. Instructive District Nursing Association, in *Public Health and Private Conscience. Boston, 1916*: 1–13, Quote is on p. 5.

27. IDNA Board of Managers' Minutes, September 25, 1918; see also: IDNA Annual Report, (1918): 32.

28. IDNA Minutes, September 25, 1918.

29. Report of the Director, IDNA Annual Report, 1918, p. 34. HG archives, BU. N34, box 11, folder 5.

30. American Red Cross New England Division, "Memo, October 3, 1918" NARA, CP Box 689, 803.11 Epi Flu, Massachusetts.

31. Eugene Kelly, *Telegram to Congressman George H. Tinkham*, September 26, 1918. NARA, CP Box 689, 803.11.

32. Alfred Crosby, *America's Forgotten Pandemic*, 51.

33. IDNA Minutes, October 23, 1918.

34. "What the Boston Metropolitan Chapter of the Red Cross Accomplished," November 18, 1918: 2–3. NARA-CP. Box 689, 803.11 Epi Flu. See also: Keeling, "Midway Between the Pharmacist and the Physician"

35. "How to Care for Influenza and Pneumonia Patients," *The Public Health Nurse* 10, 7 (November 1918): 238–245. Quote is on p. 244.

36. Ibid.
37. "What the Boston Metropolitan Chapter of the Red Cross Accomplished."
38. "Vigorous Action to Stamp Out Grippe."
39. "How to Care for Influenza and Pneumonia Patients," 244–245.
40. IDNA Board of Managers' Minutes, (November 13, 1918). HG Archives, BU. N34, box 11, folder 5.
41. 1918 Annual Report, IDNA, Box 13, N34, folder 11, p. 32. HG Archives, BU.
42. Ibid.
43. IDNA Board of Managers' Minutes (February 5, 1919): 1. HG Archives, BU, N34, box 11, folder 5.
44. IDNA Board of Managers Minutes (December 4, 1918). HG Archives, BU. N34, box 11, folder 5.
45. Ibid.
46. IDNA Annual Report (1918): 15.
47. "Vigorous Action to Stamp Out Grippe."

CHAPTER 7

The 1921 Tulsa Race Riot and the "Angels of Mercy"

Barbra Mann Wall

At that hour we mistrusted every person having a white face and blue eyes. Since, we have learned that the Red Cross workers came like angels of mercy to heal and help suffering humanity.[1]

Mary E. Jones Parrish recalled these words after surviving the destruction that resulted from a riot between Blacks and Whites on the night of May 31 and morning of June 1, 1921, in Tulsa, Oklahoma. Armed White men looted, burned, and devastated the Black community of Greenwood. Parrish wrote, "The firing of guns was renewed in quick succession. People were seen to flee from their burning homes, some with babes in their arms and leading crying and excited children by the hand. Others, old and feeble, all fleeing to safety."[2] Scores of the badly wounded were sent to makeshift hospitals, and estimates of the final death count approached 300.[3]

The American Red Cross responded and, for the first time in its history, cared for survivors of a disaster brought on by purposeful acts of human hands rather than the random hand of nature. In its response, the Red Cross followed a policy issued in 1919, which stated that, in the event of race riots, care would be extended impartially to all survivors regardless of faction or party.[4]

Referring to the incident in a later memoir, Maurice Willows, director of the Red Cross relief effort in Tulsa, called it a *disaster* rather than a riot. To him, *riot* was an inadequate term to describe what took place—the elements of a race riot were present, but because of the wholesale destruction of property and the fact that many more Blacks were killed than Whites, it was "an unequal battle." Furthermore, the same elements of distress brought by fires, floods, tornados, or other disasters were present, with the additional complication of racial discord that produced an outcome in which "the morale of the affected population was destroyed."[5] The Red Cross sent nurses, physicians, and social workers to treat and care for all the survivors, but their efforts centered mainly on Blacks whose homes, businesses, and hospital, built over many decades, were, in a matter of hours, completely obliterated by a White mob.[6]

Several books have been written that analyze the mob violence, the racism of the White rioters, and the complicity of the National Guard and police.[7] Few have focused on the work of Red Cross nurses and other personnel, the tensions inherent as they cared for the wounded in a highly charged atmosphere of a race riot, and the factors that impinged upon their work. The activities of Director Willows and the Red Cross nurses laid the foundation for the establishment of a permanent hospital for Blacks in Tulsa.

Although the Tulsa riot was ostensibly motivated by an alleged attack on a White woman by a Black man in a downtown building elevator, other tensions provided fuel for the violence.[8] Tulsa's growth between 1910 and 1920 had been dramatic due to the discovery of oil a few miles from the city, and by 1915 it had become one of the largest cities associated with the oil boom. As such, it attracted large numbers of Whites and Blacks, all looking for work in the oil industry. Thus, by 1921, Tulsa's Black population had grown to nearly 11,000. Like other states, Oklahoma had laws providing for the segregation of Black and White populations. In Tulsa, most Blacks lived in the Greenwood section of town, which boasted 2 Black schools, 2 theaters and newspapers, 13 churches, a public library, and a hospital. At the heart of the area was a thriving commercial district. In fact, two- and three-story brick business buildings, hotels, barbershops, dry cleaners, and cafes lined Greenwood Avenue. Although White newspapers callously dubbed it "Little Africa," others knew it as "Black Wall Street." As historian Scott Ellsworth asserted, Greenwood "was assuredly one of the finest Black commercial districts in the entire Southwest," although Whites owned a large portion of the land[9] (see Figure 7.1).

Racial tensions were not unique to Tulsa. Between 1917 and 1919, a series of race riots had broken out across the entire United States as an aggressive White supremacy movement grew. In East St. Louis, Illinois, in 1917, for example, a White mob had stormed the streets of the city looking for Blacks to lynch.[10] Indeed, lynching of Blacks was common, and W.E.B. DuBois and other national Black leaders increasingly asserted that Blacks should protect

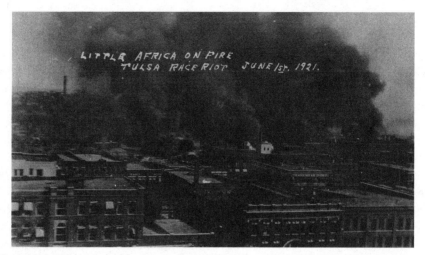

Figure 7.1   Greenwood burning. Courtesy: Tulsa Historical Society.

themselves and their homes, using the force of arms if necessary. In lieu of the ongoing unrest, Red Cross leaders at the national office developed a formal policy to guide its response to race riots and strikes. In a memo in November 1919, Red Cross General Manager F.W. Monroe emphasized the agency's "obligations to maintain a position of impartiality" as it meets "needs in forms of first aid, medical assistance, nursing services, etc. to those injured in disturbances regardless of faction to which they may belong." Furthermore, "There are also possible situations where widespread distress may develop as a result of conflict between elements in communities, affecting in some cases other than those a party to the disturbance." Although the Red Cross may act in these situations, no decision "can be made in advance as the possibilities are too various and intricate."[11]

In Tulsa, many of the Blacks were World War I veterans who had experienced respect by European allies and who believed they had earned the rights of full citizenship. They also were increasingly frustrated with the postwar wave of violence, and they were affected by DuBois and the intellectual dialogue sweeping across Black America at the time. For their part, some Whites thought Blacks were "getting above themselves."[12] It is in this backdrop that nurses' work after the Tulsa riot should be understood.

THE RIOT

On the morning of May 30, 1921, a young Black man, Dick Rowland, was accused (falsely) of attempting to attack a White woman, Sarah Page, in an elevator. That same morning, Rowland was arrested. The next day, alluding to an attempted rape, the *Tulsa Tribune* printed the story of the alleged attack under the inflammatory title, "Nab Negro for Attacking Girl in Elevator." This article has since disappeared, but it helped incite rumors of a lynching that eventually reached the Black neighborhood of Greenwood. There, a crowd of armed Blacks set out to the courthouse and offered to help protect the prisoner. Authorities at the scene apparently convinced them that their services were not needed, and they left. However, reports of the happenings spread through the city, and a group of 1,500 to 2,000 Whites also gathered at the courthouse. Others went to the Tulsa National Guard armory to demand guns. Consequently, more Black men returned to the courthouse, this time around 50 to 75; a shot was fired, and the race war was on.[13]

Outnumbered, Blacks began retreating to Greenwood. As reports of violence poured in to state authorities in Oklahoma City, the governor called in the Oklahoma National Guard, which arrived as fighting continued through the night. In the meantime, Police Chief John A. Gustafson commissioned scores of White men and armed them as deputies. Subsequently, these men made a mass attack on Greenwood, with the *Tulsa World* later reporting that "they planned to range through the negro [*sic*] settlement and 'clean it out.'"[14] With machine guns and other weapons, White citizens in and out of uniform began the attack, burning and looting the homes and businesses of the Black residents.[15]

As noted in Figure 7.2, armed White rioters rode around the neighborhood in cars and shot at houses where snipers were observed. Two thousand or more Blacks began leaving the area on foot. Many trying to escape were killed, whereas others had various medical emergencies. For example, Dimple L. Bush, a Black resident of Greenwood, recalled nurses' reports of several women delivering babies prematurely that day.[16]

By 9:00 a.m. on June 1, much of the gunfire had abated, and the governor declared martial law. Units of the Oklahoma National Guard arrested, en masse, nearly all of Greenwood's residents and marched them through the streets at gunpoint with their hands held above their heads (see Figure 7.3). The guards detained them in holding centers at the Convention Center, the

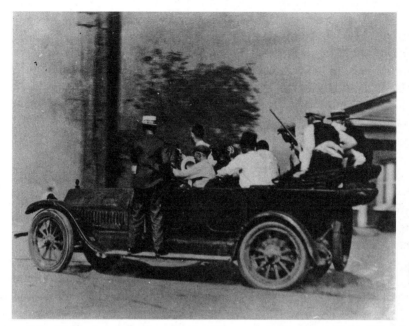

Figure 7.2   Vigilantes with shotguns in Greenwood. Courtesy: Tulsa Historical Society.

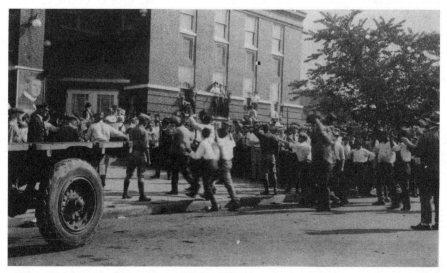

Figure 7.3   National guardsmen leading Blacks into Convention Center. Courtesy: Tulsa Historical Society.

local ballpark, and the fairgrounds while White rioters continued to loot and burn the Black residents' property. National Guardsmen also disarmed Whites, and while some were arrested, most were merely sent home. White citizens assumed that Blacks had started the riot; on June 1, more than 6,000 Black Tulsans were interned, whereas others fled the city only to return later. In the wake of the riot, 35 square blocks and 1,200 Greenwood homes and businesses lay in ruins.

According to Willows's 1921 Red Cross disaster report, the number of dead approached 300. It is unclear exactly how many were White and how many were Black. Many Whites did not give their names for fear of legal ramifications later. In other cases, bodies were hurriedly buried and, later, burial records could not be found. Furthermore, many of the dead were believed to have been buried in mass graves.[17] More recently, a forensic anthropologist for the Tulsa Race Riot Commission, which originated in 1997, was able to identify 39 confirmed dead (one a stillborn baby) based on death certificates and mortuary records. Most died from gunshot wounds. All 39 were males, of whom 26 (66%) were Black. Blacks averaged 35 years of age, typically were of the middle class, and had been long-time citizens of the Greenwood community. By contrast, the median age of the 13 Whites was 27 years, and all were of lower socioeconomic status except one, who was a junior executive of an oil company. Typical of the population of oil-boom days when young single, nonprofessionals came to the city looking for jobs and money, single men from outside Tulsa accounted for the majority of deaths.

Some of the deaths occurred from lack of care. Blacks were denied adequate treatment facilities until the late morning or early afternoon of June 1. By contrast, records revealed that several Whites' deaths were recorded before midnight on May 31, indicating they were promptly taken to hospitals. None of the Blacks' death certificates were signed before June 1, indicating that notice of their deaths had been delayed by at least 12 hours. One Black man, a well-respected physician, was shot as he walked out of his home with his arms upraised; he lay unattended for several hours before he bled to death.[18]

The riot made front-page news across the country. The *New York Times* reported 85 or more killed, although it eventually revised that number downward. A check of the hospitals showed that nurses and physicians had treated nearly 40 White citizens for injuries, and 50 Whites had already been treated and discharged without giving names. Most had arm and leg wounds obtained by hand-to-hand street fights.[19] Whites blamed Blacks and Blacks decried Whites for the violence. Parrish referred to the Black men involved as "brave and loyal . . . [They] were willing to give their lives, if necessary, for the sake of a fellow man."[20] Other Tulsans and editors of the newspapers blamed the police and sheriff for not bringing order soon enough. The *New York Times* reported:

> There has been a tremendous revulsion of feeling as the result of the outbreak, which Adjutant General Barrett, commanding the military forces, bluntly declares was caused by "an impudent negro, a hysterical girl and a yellow journal reporter." In the meantime, the City Government, the police and the Sheriff's office, are under heavy fire as having by incompetent handling of the situation brought shame upon the community.[21]

DISASTER RELIEF WORK

The Red Cross responded within 24 hours, and by the evening of June 1, local women had made special insignias of red crosses on white material to place on ambulances, motor vehicles, and trucks that eventually transported nurses, physicians, supplies, and other relief workers to hospitals and distribution centers. Local Red Cross authorities wired James Fieser, manager of the Southwestern division in St. Louis, Missouri, for help. In his response, he quoted Monroe's 1919 policy emphasizing medical and nursing service in the form of first aid regardless of faction. He also sent a division representative, Maurice Willows, who was well trained in relief work.

In addition to the Red Cross, many White Tulsans and their churches offered protection, food, and clothing to hundreds of Blacks who were left homeless. Volunteer doctors and nurses cared for the wounded in church basements. Often, White families took in Blacks who were domestics in their homes.[22] The bulk of the relief work began after martial law was declared around 11:30 a.m. on June 1. Because the all-Black Frissell Memorial Hospital had been burned to the ground, wounded Blacks initially were taken to the armory. There, the surgeon of the Third Infantry of the Oklahoma National Guard, Maj. Paul R. Brown, and his assistants gave first aid and dressed wounds until facilities at local hospitals could be assembled. There were not enough personnel to tend to the many wounded men and women, and Brown had to triage the patients, tagging each according to the seriousness of his or her wounds. He eventually sent them to the all-White Morningside Hospital, the most severely injured transferred first.

MORNINGSIDE HOSPITAL

In 1909, when the nursing professional associations affiliated with the Red Cross and a national committee on the Red Cross Nursing Service was established, the *American Journal of Nursing* had announced that "race, creed, and color lines are obliterated in this work."[23] This ideology was put to the test in 1921 in Tulsa.[24] Black nurses did work in emergency hospitals during the Tulsa riot, but whether they officially worked for the Red Cross is unclear. According to the Red Cross Nursing Service report, the total number hospitalized the first day was 163, with 80 Black patients taken to Morningside, where officials had set up a makeshift ward and surgery facility for them in the basement. The local Red Cross sent in nurses who also helped equip another emergency hospital in the basement of the Boulder M.E. Church, where 125 Blacks were transferred.[25]

Wounded White citizens had already been taken to the all-White Tulsa and Oklahoma hospitals yet Maj. Brown reserved some beds there for Black expectant mothers, also to be tended by Red Cross nurses. At the Oklahoma hospital, other Black patients were placed in the basement, where a White graduate nurse from the training school supervised nurses' aides furnished by the Red Cross. Cots crammed the crowded space, and Black women (one a nurse) and three Black men assisted in tending to the wounded. Throughout the next two days, a steady stream of White citizens came to inquire about their domestic employees and chauffeurs, whereas Black Greenwood residents sought relatives and friends. In one room was a Black woman who had been injured as she carried a patient from the burning Frissell Memorial Hospital, where she herself had been a patient.[26]

CINNABAR HOSPITAL

On June 3, Maj. Brown commandeered the old Cinnabar Hospital—which was being used as a boarding house—to be equipped as an emergency hospital, and the patients remaining at Morningside and the Boulder M.E. Church were transferred there. Because of Cinnabar's close proximity to

Morningside Hospital, staff could transfer patients requiring surgery to Morningside, which, unlike Cinnabar, had surgical services. According to Red Cross records, nurses working at the various hospitals assisted in 163 operations during the first week.[27] By June 4, the seriously injured patients in the Cinnabar Hospital totaled 150.[28] Miss E.W. Winn, an experienced Navy nurse enrolled in the Red Cross, took charge of the Red Cross nurses there.[29]

Other agencies also began relief efforts, but some were denied the chance to help. The national Black YWCA, headed by its field secretary, Miss Cordella Wynn, worked diligently with survivors. In contrast to this close cooperation between Blacks and Whites, the governor of Oklahoma refused the help of 50 Black Cross nurses from the Chicago chapter of the Universal Negro Improvement Association. The Black Cross nurses auxiliary was modeled on the Red Cross, with nurses organized on the local level. Although some of these women did not have formal nurses' training, they had practical experience in first aid and nutrition that would have been useful in the aftermath of this disaster.[30]

RED CROSS RESPONSE

Women such as Clara Barton and Mabel Boardman, who had previously occupied central leadership roles in the Red Cross, had been pushed to the side during World War I, although women did maintain leadership roles in nursing.[31] Much the same occurred in Tulsa, where Willows and other men led the relief effort, working from the local Red Cross headquarters at the Booker T. Washington High School.[32] When he arrived to direct the operation on June 4, Willows found 6,000 to 8,000 people homeless. He turned over the entire nursing service to State Supervisor of Nurses Rosalind MacKay. One of her duties was to account for nurses' salaries, which amounted to $150 a month plus expenses. In addition to working in hospitals, nurses manned a first aid and infant welfare station at the fairgrounds and a first aid station at Red Cross headquarters. These stations were under the direction of Mrs. W.D. Godfrey.[33]

The Red Cross nurses' work at the fairgrounds camp was varied. They saw patients with urgent problems individually and accompanied physicians on obstetrical cases. Trained in home hygiene and family health care, they carried out their teaching roles through demonstrations in bed making, first aid, bathing babies, and preparing infant food. Another major responsibility was the daily inspection of the fairgrounds camp for contagious diseases. Also at the camp, they assisted with 451 surgical dressings and tended 240 patients who received medical care. Both nurses and physicians vaccinated 841 people for tetanus, typhoid, and smallpox, giving 500 vaccinations on the morning of June 4. Nurses and other helpers prepared special feedings for 144 children and cared for 125 people with dysentery, which cleared after 3 days. Eventually the Red Cross set up a day nursery for Black children whose mothers had to go to work, often as domestics in White homes. A Black woman supervised the nursery, and nurses prepared the children's feedings.[34]

Bessie Richardson, from the Tulsa County Public Health Association, took charge of Red Cross field services outside the fairgrounds camp, which involved Red Cross and local public health nurses canvassing the city to find those who needed medical and nursing services. They made 4,512 calls and 34 emergency visits for the thousands of displaced survivors (see Table 7.1).[35] After the survey, the nurses set up medical, tuberculosis, dental, and venereal disease clinics and a dispensary, which the Red Cross turned over to the Tulsa County Public Health Association nurses. A physicians' committee of both Black and White doctors worked in conjunction with the nurses in all these areas. Black doctors, in particular, provided continuous coverage at the fairgrounds and other temporary quarters.[36]

White nurses working for the Red Cross had to prove to their patients that they could be trusted, because the Black community did not always perceive them as "angels of mercy." W.E.B. DuBois reported to Willows that U.S. Black citizens were bitter toward the Red Cross because of

Table 7.1 Survey Results of the Work of Six Nurses Over 5 Days

No. calls of the investigation	4,512
No. patients found	531
Classification of cases:	
Prenatal	38
Infant welfare	359
General	154
Referred to dispensary	80
No. emergency calls	34
No. nursing care	69
No. referred to relief department	551

Source: Disaster report by Maurice Willows, December 31, 1921.

reports from soldiers returning from World War I alleging that American Red Cross nurses in army hospitals in France had discriminated against Black officers. The soldiers claimed that Jim Crow laws had been in effect during the war when nurses had sent Black officers to hospitals for privates. DuBois personally traced down some of these complaints and found that it was hard to fix responsibility. Both the Red Cross and the Army "passed the buck" to each other. Nevertheless, DuBois was willing to use his magazine, *The Crisis*, to highlight the positive work of the Red Cross toward Tulsa sufferers.[37]

By June 7, many of the refugees had found jobs, but by then all Blacks had to carry proper identification in the form of green cards when they went out in public. They found this humiliating, but they would be arrested otherwise.[38] On June 11, Willows wrote that the situation was extremely tense. Refugees who initially left Tulsa began returning, which strained existing resources.[39] It was important to Willows, however, and to the Black people themselves not simply to give or receive handouts. Rather, as he wrote, "We furnished all necessary items for the negroes [*sic*] to rehabilitate themselves, requiring themselves to work it all out!"[40]

It was not until June 17 that Red Cross officials moved the emergency hospital at Cinnabar to Booker T. Washington High School (see Figures 7.4 and 7.5). After indoor plumbing and electric lights were installed, four rooms housed the injured, with one reserved for maternity care. Parrish provided a picture of the kinds of patients nurses attended:

> I can never erase the sights of my first visit to the hospital. There were men wounded in every conceivable way, like soldiers after a big battle. Some with amputated limbs, burned faces, others minus an eye or with heads bandaged. There were women who were nervous wrecks and some confinement cases.[41]

At the Booker T. Washington facility the nurses improvised by using the domestic science room to accommodate a kitchen and dining room, and they outfitted a screened porch to house tuberculosis cases. As the Red Cross nursing report stated, "The moving of patients so many times during the last two weeks and equipping of two hospitals was [a] fair-sized task and too much praise cannot be given to the nurses who so cheerfully served under these trying conditions." By June 21, the hospital service was thoroughly organized. Both Black and White physicians worked at the

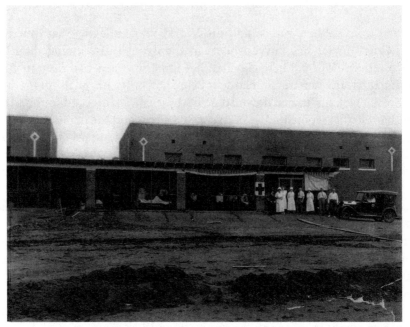

Figure 7.4 Booker T. Washington School, used as a Red Cross Hospital.
Courtesy: Tulsa Historical Society.

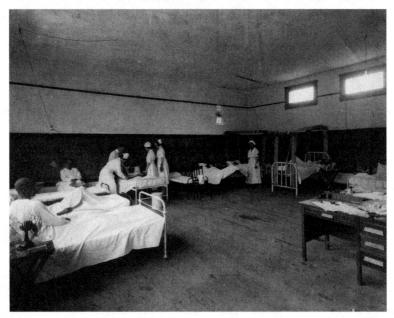

Figure 7.5 Inside of Booker T. Washington School, used as a Red Cross Hospital.
Courtesy: Tulsa Historical Society.

emergency hospital and saw the patients whom nurses referred to them from the field survey.[42]

At the Red Cross's insistence, the city and county government bore much of the cost for the Red Cross relief. On June 1, the Chamber of Commerce and other city agencies appointed a public welfare board consisting of leading White businessmen to assist with finances, food, housing, and hospital care. This committee met with Red Cross representatives and, along with the mayor, on June 2, designated the Red Cross as the official relief agency. The Public Welfare Board announced that it would not appeal for outside help for contributions but started its own campaign, collecting $26,000 at first, with more promised. The Red Cross national headquarters assumed responsibility for payment of Red Cross personnel.[43]

Much to Willows's dismay, however, neither the city nor county contributed substantially to Greenwood's rebuilding. On June 2, the National Guard, rather than assisting with the cleanup, required "all able-bodied" Black men to do so. The Black Citizens Relief Committee and the East End Welfare Board assisted in relief efforts. The latter was a group of Black leaders who primarily worked to coordinate activities and collect funds for rebuilding. Parrish wrote of them, "These men worked faithfully and have fought many battles for their fellow man," and they helped meet both physical and legal needs.[44] Eventually, the Red Cross demanded that $40,000 in the 1921–1922 city budget be delegated to finish the relief program, and the mayor acceded.

The Red Cross position soon went beyond the cautious role of providing "first aid, medical assistance, and nursing services" that Fieser had originally instructed. The many tents that the Red Cross had initially provided were inadequate for long-term use, and by September, Willows was developing a housing plan. It involved a more permanent kind of tent consisting of a 3-foot boarded wall and floor with screened side flaps and necessary household equipment (see Figure 7.6). The Red Cross remained in Tulsa for seven months following the riot, and it provided the most sustained relief effort at a cost of more than $100,000.[45]

Municipal authorities, however, initially impeded any rebuilding by making plans to convert Greenwood into an industrial district and relocate the Black community further north. They passed a fire ordinance that required new buildings in the burned district to use fireproof materials that essentially prohibited residents from rebuilding because they were unable to afford the costs. In response, the Black law firm of Spears, Chapelle, and

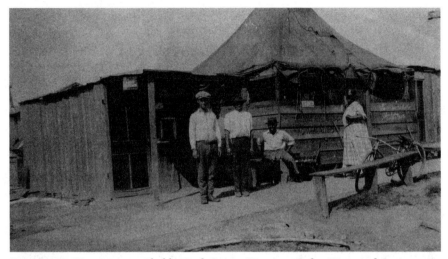

Figure 7.6   Housing provided by Red Cross. Courtesy: Tulsa Historical Society.

Franklin filed lawsuits in August and again in September and finally won when judges granted a permanent injunction against the ordinance.[46] In a personal account written years after the riot, Willows indicated his deviation from official Red Cross policy to advocate for Black people in this issue, knowing that they could not afford the more expensive houses. Showing a comradeship with Black citizens, Willows wrote, "Our attorneys, headed by a wonderful judge (Eakes) fought the council and WON hands down!"[47]

MAURICE WILLOWS HOSPITAL

Once the city ordinance was defeated, by the end of September the rebuilding of Greenwood was significantly underway. The goal was to replace the 1,200 houses that had burned. As the *Black Dispatch* noted, Black families were working together to "take care of themselves." In addition, charges against Dick Rowland had been dismissed.[48] Because Booker T. Washington School was needed for classes that fall, the Red Cross commenced to build a more permanent hospital to continue caring for those wounded during the disaster and to provide care for Black patients who had become sick with other diseases. For example, lack of suitable housing created conditions conducive to pneumonia, and other Blacks became ill while working outdoors clearing debris. Tuberculosis and venereal disease also were prevalent. County commissioners and the Board of Education jointly provided property on which Black laborers constructed a 9-room, 30-bed hospital, aptly called the Maurice Willows Hospital (see Figures 7.7 and 7.8). The hospital had male and female surgical wards, a maternity ward, a women's general medical ward, a fully equipped operating room, and a large porch for convalescent patients. The Red Cross furnished the building material and the East End Relief Committee the labor, and it cost approximately $68,000. On September 1, nurses once again packed up and moved their patients and equipment to the new facility. By the middle of the month, the new hospital still housed 14 riot cases.[49]

In the end, the city and county spent nearly $200,000 of tax money for relief and rehabilitation. In the seven months that the Red Cross was in Tulsa, medical and nursing personnel provided care to 233 people; emergency dressings and supplies to five hospitals; and tents, clothing, cooking utensils, and bedding to 2,056 families and 8,200 people. Nurses were

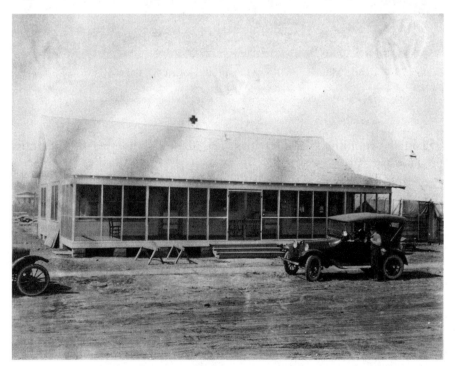

Figure 7.7   Maurice Willows Hospital. Courtesy: Tulsa Historical Society.

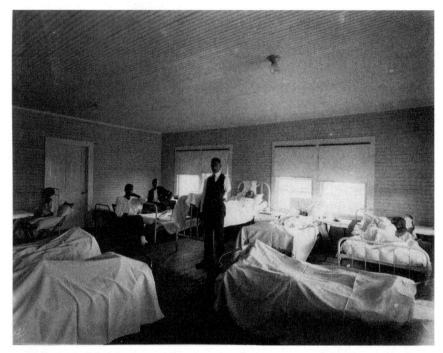

Figure 7.8   Inside Maurice Willows Hospital. Courtesy: Tulsa Historical Society.

essential to fulfilling these activities. The Red Cross reimbursed each hospital for its costs.[50]

Table 7.2 reveals a summary of the Red Cross medical and surgical relief as of December 31, 1921, when the agency officially ceased its operations.[51] Significantly, 18 deaths occurred, which did not become part of the official death count of 39 noted earlier. Some people likely died of complications from injuries sustained during the riot. Other deaths, such as those of elderly persons or children, could have been caused by diseases as a result of exposure when their homes were destroyed. The last Black person to die of wounds from the riot occurred on August 20, 1921, at Maurice Willows Hospital. Nurses had cared for this 21-year-old man for 11 weeks before he succumbed to complications.[52] Nurses continued to care for Black patients in the hospital and to help needy families in the community until December 31, 1921 (see Figure 7.9).

Table 7.2 Summary of the Medical and Surgical Relief as of December 31, 1921

No. wounded Whites hospitalized during and after riot at Red Cross expense	48
No. wounded Blacks hospitalized during and after riot at Red Cross expense	135
No. Blacks hospitalized since riot	98
Total no. receiving hospital care	233
No. patients still remaining in hospital	22
No. deaths	18
No. discharges	193
No. first aid cases during and after riot	531
No. patients receiving vaccinations	1,800
No. Black physicians used by Red Cross in treatment of sick since riot	11
No. White physicians whose services were paid for by the Red Cross	11
No. nurses employed by Red Cross during and after riot	38 (hospital) 8 (field)

Source: Disaster Report by Maurice Willows, December 31, 1921.

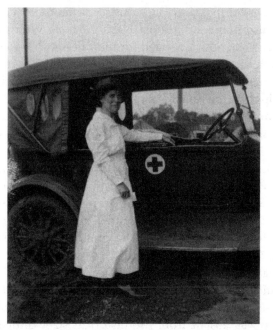

Figure 7.9   Red Cross nurse at Maurice Willows Hospital. Courtesy: Tulsa Historical Society.

The Red Cross opted to stay until the end of the year because there was no agency equipped for record keeping and casework to deal with dependent families in Tulsa. By then, Black leaders had incorporated the Colored Hospital Association to assume the management of the Maurice Willows Hospital. It would be directed by a board of representative Black citizens. However, Willows did not view Blacks as capable of finishing the hospital "unless some White guiding hand is available."[53] An all-White nursing staff remained until the new association began functioning on January 1, 1922, when Black nurses and physicians assumed responsibility.[54] In 1924, there were 17 Black doctors in Tulsa. Hospitals in Kansas City and St. Louis provided most of the Black nurses who eventually worked in Oklahoma.[55]

CONCLUSION

As a legacy of its work after the 1921 race riot, the Red Cross was recognized in Tulsa and across the country as the primary response agency for both natural and human-made disasters. Despite its claims of impartiality, the Red Cross response in Tulsa was not neutral. In an era of widespread racial discrimination against Black citizens, Willows and the Red Cross nurses consistently advocated for their needs after the riot. This was evident through their interactions with local committees; the provision of building materials for homes; the support they gave to helping men and women to help themselves; and, most important, the provision of needed medical and nursing care. As Marian Moser Jones asserts, by ostensibly providing *disaster relief*, as Willows labeled it, the Red Cross could mask its true position of supporter for the Black community.[56]

Parrish viewed the Maurice Willows Hospital as "the most constructive piece of work done by the Red Cross" in Tulsa.[57] The city operated it until 1937, when the county took it over. Then, from 1941 to 1967, it was known as the Moton Memorial Hospital and was administered by Mrs. Dimple Bush. It was the largest Black hospital in Oklahoma and the last to be phased out in the 1960s.[58]

Unfortunately, what John Hope Franklin and Scott Ellison have labeled *historical amnesia* occurred after the riot. Although the disaster made headlines for several weeks, it soon moved to the shadows of Tulsa history and eventually was absent from the historical stage altogether. The riot became a source of local embarrassment as city boosters and others were

more and more fearful of what the riot would do to the young city's reputation.[59] In 1997, however, after attention was given to the riot during its
75th anniversary, the Tulsa Race Riot Commission was created to develop
a historical account of the event. Its charge was to determine the cause of
the riot, assign responsibility, and determine if reparations should be recommended. The Oklahoma state legislature passed the "1921 Tulsa Race
Riot Reconciliation Act" in June 2001. It did not carry out all of the commission's recommendations, but it did provide for more than 300 college
scholarships for descendants of Greenwood residents. It also mandated the
creation of a memorial to those who died in the riot and called for new efforts to promote economic development in Greenwood.[60] As the country
currently struggles to understand America's racial past, it is helpful to look
back at the legacy of nurses and other health care workers who tended to
all survivors of the Tulsa riot in 1921, regardless of race.

STUDY QUESTIONS:

1. Consider the Red Cross response to the 1921 Tulsa race riot. What
   factors came into play that altered their rule of impartiality?
2. Discuss Willows's use of the term *disaster relief* as a means of infrastructure support for Blacks. Relate that to the Red Cross's stance
   on neutrality.
3. John Hope Franklin and Scott Ellison describe *historical amnesia*
   after the riot. Discuss this label in reference to this riot. Compare
   it to the silence after the 1918 influenza pandemic. How did the
   responses differ after the 9–11 tragedy? Why?

NOTES

1. Mary E. Jones Parrish, *Race Riot 1921: Events of the Tulsa Disaster*, rev. ed.
   (Tulsa, OK: Out on a Limb Publishing, 1998), 23. This is a reprint of the
   original book written in 1922 by Mrs. Parrish, who recorded the events
   and feelings of others who experienced the riot first hand.
2. Ibid., 20.

3. "Scores Badly Wounded Removed to Hospitals: Three Die on the Way," *Tulsa World*, June 1, 1921, 1.

4. Copy of James L. Fieser, manager, Southwestern Division, to A. L. Farmer, chairman of the Tulsa County Chapter of the American Red Cross, June 1, 1921, and copy of F. C. Munroe to Alfred Fairbank postal telegram, Washington, DC, November. 4, 1919. These copies are located in Bob Hower, *1921 Tulsa Race Riot and the American Red Cross "Angels of Mercy"* (Tulsa, OK: Homestead Press, 1993). This book is a compilation of the memorabilia of Maurice Willows, director of Red Cross relief in Tulsa during the riot, by his grandson. It contains newspaper clippings, original letters, and photographs that the author inherited from Willows's daughter, the author's mother.

5. Maurice Willows, director, "Disaster Relief Report," December 31, 1921, located in Rudisill Regional Library, Tulsa, OK (hereafter cited as RL). For the second quotation, see Maurice Willows to A. L. Farmer, "Disaster Relief Report for Tulsa County Chapter, American Red Cross, September 14, 1921," box 716, RG 200, National Archives Gift Collection, Records of the American National Red Cross, 1917–1934, College Park, MD (hereafter ANRC).

6. Noted in Hower, *1921 Tulsa Race Riot*.

7. Scott Ellsworth, *Death in a Promised Land: The Tulsa Race Riot of 1921* (Baton Rouge: Louisiana State University Press, 1982); James S. Hirsch, *Riot and Remembrance: The Tulsa Race War and Its Legacy* (Boston: Houghton Mifflin Co., 2002); and Alfred L. Brophy, *Reconstructing the Dreamland: The Tulsa Riot of 1921, Race, Reparations, and Reconciliation* (New York: Oxford University Press, 2002).

8. Willows, "Disaster Relief Report"; Ellsworth, *Death in a Promised Land*.

9. Ellsworth, *Death in a Promised Land*, 16. See also *Tulsa Colored Business Directory*, January 22, 1921, 1989-004-2-1-7; and *City Directory 1921*, 1989-004-2-3, Tulsa Race Riot 1921 Archive, McFarlin Library, University of Tulsa, Tulsa, OK.

10. Malcolm McLaughlin, "Ghetto Formation and Armed Resistance in East St. Louis, Illinois," *Journal of American Studies* 41, 2 (2007): 435–467.

11. Munroe to Alfred Fairbank postal telegram.

12. Ellsworth, *Death in a Promised Land*; Frances W. Prentice, "Oklahoma Race Riot," *Life in the United States* (New York: Scribner's Sons, 1933), 151. See also Marian Moser Jones, "Confronting Calamity: The American Red Cross and the Politics of Disaster Relief, 1881–1939," PhD Diss., Columbia University, 2008. Proquest Dissertations and Theses, Publication #AAT 3317567, 444.

13. "Whites Advancing into 'Little Africa': Negro Death List Is About 15," *Tulsa World,* June 1, 1921, 1; "Dead in Race Riot," *Tulsa Daily World,* June 1, 1921, 1.

14. Ibid.

15. Parrish, *Race Riot 1921.*

16. Ibid., 106.

17. Willows, "Disaster Relief Report"; Ellsworth, *Death in a Promised Land.*

18. Clyde Collins Snow, "Confirmed Deaths: A Preliminary Report," in *Tulsa Race Riot: A Report by the Oklahoma Commission to Study the Tulsa Race Riot of 1921,* 109–122. This report can be accessed at http://www.tulsarepara tions.org/FinalReport.htm (accessed July 25, 2009). See also "Loot, Arson, Murder," *The Black Dispatch,* June 10, 1921, 1. This was the Black news-paper in Oklahoma City. The office of the *Tulsa Star,* a Black newspaper in Tulsa, was burned during the riot.

19. "Series of Fierce Combats," *New York Times,* June 2, 1921, n.p.

20. Parrish, *Race Riot 1921,* 18.

21. "Tulsa in Remorse to Rebuild Homes; Dead Now Put at 30," *New York Times,* June 3, 1921, n.p.; "Press Scolds Tulsa; Editors Blame Police," *Tulsa Tri-bune,* 5 June 5, 1921, n.p.

22. Willows, "Disaster Relief Report"; "Local Red Cross Is Reorganized," *Tulsa World,* June 3, 1921, 1, 3; and "Tulsa Churches in Mercy Work," *Tulsa World,* June 3, 1921, 9. (RL).

23. Editorial Comment, "The Red Cross," *American Journal of Nursing* 10, 2 (1909): 79.

24. Joyce Ann Elmore, "Black Nurses, Their Service and Their Struggle," *Ameri-can Journal of Nursing* 76, 3 (1976): 435–437. During World War I, the Red Cross had voted to accept Black nurses, but only if the sur-geon general of the army would allow them. This did not occur until the flu epidemic of 1918 and 1919, when nurses were overwhelmingly needed.

25. Paul R. Brown, Maj. M.C. Commandg. San Det. 3rd Inf. to Adjutant General of Oklahoma, "Work of the San Det. During Riot in Tulsa: July 1, 1921." Tulsa Race Riot 1921 Archive, 1989-004, McFarlin Library, University of Tulsa; "Nursing Service Report, June 21, 1921," in ANRC.

26. Willows, "Disaster Relief Report"; "Many Dismissed From Hospitals," *Tulsa Daily World,* June 3, 1921, 13. For patients with burns and gunshot wounds, nurses administered opiates to relieve pain.

27. Willows, "Disaster Relief Report."

28. Interoffice memorandum, James L. Fieser to W. Frank Persons, June 23, 1921, ANRC.

29. During World War I, more than 29,000 American Red Cross nurses had volunteered with the Army or Navy Nurse Corps. See Cheryl K. Schmidt, "American Red Cross Nursing: Essential to Disaster Relief," *American Journal of Nursing* 104, 8 (2004): 35–38.

30. Hirsch, *Riot and Remembrance*, 130. For more information on Black Cross Nurses, see http://www.pbs.org/wgbh/amex/garvey/peopleevents/e_womenunia. html (accessed July 27, 2009).

31. Jones, "Confronting Calamity." Clara Barton resigned in 1904, and Mabel Boardman succeeded her. See also "General Information, Mabel Boardman," at http://www.wcredcross.org/general/mabel.html (accessed September 29, 2009).

32. Ibid.

33. "Nursing Service Report"; "Hostess House for Negroes Is Being Erected," *Tulsa Tribune*, June 4, 1921.

34. "Nursing Service Report."

35. "Disaster Report by Maurice Willows," December 31, 1921, ANRC. See also Hower, *1921 Tulsa Race Riot.*

36. "Nursing Service Report"; "Hostess House for Negroes."

37. M. Willows to James L. Fieser, November 25, 1921, and W. Frank Persons to James L. Fieser, November 22, 1921, ANRC.

38. "Thousands Leave Tulsa," *The Black Dispatch*, June 17, 1921, p. 1.

39. Inter office memorandum, Fieser to Persons. June 11, 1921, ANRC.

40. Willows, "Disaster Relief Report."

41. Parrish, *Race Riot 1921*, 29.

42. "Nursing Service Report."

43. Willows, "Disaster Relief Report" and "Red Cross in Field Until All Are Well," *Tulsa Tribune*, June 4, 1921, 1.

44. Parrish, *Race Riot 1921*, 32.

45. Danny Goble, "Final Report of the Oklahoma Commission to Study the Tulsa Race Riot of 1921," in *Tulsa Race Riot: A Report*, 1–20.

46. "Blacks Seek Injunction Against Illegal Ordinance," *Black Dispatch*, August 19, 1921, 1; and "Tulsa Negroes Win Permanent Injunction," *The Black Dispatch*, August 26, 1921, 1.

47. Willows's personal account, in Hower, *1921 Tulsa Race Riot*, 112.

48. "Rebuilding of Greenwood Almost Accomplished," and "Release Dick Rowland," *The Black Dispatch*, September 29, 1921, n.p.

49. Willows, "Disaster Relief"; "Third Report of the Tulsa Relief Committee," *The Black Dispatch*, November 19, 1921, n.p.; and Hower, *1921 Tulsa Race Riot*, 91.

50. Willows, "Disaster Relief Report"; "Summary of Red Cross Work in Tulsa," ANRC.

51. "Disaster Report by Maurice Willows, December 31, 1921," ANRC. See also
    Hower, *1921 Tulsa Race Riot.*

52. Snow, "Confirmed Deaths."

53. Maurice Willows, "Full Social and Medical Relief Report Up to and Including
    December 31st, 1921," RL.

54. "Disaster Relief Report for Tulsa County Chapter," September 14, 1921, ANRC;
    Willows, "Disaster Relief Report"; and Hower, *1921 Tulsa Race Riot,* 175–
    177.

55. Charles James Bate, *"It's Been a Long Time" and We've Come a Long Way* (Musko-
    gee, OK: Hoffman Printing Co., 1986). Few Black nurses graduated in
    Oklahoma schools of nursing up to the 1970s. In 1980, the historically
    Black Langston University opened a baccalaureate in nursing program. See
    M. Elizabeth Carnegie, *The Path We Tread: Blacks in Nursing Worldwide,
    1854–1994* (New York: National League for Nursing Press, 1995).

56. Jones, "Confronting Calamity."

57. Parrish, *Race Riot 1921,* 70.

58. Bate, *"It's Been a Long Time."* Today, the facility is a clinic.

59. John Hope Franklin and Scott Ellsworth, "History Knows No Fences: An Over-
    view." In *Tulsa Race Riot: A Report,* 26.

60. http://www.tulsareparations.org/FinalReport.htm (accessed July 26, 2009).

CHAPTER 8

The New London, Texas, School Explosion, 1937: "Unparalleled Disaster"

Barbra Mann Wall

This unparalleled disaster is remarkable for the speed and smoothness with which the operating companies interested in this field coordinated their rescue and aid work.[1]

Four days after a natural gas explosion in the East Texas town of New London leveled a school, Albert Evans wired these words to James Rieser, Vice Chairman of the American Red Cross in Washington, DC.[2] At about 3:15 in the afternoon of March 18, 1937, a blast occurred that eyewitnesses described as "one loud rumbling noise." The arc of an electric switch in the manual training room ignited a gas leak from pipes under the New London school at the moment that a teacher plugged a portable sander into a wall socket. The eyewitnesses reported that school walls bulged and rooms crashed down as a huge wing of the school collapsed.[3] One young seventh grader was walking toward his teacher at the time of the explosion. He recalled, "I had barely reached the teacher and sat down when the room went *whoom!* A blast came across straight horizontal. All these steel lockers that had been embedded in the wall blew kids out of their seats and fell on top of us." Other children remembered being knocked under counters, stumbling over injured children, and pushing each other out of windows to safety.[4] The disaster killed more than 300 children and 14 teachers. The local response to the explosion was quick and efficient, but the psychological trauma lingered, as few spoke of the grim events for many years.

Survivors and other eyewitnesses constructed narratives or stories afterward, which provided them a means of healing and restoration. In their stories, it is clear that the contextual factors of time and place—East Texas in 1937—shaped the ways in which people made sense of their disaster experiences. Factors included not only the influence of geography but also economics, social position, and religious beliefs. The narratives add to theoretical formulations about collective memory as survivors found ways to pass their memories of the disaster to others.

A focus on Texas allows race to be considered in the analysis, because during the first half of the twentieth century Jim Crow laws were in effect in the southern and border states. These laws legally sanctioned racial segregation, especially of Blacks, in all public facilities. In New London, segregation of schools and housing directly influenced casualty lists. At the same time, this disaster also led to the collapse not only of physical structures but also of social boundaries, and it brought about a major policy change in the oil and gas industry.

THE INITIAL RESPONSE

At present, New London is a small town in East Texas with a population of less than 1,000. When the explosion occurred, however, it was a prominent center in the state. Located in northwest Rusk County, it had what some called the richest rural school in America. The consolidated junior and senior high school served residents in the East Texas oil fields, and its growth had taken off after the discovery of oil in 1930 in Rusk County. Thousands of derricks surrounded the school. In most of the oil fields, natural gas was also produced. Rather than using a boiler for heat, as most schools did, the New London school relied on free gas. This was especially appreciated because people were still in the midst of the Great Depression, but it was a leak from this gas that led to the blast.

Oil workers several miles away heard the rumble and then saw a huge cloud of dust fill the sky. They immediately jumped in their trucks and rushed to the scene. Many of the casualties were their children. Significantly, all the children were White because segregation prevented Blacks from attending the school. The importance of time and place affected not only who was injured but also the quick response of workers in the nearby oil fields. They brought their heavy trucks, draglines, portable generators, and shovels with them and cleared the debris within 17 hours, a feat that did not go unnoticed by local residents. One doctor, writing about the disaster to his parents, noted that the school was "one of the wealthiest and biggest rural schools in the world—right in the middle of the oil field." Had it "not been for the big oil companies, who immediately sent all their big 10-ton trucks and [C]aterpillars, and oil field men who knew how to work, they would still be digging in the ruins."[5] Years later, however, one of those workers remembered a different aspect of the past: "Most of the rubble was moved with bare hands, not machinery. A guy came by with a truckload of peach baskets, and the workers formed a line and passed the baskets" full of body parts and debris.[6]

After nightfall, martial law was declared, with only doctors, nurses, police officers, rescue workers, and relatives allowed near the area. The whole scene was lighted up with floodlights. It was reported that, sometime in the night, a worker discovered a blackboard with writing that reflected a macabre irony: "Oil and natural gas are East Texas' greatest mineral blessing. Without them this school would not be here and none of us would be here learning our lessons."[7]

The disaster made national and international headlines, and regional variations in disaster coverage were evident. East Texas newspapers focused on photographs of disaster scenes and stories of survivors who just missed being killed.[8] Emotional language was especially evident when reporters wrote personal accounts of well-known community residents who had died. The *New York Times* testified to the importance of the place on page 14, where it showed a Texas map with New London's location. To excite the imagination of its readers, a reporter contributed to the mystique of oil-rich Texas in describing "the inevitable oil-well derricks, which, having provided tax money from which the school was built encroached even on the playgrounds." Then, the article highlighted the largest oil fields in the area: Humble Oil, Gulf, and the Tidewater Oil Company, which sent more than 1,000 workers for rescue operations.[9]

As the school collapsed, the disaster also brought about a crumbling of social boundaries. Texas newspapers reported the huge outpouring of support. Race emerged as an issue in one newspaper when it noted that "many Negro ambulances were used and several Negro doctors assisted with the relief work." They worked alongside members of the American Legion, Texas Rangers, National Guard, and Boy Scouts.[10]

Social class was highlighted in the *New York Times* report: "Oil field workers, farmers, and White collar men from the communities surrounding New London" all participated in the rescue operations.[11] Telegrams and letters came to New London from schoolchildren as far away as Japan and South Africa, and President Franklin Roosevelt and even Adolf Hitler sent condolences.[12]

THE RED CROSS RESPONSE

Bulletins from local radio stations, which had erected temporary microphones at the disaster scene, helped direct the emergency response. As radio messages spread the news of the disaster, doctors, nurses, and ambulances responded from all over the state. Newspapers reported "hundreds of white-clad nurses with doctors and interns from scores of hospitals" at the scene along with morticians and hearses. The highways leading into the small town were filled with automobiles.[13] The American Red Cross arrived by 4:00 a.m. Drugstores and hospitals drained their stores of bandages and disinfectants and sent them to the wreckage site. Rescue workers gave first aid to survivors, carried them to the highway, and put them in passing automobiles, which rushed them to nearby hospitals. All of the small towns surrounding New London had clinics, and they also were full of casualties.[14]

The medical director of the national office of the Red Cross flew to the scene along with other regional and national personnel. The Red Cross often found itself in competition with local agencies over just who would be in charge of the relief operations. William Baxter, head of the Midwestern branch office, wired the national office: "Although our problem of stepping in and gaining recognition as the official relief agency is much simpler today than it was 10 or 15 years ago, we still find instances in which city or county officials, or even other organizations wish to assume responsibility for relief activities." Because he expected such a large outpouring of relief, he staffed the job with more national workers than usual.[15]

Along with local responders, 50 Red Cross nurses from Texas and the national association gave initial first aid at the scene and rushed survivors to nearby hospitals and clinics in Tyler, Overton, Kilgore, Jacksonville, and Henderson. Other Red Cross nurses assisted regular hospital personnel with more than 80 patients who were suddenly hospitalized, including four workers, and they visited patients remaining in their homes. Injuries to survivors included fractures of the back and extremities, eye and other lacerations, and head injuries. Skull fractures predominated, and nearly all the survivors with severe injuries were in a state of shock. Some were unconscious, whereas others were semicomatose.[16]

The Red Cross assigned 14 nurses to accompany prostrated parents and other grieving friends and relatives to gravesites to administer whatever care they could. Mothers wept on nurses' shoulders, and fathers tried to take whatever comforting words the nurse could offer. When six different families lost three children each, nurses were sorely needed. According to the Red Cross medical director, "This disaster represents the first experience to my knowledge where the gravity of the situation necessitated nurses in attendance at burial places." The Red Cross also furnished sheets for improvised hospitals and morgues, transportation, food for homes that were unprepared for the huge numbers of relatives coming in, and flowers for the graves. It also arranged for clergymen to visit homes over the next several days.[17]

Red Cross hospital reports noted nervous parents who, in the Red Cross reporter's words, were problematic for the hospital staff. One mother insisted on remaining with her son at all times and was considered "over solicitous," which "prevented the boy from being cooperative." Another mother held firm that she wanted to take her son's temperature and pulse. He had suffered a comminuted fracture of the leg and was in severe shock for days. In an era before antibiotics, his wound developed gangrene that required several operations, and at one point he was not expected to live. The hospital staff called someone from the Texaco Oil Company, presumably the employer of the woman's husband, to keep her out of the room "so the boy could rest."[18] After transfusions of glucose and other measures, physicians eventually amputated the young man's leg; he survived and was fitted with a prosthesis. He did not go home until July 23, four and a half months after the explosion. The Red Cross assumed all costs. That parents were "nervous" could be quite expected under the circumstances, and staying in the rooms with their children was understandable, as seen in today's hospitals. However, hospital policies differed in the 1930s, when strict visiting hours often kept sick children from seeing their parents except a few times a week.

Another case involved a 19-year-old woman who suffered a compound fracture of her leg and severe shock. She was taken to a local clinic in critical condition. There, she received antitetanus serum, glucose, and oxygen. She was then transferred to Mother Frances Hospital in Tyler. Owned and operated by the Sisters of the Holy Family of Nazareth, the new Mother Frances Hospital had opened its doors on the day of the explosion, one day before its scheduled opening. While there, the patient developed pneumonia. Writing about her experiences several months later, she said, "The first two weeks were terrible especially for my folks not knowing whether I was going to live or not; and had it not been for the prayers to God to spare my life I would have been taken too." Two special-duty nurses stayed with her, a day nurse until May 1 and a night nurse until May 28. She recalled the day nurse working constantly, "fearing if she stopped I would die." It was a month before she could sit up in a wheelchair. The principal of the high school brought graduation gowns for her and the young amputee, and they both received their high school diplomas while in the hospital.[19]

This student went home on May 28, where she received follow-up care from a special Red Cross nurse who remained in the community for several months to check on patients after their hospital discharges. For this young woman, the Red Cross purchased a firm mattress for home use, crutches, and a wheelchair, and the nurse visited frequently to encourage proper leg exercises. Again, the Red Cross paid all the bills. Milk and fruits were typical diets for convalescence, and the Red Cross provided them to families both in the hospital and at home. The agency also furnished materials for dressing changes, including gauze bandages, adhesive tape, peroxide, silver nitrate, and alcohol. Expenditures for the disaster operation eventually totaled $52,150.02.[20]

CONSTRUCTING NARRATIVES TO MAKE SENSE OF DISASTERS

After the initial response was over, the disaster became the impetus for reflection by city leaders, reporters, newspaper editors, filmmakers, survivors, and health care workers in the form of letters, memoirs, oral histories, newspaper stories, and professional publications. Examination of these narratives can enhance nurses' understandings of the ways in which people perceive disasters that have befallen them, how region affects perceptions, and how people try to heal and restore their shattered lives even as they rebuild their physical structures.

Narrative theory, according to Kevin Rozario, posits that humans like to tell stories to "make sense of that which seems most senseless." Narratives supply "comforting illusions of order," and "part of the attraction of disaster narratives lay in their power to settle those who have experienced the unsettling of their lives."[21] In her discussion of narrative inquiry for nurses, Maureen Duffy asserts that narratives or stories "are the primary way that people make sense of their experience and through some form of oral or written conversation reveal and share that experience with others."[22]

Analysis of the New London disaster also relies on Edward T. Linenthal's scholarship on trauma and commemoration. In particular, he describes progressive, redemptive, and toxic narratives of survivors of the 1995 Oklahoma City bombing, and a historical parallel can be seen in the New London community in 1937. Progressive narratives are often constructed to make sense of the horror by emphasizing reassuring rhetoric of civic reconstruction. Redemptive narratives mobilize religious traditions as a means of healing and restoration, and toxic narratives focus on the persistence of intense mourning and strained relationships.[23] Although many similarities can be found between the New London disaster and Linenthal's work, in other areas, the stories diverged due to differences in time and place.

This disaster was an accident related to changes that reflected the growth of the oil industry in Texas in the first half of the twentieth century. The death toll alone, however, does not account for the disaster's full impact on the town. The explosion dramatically altered the lives of all the residents involved. It was through popular expressions of mourning and public commemoration that survivors were able to make sense of the tragedy during the course of grieving and healing.

In this predominantly rural evangelical Protestant community, many people relied on their faith to get them through the hard times. One woman's redemptive narrative revealed that she saw her escape from death as an act of God, although she could not understand why she lived and others did not.[24] In expressing its sympathy, the local Masonic lodge focused on God's will "in removing from our midst a great many of the dearest of our brethren."[25] The religious scene was prominent as local churches held funeral services and religious leaders mobilized resources to help people deal with the tragedy. Overton Baptist Church became a temporary hospital. On Easter Sunday following the tragedy, Protestant churches in the area held a combined memorial service at the disaster site that was nationally broadcast by radio. The governor of Texas spoke, and pastors of a Methodist church, a Church of Christ, and two Baptist churches gave messages.[26]

Doubts concerning culpability for the school disaster lingered. A court of inquiry heard testimony regarding the cause of the explosion, and several government agencies also investigated. Each inquiry agreed that the explosion resulted from a gas leak in the heating system under the building, but none held any one group or person ultimately responsible. This was especially difficult for families, who blamed the local school board and gas company. Their anger was highlighted in a narrative in which a survivor recalled, "One lady told my dad to talk to her husband, who was getting ready to shoot the superintendent or whoever let this happen." The father calmed the man down.[27]

In a commemorative edition of a local newspaper, some of the eyewitnesses remembered that fateful day. Several of the oil field laborers who rushed to the scene eventually fought in World War II, and their memoirs of 1937 made analogies to the battlefield. One recalled, "I was in the South Pacific Theatre and saw a lot of death, but never anything like that night in London. Those were children. . . . I'll never get over it." Another wrote, "You know, we were known as 'oil field trash,' but that night we all worked together. I saw a lot of bad things in the war, but it wasn't the same."[28]

In 2005, and again in 2007, various journalists asked survivors to share their memories for other commemorative publications. Questions focused on where people had been and what they had heard and felt at the time of the explosion. One woman recalled looking at her dead sister in her casket. "It didn't look like her at all. That stays with you a long time."[29] Another survivor remembered, "People were afraid to talk about it, almost no family in this community was unaffected, and whenever people would tell us about the explosion it would be sort of in whispers and don't say anything in front of so-and-so because they lost a sister."[30] These narratives reveal the lasting impact of mass death, similar to Linenthal's "toxic" narrative in which people continued to struggle with enduring pain and loss.[31] They do not represent an ideal model for recovery because, although the town's recovery was remarkable, it came with huge costs. Survivors internalized the event for many years.

COMMEMORATION AND MEMORIALIZATION

In the immediate aftermath of the horrible tragedy, the townspeople, perhaps partially in an effort to keep their personal traumas at bay, directed their energies into rebuilding the school close to the site of the old one. Attachment to this particular place overcame any concerns to build elsewhere. The building was not constructed directly over the original site, however, due to reminiscences of so many bodily remains scattered over the area. To be sure, optimistic narratives surfaced. One author writing about the disaster in 1938 stated: "Anywhere you touch this school, there is a feeling of confidence. The great throngs that often packed the auditorium, even to the overflowing point, inspired absolute confidence that the New London community still has its old spirit of confidence."[32] This rebuilding project served survivors and their families well, giving people a collective purpose and reducing their sense of powerlessness.

In 1938, city leaders, together with an executive committee and architectural firm, began planning the first permanent memorial site on the main street's median, a cenotaph that had each person's name inscribed on it to honor the dead. A cenotaph is a monument for persons whose remains are elsewhere, and townspeople deemed this the most appropriate form of commemoration. To pay for it, individuals (including children) donated money. Erected in 1939, the cenotaph is made of Texas pink granite. Stones face the structure with engraved names of the known dead by school grade.[33]

Inevitably, however, that temporary respite from the full brunt of grief would end. It was then that the tragic memories became, for most of the townspeople, literally unspeakable horrors. Thus, even as physical rebuilding occurred, emotional recovery was delayed. For the next 40 years, most people consciously chose not to speak in depth again of the event, as if doing so would resubject them to extreme emotional pain they felt they could neither escape nor personally endure.

In 1977, two survivors organized the first reunion of former students, and they finally were able to discuss their childhood traumas. One woman remembered, "None of us could even cry when it happened. We didn't for years. At that reunion, we finally talked and cried, you know?" Another noted, "When I got the invitation for the 40th anniversary, I thought, 'Okay. I'm ready.' That's the first time I cried. Before that, I wouldn't think about it. I blocked the memory out of my life."[34]

One of their greatest needs was for expunging guilt. One man recalled that, as a fifth grader at the time, "I asked a student to change seats with me so I could flirt with a little girl in front of her." The first girl died in the explosion, whereas the boy survived. He buried his guilt feelings all those years, and it was not until the reunion that he could admit to her sister what he had done. "I had to unburden myself of this guilt," he stated. Like many other survivors, he found the reunions to be a place for healing.[35]

The urge to memorialize took another form in 1998. One woman, who by chance had left school early that day in 1937 and survived, was instrumental in developing a museum. Visitors could see the cenotaph and the reconstructed school located across the street.[36] As news of the planned museum spread, survivors and their family members donated items and told their stories. To remember and retell the past, the artifacts that townspeople chose for display included actual debris found at the scene, such as children's shoes, books, clothes, photographs, and one of the peach baskets used in the rescue. These tangible artifacts rekindled memories and commemorated those who died.

The cenotaph memorial, the museum, and the oral histories are similar to what Linenthal calls a "language of engagement, not just a language of commemoration."[37] Those whose lives were intimately connected to the disaster told stories of individual courage and grief. Today, along with some of the remaining survivors and their family members, volunteers lead visitors through the museum's halls and tell stories about particular people who died. The museum also has videotapes in the *Americana Histories* series, among them a 1937 newsreel that focuses on emotional eyewitness' accounts and recovery scenes, a tape of survivors at one of the reunions, and the voice of Walter Cronkite, who reported on the disaster. These tapes can help present-day visitors experience the emotions felt by eyewitnesses and survivors, thereby facilitating a greater appreciation of the tragedy in ways not possible with traditional exhibits.

Some families left East Texas after losing one or more children in the disaster, and others moved away when the economic base of support changed as the oil industry in East Texas declined. Commemoration of the 1937 disaster remains, however. The next generation of students after the explosion interviewed survivors, rescue workers, and National Guardsmen, who initially responded. Then in 2000, an anniversary newspaper focused attention on the progressive narrative with its headline, "School Blends Hope for Present, Respect of Past."[38] Today, third-generation students learn the history of their school and participate in memorial events. The museum has brought an event that happened many years ago into clearer focus.

THEORETICAL DISCUSSION

Collective memory about the New London disaster was represented in the memorials that the survivors chose to erect. Cultural historians have theorized that *collective memory* is a contested term, however. For the purposes of this discussion, it is defined as memory constructed by a group and passed on to others.[39] As the school disaster entered people's memories in different ways, individuals also constructed various stories or narratives to help them deal with the trauma, and these stories became a part of the community's collective memory.

As people constructed their memories and tried to rebound from the disaster, parallels and disjunctures occurred.[40] In this Texas disaster, the outpouring of generosity and selflessness was moving, and progressive narratives of courage and heroism were evident. In addition, religious understandings based on rural evangelical values shaped some responses. Other people, influenced by recent wartime experiences, drew dramatic parallels to war scenes. Family members and survivors also lived out stories that were traumatic.

These findings expand theoretical formulations about disasters, however, by arguing that contextual factors of time and place influence the realities and perceptions of those who live through disasters. "Place" includes not only the influence of geography but also culture, economics, class, race, and religion. A major argument has been that as physical structures collapsed, so did social barriers. Indeed, some survivors remembered that these disasters blurred racial and social class boundaries, even if only temporarily.

Geography also was significant, as the disaster occurred in a section of the country rich in oil and gas reserves. In 1937, New London was a small East Texas town rooted in evangelical Protestantism. It originally had an agricultural economy but was transformed by the discovery of oil and gas. It was tragic irony that the industry that brought wealth and prosperity to many citizens also led to the death and misery of many others when a gas leak resulted in a devastating explosion. Arguably, it was a disaster waiting to happen.

The difficulty and pain of reconstructing an event can be seen in the survivors' responses. Although they constructed a memorial within a year of the tragedy, this was before the days of grief counseling at the scene. East

Texas in the 1930s was an area permeated with rural values, and survivors relied on their tenacity and their faith in God to help them get through the tragedy. Rather than dwelling on the past, they chose to remain silent. It was not until many years later that they met to discuss the tragedy. They risked having to face the pain of old memories and accompanying negative feelings, but what they found instead was relief of no longer having to run from them. Their accounts were narratives that had cathartic and healing purposes. After many years, community bonds were restored; these were rooted in shared memories, as defined by the reunions that the survivors and family members established, the cenotaph they erected, the museum they built where they preserved their remembrances, and their willingness to participate in oral histories. This made a strong statement that dialogue with the past is still important.

In 1937, the racially segregated society within which the Texans lived affected who would write narratives, whose narratives would be heard and remembered, and who would be considered heroes and heroines.[41] Special attention was given to rescue workers from the oil fields who rapidly cleared the debris after the New London school explosion. Perhaps in an effort to lessen racial barriers, one local reporter in New London pointed out that Black doctors also worked as rescuers, even though school segregation meant that only Whites were the casualties of the explosion. Without each of these narratives, one would get an incomplete picture of the disaster response.

Through their narratives, people discussed a web of feelings behind their stories. These included not only guilt but also pride in the rebuilding of the new school. Private narratives became public memories through newspapers, commemorative publications, professional journals, videos of reunions, and a museum. It must also be pointed out that the construction of memoirs and oral histories was affected by many factors, including questions that interviewers asked. For example, publications after the disaster focused on what the person remembered about the disastrous event.[42] Written after the fact, time may have allowed survivors to rework the disaster in their recreations.

This disaster also influenced the broader social and political community. Media reports, personal testimonies, and congressional hearings after the New London school explosion fed into policy changes. Although no one person or group was found culpable, the urge to "do something" remained strong. New Londoners petitioned the state legislature to require that a malodorant be used in all gases so that future leaks could be detected. They were successful.

CONCLUSION

This chapter has not only revealed the initial response to the 1937 New London school explosion but has also highlighted how a collective memory of the disaster has been maintained.[43] It has argued that collective memory is more than just an aggregate of individuals' personal memories; it includes many different ways of remembering. The cenotaph memorial is an expression of collective memory by the community at large. As well, New Londoners preserved the memory of the disaster by saving artifacts in the museum, which became a powerful form of remembrance.[44]

Finally, a history of the New London school tragedy suggests a way for nurses to think about healing and restoration after current disasters. Peggy Chinn reminds us that nurses are "concerned with interactions between environment and human experience." This is what distinguishes nursing from disciplines that focus only on a medical model.[45] As greater attention is being paid to the ability of affected communities to recover from disasters, it is important to understand that part of the restorative process for survivors is to establish meanings to help them regain control over their lives and futures. How people make sense of their experiences can provide significant information about culture, community, and self-identity.[46]

STUDY QUESTIONS:

1. For what purpose did the specific narratives described in this chapter function? How might the stories of the chaos after the disaster provide a release for fears? How might they define or contest certain values?
2. How does a regional focus shape disaster narratives? More specifically, how did the nature of "place" affect people's attempts to impose order after disasters?
3. At what point in time do people choose to create an infrastructure for memorializing? What might they choose to include? Consider items commonly placed in makeshift memorials as a starting point for discussion.
4. How might the ideas in this chapter concerning commemoration help one to understand plans for memorializing the 9/11 disaster?

NOTES

1. Albert Evans to James L. Fieser, Vice Chairman American Red Cross, Washington, DC, Western Union telegrams, March 20 and March 22, 1937; in DR 745, RG 200, National Archives Gift Collection, Records of the American National Red Cross, College Park, MD (hereafter ANRC).
2. Ibid. The town of New London was incorporated in 1963. For the purposes of this chapter, it will be referred to as New London.
3. "And Then the Dust Lifted," *Henderson Daily News*, March 19, 1937, 8; "Survivors Remember New London School Explosion, http://web. archive.org/web/20080219004649/, http://www.ketknbc.com/news/ local/6562857.html; "When Even Angels Wept," http://www.vimeo. com/1695931?pg=embed&sec=1695931; http://www.youtube.com/watch? v=aKt01p3DJRw (accessed April 2, 2010).
4. K. Vine, "'Oh, My God! It's Our Children,'" *Texas Monthly* (March 2007), 130–131.
5. Dr. C. G. Engle to Mother and Dad (n.d.), New London Museum and Tearoom, New London, TX.
6. Vine, "'Oh, My God!,'" 130, 273, 278. Scenes can be viewed at http://www. youtube.com/watch?v=aKt01p3DJRw (accessed April 2, 2010).
7. Memory of Mollie Ward in Vine, "'Oh, My God!,'" 274; "School Blackboard Discloses Stark Irony of Lesson," Special Edition, *Overton Press*, n.d. A replica of the blackboard is displayed in the New London Museum and Tearoom, New London, TX.
8. http://www.youtube.com/watch?v=jf2OwBvdKEk (accessed April 2, 2010).
9. "500 Die in Blast at Texas School," *New York Times*, March 19, 1937, 14.
10. "Highlights in Disaster," *Henderson Daily News*, March 19, 1937, 5.
11. "Ruins Illuminated, *New York Times*, March 19, 1937, 1.
12. "Identity of Dead Children Becomes Gigantic Task for Workers in London School Tragedy," *Henderson Daily News*, 19 March 1937, 1.
13. Ibid.
14. Evans to Fieser, Western Union telegrams, March 20 and March 22, 1937, ANRC.
15. William M. Baxter to Fieser, April 14, 1937; and Evans to Fieser, Western Union telegram, March 29, 1937, ANRC.
16. William DeKleine, "Medical Report: New London School Disaster," March 27, 1937; Evans to Feiser, Western Union telegram, March 22, 1937, ANRC.
17. Howard J. Simons to William M. Baxter, May 8, 1937; DeKleine, "Medical Report," ANRC.
18. Cases III and IV, box 1271, folder titled "Texas Explosion," ANRC.

19. Case VI; "The New London School Disaster," by (name omitted for confidentiality), ANRC.
20. "The New London Texas, School Explosion," American Red Cross, Washington, DC"; and Harriett Keller, Red Cross nurse, to DeKleine, April 2, 1937, ANRC.
21. Kevin Rozario, "Making Progress: Disaster Narratives and the Art of Optimism in Modern America," in *The Resilient City: How Modern Cities Recover from Disaster*, eds. Lawrence J. Vale and Thomas J. Campanella (New York, NY: Oxford University Press, 2005), 33.
22. Maureen Duffy, "Narrative Inquiry: The Method," In *Nursing Research: A Qualitative Perspective*, ed. Patricia L. Munhall (Boston, MA: Jones & Bartlett Publishers, 2007), 401.
23. Edward T. Linenthal, *The Unfinished Bombing: Oklahoma City in American Memory* (New York, NY: Oxford University Press, 2001).
24. "Kennedy Recalls Tragedy in the Sixth-Grade Class," *Overton Press*, March 16, 2000, 1.
25. "Local Masonic Lodge Adopts Resolutions," *Overton Press*, March 26, 1937, n.p.
26. "Memorial Service Sunday on Nation-Wide Hook-Up," *Overton Press*, March 26, 1937, n.p.
27. Vine, "'Oh, My God!'," 278.
28. Newspaper clipping, "Out of the Ashes," *Henderson Daily News*, n.d., New London Museum and Tearoom, New London, TX.
29. Vine, "'Oh, My God!'," 276.
30. http://www.kltv.com/Global/story.asp?S=6244436 (accessed April 1, 2010).
31. Linenthal, *The Unfinished Bombing*.
32. R. L. Jackson, *Living Lessons From the New London Explosion* (1938; repr., New London, TX: London Museum, 2005).
33. http://www.texasbob.com/travel/tbt_london.html (accessed July 16, 2009).
34. Vine, "'Oh, My God!'," 280.
35. Vine, "'Oh, My God!'"; special commemorative edition of *Overton Press*, March 16, 2000, reprinted from *Overton Press* dated in 1937; and *Overton Press*, March 15, 2001 and March 17, 2005.
36. K. Straach, "Museum Helps New Londoners Work Through the 'What Ifs,'" *Arkansas Democrat-Gazette*, May 3, 1998.
37. Edward T. Linenthal, "The Predicament of Aftermath: Oklahoma City and September 11," In Vale and Campanella, *The Resilient City*, 55.
38. "School Blends Hope for Present, Respect of Past," *Overton Press*, March 16, 2000, 5.
39. Maurice Halwachs, *On Collective Memory* (Chicago, IL: University of Chicago Press, 1992).

40. Linenthal, *The Unfinished Bombing*; and Rozario, "Making Progress," 27–54.

41. Rozario, "Making Progress."

42. "Kennedy Recalls Tragedy"; "Out of the Ashes"; and special commemorative edition of *Overton Press*, March 15, 2001 and March 17, 2005.

43. B.C. Brower, "The Preserving Machine: The 'New' Museum and Working through Trauma—The Musee Memorial Pour la Paix of Caen," *History & Memory* 11, 1 (1999): 77–103.

44. Kirk Savage, "History, Memory, and Monuments: An Overview of the Scholarly Literature on Commemoration," http://www.nps.gov/history/history/resedu/savage.htm (accessed April 1, 2010).

45. Peggy L. Chinn, "From the Editor: Healing and Restoration," *Advances in Nursing Science* 31, 3 (2008): 183.

46. Peter Burke, *What Is Cultural History?* (Cambridge, England: Polity Press, 2004).

The 1942 Cocoanut Grove
Nightclub Fire: Out of the Ashes

Patricia A. Connor Ballard

400 DEAD IN HUB NIGHTCLUB FIRE! Hundreds Hurt in Panic as the Cocoanut Grove Becomes Wild Inferno! The worst fire in Boston's history last night snuffed out the lives of 399 merrymaking men and women in the blazing inferno of the famous Cocoanut Grove nightclub amid scenes of utter panic and horror. Crushed, trampled, and burned as nearly 1000 patrons, entertainers, and employees fought desperately to gain the exits through the sheets of flame, scores of victims were left on the floor helpless. Others reached the street enveloped in fire, only to die in agony in the street or in hospitals.[1]

On a cold and rainy Thanksgiving weekend in wartime 1942, a popular Boston nightclub became engulfed in flames within 12 minutes, killing nearly 500 people. In contrast to previous disasters, the dead greatly outnumbered the survivors.[2] The Cocoanut Grove fire remains one of the worst catastrophes in U.S. history. The long list of the dead victims was read over the radio for hours and published in the city's newspapers next to Christmas advertisements.

Prior to 1942, the care of burn injuries was difficult and often unsuccessful. Burn injury was seen as a local injury, not systemic trauma as it is viewed today. Prognosis was poor if burns covered more than one-fifth of the body. Technology for sustaining the life of a critically ill burn patient was nonexistent; as one former physician noted, "We had so little technology . . . one respirator on each floor at best. The technology for studying blood gases and chemistries didn't exist anywhere. We were giving oxygen directly through green rubber tubes (nasal catheters)."[3]

Following burn injury, many patients died of hypovolemic shock or overwhelming infection. Burn shock was believed to be the result of toxins absorbed from the traumatized skin surface. Fluid replacement was inadequate to fully compensate for intravascular fluid loss through edema and drainage. Topical wound care was often ineffective in preventing infection. Smoke inhalation injury had not yet been recognized as a life-threatening complication. For those who survived their burn injuries, severe disfigurement was common despite attempts at reconstructive surgery.

Burn wounds were a common war wound in World War II, and the U.S. government was in haste to identify a simple and effective burn dressing that could be quickly implemented in the battlefield by military personnel with limited medical training. Federal research funding was awarded by the National Research Council (NRC) and the Office of Scientific Research and Development to Dr. Oliver Cope of Massachusetts General Hospital (MGH) and Dr. Charles Lund of Boston City Hospital (BCH) for this purpose.[4] Cope was both a surgeon and an endocrinologist, with expertise in the management of hyperparathyroidism and a growing side interest in the management of burns. Lund was chief of surgery at BCH. These two physicians were experts in burn care. Cope received his research funding earlier than Lund, and Cope's regimen using a petroleum dressing was already established at the time of the nightclub fire. In addition to research on burn injury, wartime activities also included preparing the city of Boston for potential German attack. For example, MGH had established a blood bank; developed and published a disaster manual; and put aside emergency supplies, such as sterile surgical dressings, extra shock blocks, wooden intravenous poles, and sawhorses for stretchers.[5] The city had implemented a mock blitz drill the week prior to the nightclub fire, stockpiled and inventoried emergency supplies, and developed a disaster tagging system for victims. The multidisciplinary disaster planning resulted in a group identity for a common cause. Hospital staff became more unified and collaborative in their practice. All of these preparations were useful at the time of the nightclub fire.

THE DISASTER

Located near Boston's many theaters and restaurants, the Cocoanut Grove Nightclub offered cocktails, dinner, and dancing. Open illegally at the peak of Prohibition, it also offered the mystique of a dubious past with long-standing gossip about its connections to both mobsters and politicians (and Boston had its share of both). It was the most popular American nightclub of that era. The tropical paradise environment of the nightclub included false palm trees, artificial tropical plants, bamboo, paper decorations, and low cloth-draped ceilings. The walls of the nightclub were covered in imitation leather. Its movable ceiling roof, which could be rolled back in good weather, allowed for dancing under the stars.

On November 28, 1942, Bostonians took a short break from war to focus on the big game . . . Boston College (BC) faced Holy Cross College of western Massachusetts in the annual football rivalry game at Fenway Park before a sellout crowd of 44,000. Boston College was established in the late 1800s to educate the sons of Boston Irish Catholics as an alternative to the elite but Protestant Harvard University. Although also Catholic, Holy Cross College was viewed by working-class Bostonians to be beyond their means. Undefeated that season, BC expected a Sugar Bowl invitation after their anticipated win over Holy Cross. Confident of their success, BC supporters planned a massive postgame party at the nightclub, with local politicians and members of the city's social elite in attendance.[6] Holy Cross, however, blatantly handed BC its only defeat of the season, 55–12. A few BC supporters decided to go to the nightclub anyway, but most stayed home or chose to drown their sorrows at the bar of the nearby Statler Hotel. Ironically, a BC victory would have led to disaster on a much larger scale.

That evening, an estimated 1,000 guests crowded into the nightclub, far exceeding the 460 recommended occupancy guidelines.[7] The guests included more than 200 sailors and soldiers, the Boston police commissioner, and the city's director of Civil Defense. A fire started among the highly combustible decorations of the downstairs Melody Lounge around 10:00 p.m. A teenage busboy observed a soldier remove a light bulb in an effort to secure romantic privacy with his girlfriend. The busboy lit a match in an attempt to locate the removed light bulb, and a burst of blue flame was observed soon after in a nearby false palm tree. 50 years later, the Boston Fire Department concluded that the fire was actually the result of a leaky ventilation system in the Melody Lounge. Freon gas, used in cooling systems of the time, was in limited supply owing to the war, and a flammable gas called methyl chloride was being used at the nightclub instead.[8] Methyl chloride was odorless and produced toxic fumes and a blue flame when burning. A former refrigeration worker commented later:

It was common knowledge among workers at National Sales and Miller Seddon [which handled domestic refrigeration accounts and serviced the cooling system for the Cocoanut Grove nightclub] that the Cocoanut Grove was cooling beer, food—and people in the summer—with methyl chloride. . . . It was dangerous stuff, but you've got to remember, there were almost no fire codes back then.[9]

Guests were initially amused by busboys trying to extinguish the flames using seltzer bottles from the bar. Others misinterpreted the cries of "fire!" as "fight," which was not an uncommon occurrence in the nightclub, or delayed leaving in order to pay their bill or retrieve their fur coats from the coat room. The fire spread quickly. General mass panic set in when burning fabric and decorations fell from walls and ceiling. The ventilation system circulated hot smoke and fumes. As flames ate through the building's electrical system, the interior of the nightclub was plunged into total darkness.

Guests competed with each other for space on the only visible exit out of the downstairs lounge, a narrow dark stairway leading upstairs to the main floor of the nightclub. The fire moved upstairs faster than guests could escape. There were no marked emergency exits or posted plans for emergency escape, and secondary exits were known only to employees of the nightclub. Glass–brick windows appeared to be only for decorative purpose and did not provide an access to the outside when broken. Several doors were intentionally locked to prevent nonpaying guests from leaving the nightclub. Some doors were hidden by drapery or blocked by furniture. Others were positioned to swing inward instead of outward. One door was blocked by the band's drummer, who attempted to escape while carrying the bass drum of his expensive drum set. Ironically, 8 days prior to the disaster, a lieutenant from the Boston fire department had performed a flame test on the decorations of the newly opened lounge and concluded that all regulations were met in terms of nonflammable material, adequate number of exits, and sufficient number of working fire extinguishers.[10] The lounge, however, was never assessed by the city building inspector and should have remained closed until then.

Only a small portion of guests managed to flee unharmed. Over 30 escaped the flames by crawling through a small upper level window and jumping to the street. Fifteen people survived by seeking refuge in the metal refrigerators of the downstairs kitchen, as a surviving nightclub employee later described to a local newspaper reporter:

After the fire broke out, Marra (Tony) and Rizzo (John) ended up crawling around the floor of the nightclub's kitchen to survive the smoke. At one point, Marra escaped the smoke by sticking his head in a chest containing ice cream . . . Maura and Rizzo bumped into each other in the dark, embraced, and got a bottle of whiskey to break open a window, from which they escaped.[11]

The most horrifying sight of the night was the vision of more than 200 guests pinned against the jammed glass revolving door of the club's main entrance on Piedmont Street, while rescuers watched in horror.[12] John Rizzo, the nightclub waiter who survived the fire, recalled:

> It was after ten [p.m.] when Mickey Alpert got on stage to open the show with 'The Star Spangled Banner.' Suddenly, we heard a commotion and thought it was a fight, but from the foyer, we saw a ball of flame. Frank [friend] ran twenty feet to the revolving door, and that was the last I saw of him. The revolving door was where all those people got caught, and Frank was one of the bodies stacked up there.[13]

The intense flames kept the firefighters at a distance, and attempts to release the jammed door were initially unsuccessful. Efforts to open up the movable ceiling and allow firefighters direct access to the fire were also unsuccessful.

In all, only 228 guests escaped unhurt, and 494 died. The dead included 51 military personnel, all 4 sons of a local family, newlyweds, couples celebrating their wedding anniversary, and a popular Western movie star named Buck Jones. Most died before reaching the hospital, asphyxiated by smoke or fumes from burning decorations and furniture. John Collins, a naval fire fighter assisting the Boston fire department that night, was haunted by the sight of one of the young victims found in the downstairs lounge:

> Of all the vivid impressions made upon me that evening, perhaps the most unforgettable was when we first went down into the Melody Lounge . . . there, sitting at a table was a very pretty girl. She was sitting with her eyes open and her hand on a cocktail glass, as if waiting for someone. At first I

looked at her and wondered why she was just sitting there, thinking she was okay . . . but, of course, she was dead.[14]

THE RESPONSE

By a coincidence of fate, firefighters and police were nearby dealing with a car fire when they noticed smoke from the area of the nightclub. William Doogan, a responding policeman, saw an injured sailor running down a nearby street:

> I jumped out of the car and headed toward him . . . He was hollering for help and screaming, and as he ran to me I could see that there was smoke coming out of his clothes. When I looked closer, I could see some of the skin hanging off his fingers and I could see skin hanging off the inside of his thighs. I lost track of everything around me. My only thought was to get this kid to . . . city hospital.[15]

Doogan and his partner were later reprimanded for not completing their official report on the car fire.

The initial emergency response to the disaster was chaotic and inadequate, and it lacked direction and coordination. The narrow historical streets of Boston became an obstacle to larger rescue vehicles. Crowds were everywhere, and security was insufficient. Looters persisted in scavenging jewelry and wallets from dead, unconscious, or dazed survivors collapsed on the streets. Hewson Gray, a BC supporter who escaped the burning nightclub with his wife through one of the few doors opened by firefighters, described the scene outside the burning nightclub:

> People were collapsing as they came out, having been exposed to the smoke and flames. They were dropping all around, even some that looked okay . . . [but] had soot around their faces. They were lying everywhere.[16]

A similar scenario was noted at the nearby hospitals, as survivors with visible minor injuries collapsed within hours.

Hundreds of victims were transported to nearby hospitals without warning to the facilities. Ineffective triage resulted in many of the dead being transported to the hospital for care before a team of BCH physicians arrived at the scene. Temporary morgues were set up at adjacent buildings, including a nearby parking garage. A shortage of ambulances at the scene forced officials to commandeer any available vehicle for transport of victims to the hospital. Many died en route. A policeman assigned to BCH recalled, "I saw a dump truck come into the hospital with the tail board down and four or five victims on the back. They were treated as nicely, as humanely as possible, but conditions were rough."[17] One man was working the evening post office shift that night, transporting mail to the main post office at nearby South Station. Recalling the incident decades later to family members, he remembered transporting the injured to BCH in the back of his postal truck but never knew if the persons he was carrying were alive or dead. Postal officials later reprimanded him for allowing unaccompanied civilians to be next to bags of mail and postal money orders.

Many of the rescuers burned their hands pulling the bodies out of the burning wreckage. Clergy who ministered last rites to victims at the fire scene suffered a similar fate, as the bodies were so hot. Despite protective gear, firefighters were often covered with scratches and bruises inflicted by desperate victims who clawed and grabbed their way to safety.[18] The son of an exhausted Boston firefighter recalled, "He was . . . in bed, describing how bodies were stacked up at the door to Shawmut Street, but not all of them were dead. He pulled up his trousers and showed me the scratches on his legs where people had clawed at him to pull them out."[19]

Firefighters later described persistent flashbacks of the sight, the stench of burnt flesh, and the sensation of limbs tearing apart in their hands as they recovered bodies. The horrifying nature of the disaster haunted many of them for years. Decades later, a retired firefighter recalled rescuing nightclub singer Dotty Myles, 17 years old at the time, to a newspaper reporter:

> She followed the crowd and found herself stranded at the door to Shawmut Street, crushed among a stack of people, some dead. In agonizing pain, she saw a light and gasped to [a] firefighter, "Mister, help me!". . . . But her wrists were burned and blistered and when he grabbed her, raw skin came off in his hands.[20]

Disfigured from her injuries, Myles became a radio singer but avoided going out in public without a veil for years. She recalled praying the rosary during her 6-month stay at MGH, using the circular drapery rings for counting reference, and she remained in contact with the firefighter who rescued her.[21]

The severity of injuries among the patients caused the media to impose a self-censure on the publication of their disaster photos in order to spare the public from such horror during wartime. The most horrifying of the pictures taken that night by photographers on the scene were never published in Boston newspapers but instead were locked away in office files for years.

Over the course of several hours, the Boston Fire Department received the assistance of firefighters from 25 nearby cities and towns during the five-alarm fire. The Boston Metropolitan Chapter of the Red Cross alerted more than 1,000 Red Cross workers. All state medical examiners within 50 miles were called to report to the temporary morgues set up to handle the dead. Many of the deceased were charred beyond recognition, and dental students from nearby Tufts University assisted with identification of the corpses. The U.S. Navy made available firefighters, corpsmen, and shore patrol personnel. Nurses and doctors as well as nursing and medical students within 30 miles of Boston were notified by public radio of the disaster and asked to volunteer their services. The Red Cross recruited hundreds of volunteer nurses, including those who were retired, during the first week after the fire. The Red Cross later employed additional nurses and nurse aides to care for the survivors, and it assumed the cost of hospitalization, funeral and burial fees, family travel and lodging, clothing, rent, and household expenses for many of the fire victims.[22]

THE INJURED

The majority of the injured were brought to BCH or MGH for care, presenting with burns and respiratory distress. Burns ranged from partial to full-thickness depth. Full-thickness burns appeared dark and charred, with the dry leathery eschar of a typical flame burn, or raw, with exposed underlying tissue. Burns differed between men and women, with females being more severely injured than the males. Many women wore the strapless formal dresses popular in that era, despite the New England winter weather, thus exposing their necks, arms, shoulders, backs, and legs to flame. Burns of the hands, face, and scalp were also common. Hand burns occurred as victims tried to shield their faces from the flames. Most appeared disheveled, covered in grime and soot, and suffering from hypothermia due to the cold damp weather and water from fire hoses. A large number presented with a bloated, cherry-red face suggestive of carbon monoxide poisoning. Many had been incontinent of urine or stool, and others were covered with vomitus. Anxiety and hysteria were common.

Upon admission to the hospital, injured patients who had received morphine sulfate for pain had their forehead or anterior chest marked with the letter "M" in red grease pencil or with lipstick borrowed from the nurses.[23] Several patients were overmedicated with the narcotic drug and experienced respiratory depression. In haste, morphine was often administered without first determining if the person was alive or dead. At one point, victims covered every space of the emergency ward and its nearby corridors. When stretchers became unavailable, the injured were placed on the floor. A witness at BCH later recalled:

> Space was so precious . . . we had to stack them up against the wall and drop a sheet over them . . . that would save the doctors from seeing the same victim twice . . . Bodies were piled on the floors and many of them were outside. Honest to God, they looked like some of the wood I see stacked near the fireplace.[24]

Hospital staff moved among the victims, sorting the dead from the living. They moved the deceased to one side of the hall to await transport to the morgue, while the conscious living watched a few feet away from the other side of the hall.

The injured people brought to the hospitals in the early phase of evacuation received the most attention and care, as their arrival coincided with the 11:00 p.m. shift change. With the rapid increase in the number of patients arriving at the hospital, attention then had to shift to those with the most severe and life-threatening injuries. Nurses wrapped patients in dry sterile sheets and administered oxygen, intravenous (IV) normal saline, and injections of anti-tetanus serum. The administration of IV fluid therapy, equal parts normal saline and plasma, for the treatment of shock following burn injury was based on Dr. Frank Underhill's research at Yale

University following the 1921 Rialto Theater Fire.[25] The presence of extensive limb burns and shock complicated the placement of peripheral IV catheters. Physicians performed venous cutdown as necessary, and they considered intraosseus fluid infusion using the sternum on more than one occasion. Blood and plasma transfusions were administered as needed, with more units of blood per fire victim used within the first 24 hours of the disaster than was provided to the victims of the Japanese bombing of Pearl Harbor in Hawaii. The "walking wounded" patiently watched over each other until hospital staff became free to attend to their injuries. Medical and nursing staff worked hour after hour for 2 to 3 days continuously with minimal relief.

CARE OF THE INJURED AT BOSTON CITY HOSPITAL

On the evening of the nightclub fire, a holiday party was being held at a nursing residence near BCH, with approximately 80% of the hospital's off-duty personnel in attendance. Party guests included the hospital's chief administrator. When the injured started arriving at the emergency ward, all medical staff were alerted. The holiday party quickly dissolved, and nurses and physicians immediately reported to the hospital to assist with care of the fire victims. Many did so while still in their party apparel.

BCH was closer in proximity to the fire scene, and 80% of the victims were taken there. An injured person arrived at BCH on an average of one every 11 seconds, quickly overwhelming the hospital staff.[26] 300 people were declared dead on arrival at BCH, with 131 survivors admitted for inpatient care. Hospital officials requested that additional patients be taken to MGH or one of the other nearby hospitals. All hospitals within the city of Boston were then put on alert. In addition to BCH and MGH, injured personnel were taken to Peter Bent Brigham Hospital, Saint Elizabeth's Hospital, Saint May's Hospital, Saint Margaret's Hospital, Massachusetts Memorial Hospital, Carney Hospital, Cambridge City Hospital, Mount Auburn Hospital, Faulkner Hospital, Beth Israel Hospital, Chelsea Naval Hospital, and the U.S. Marine Hospital in nearby Brighton.[27]

The patients transported to BCH often manifested respiratory distress that persisted despite traditional treatment by oxygen (administered by tent or nasal catheter), bronchoscopy, suctioning, tracheostomy, and the administration of sulfonamides. Many of the firefighters who entered the burning building also experienced respiratory distress. One physician recalled caring for fire victims with respiratory problems:

> The first point observed was that, whereas many patients had both severe burns and severe respiratory complications, there were also those who had either relatively minor burns and severe respiratory complications, or the opposite. Some of these people survived, and some did not. Thus, it appeared evident from the beginning that the respiratory complications were not necessarily parallel to the burns, and may not have been caused by direct thermal burns of the respiratory tract.[28]

Two BCH wards designated and stocked for wartime casualties housed the majority of the fire survivors, with overflow patients sent to open beds of other wards. A senior nursing instructor from the BCH diploma nursing school was dispatched with a handful of nursing students to prepare the first ward for patients.[29] In all, more than 30 wards in 8 buildings at BCH housed victims of the disaster.[30]

The BCH medical staff divided into two teams—one focusing on burn wound care, and the other on IV fluids, respiratory treatments, and medications. Large volumes of normal saline and plasma were administered for shock without inducing pulmonary edema, including 693 units of plasma, 17 units of albumin, and 149 units of normal saline.[31] It became apparent that the overwhelming needs of the patients demanded flexibility among the medical and nursing staff, and roles and responsibilities that were rigid prior to the disaster began to blend temporarily. Suddenly faced with more than 100 acutely injured patients, teams of physicians and nurses worked together to provide care, as one former BCH physician remembered:

> One of the nurses was promptly detailed to go from bed to bed and to take and record the pulse and respiratory rates and the blood pressure on each patient in rotation. Three of the nurses were assigned to the special nursing care of the sicker among the patients, each being asked to care particularly for one of the three sickest patients (Cases 100, 102, and 119). Many of the details of the nursing care were carried out by the interns and the other physicians present.[32]

BCH boasted several burn experts on its medical staff, including Drs. Charles Lund, Newton Browder, and Robert Aldrich. Dr. Aldrich, in his prior work at the Johns Hopkins University Hospital, had investigated the use of gentian violet as an alternative to tannic acid for topical burn care. Dr. Lund was already on site, treating an elderly male with burn injuries sustained while smoking in bed, as the initial wave of the disaster patients arrived at BCH. Unprepared to implement his new research protocol for burn wound care to so many patients on such short notice, Lund instructed his staff to utilize the older burn procedure that incorporated triple dye as the topical agent. The research-oriented BCH medical staff worked in a meticulous and methodical manner for months after the disaster. They documented patient status, diagnostic testing, and treatment on every patient down to the smallest detail. Lund and the BCH chief of infectious disease visited every patient on daily rounds. They presented their detailed observations and documentation later to the medical community in multiple journal articles and paper presentations.[33]

Unfortunately, the BCH nursing staff did not record their experiences in detailed journal or presentation format for public dissemination. Rather, nurses' work was limited to brief mention by physicians who authored post-disaster medical articles. For example, 50 years later, Dr. Stanley Levenson, a BCH physician at the time of the disaster, acknowledged the contribution of the BCH nurses: "You simply kept [the patients] going, kept them breathing, getting them to cough, urging them on, physically clearing their airways, lending moral support. We had great attending doctors . . . residents, medical students, and most of all, we had wonderful nurses."[34] Dr. Charles Davidson, another BCH physician at the time of the disaster, echoed Dr. Levenson's comments 3 decades after the nightclub fire: "Our rounds supplemented the superb care given by interns and residents, staff physicians, nurses, aides, and many others at the bedside, often on a 24-hour a day basis."[35]

The intensity of the injuries required a shift in the delivery of nursing care. The injured patients required one to six nurses per patient for care. The BCH staff nurses were supplemented by nursing students, medical students, retired nurse volunteers, and a large contingent of Red Cross nurses and nurse's aides. Other nurses were "on loan" from nearby hospitals, as well as from both public and private nursing agencies. This occurred at MGH as well. The Boston Committee on Red Cross Nursing Service, according to preestablished wartime policy, became the central recruiting and assignment agency for volunteer nursing personnel immediately following the disaster. After 7 days, however, the volunteer nurses returned to their primary jobs and were relieved by nurses employed by the Red Cross. The Red Cross paid approximately $15,000 for supplemental nursing care within the first two-and-a-half months following the disaster.[36] Extra BCH supplies had been put aside for disaster and war purposes; however, the disaster quickly depleted the hospital's supplies of narcotics, plasma, triple dye, oxygen equipment, dressing material, syringes, and bed linen. In addition to supplemental personnel, the Red Cross also provided BCH with additional supplies and financial funding for the care of the disaster victims.

The nurses' aide played a significant role in the care given to the nightclub fire victims. The volume of nursing care necessarily was monumental, even with supplemental nursing personnel, and the aides met the challenge successfully. Many were homemakers who had volunteered to take brief courses offered by local hospitals or the Red Cross to assist with the nursing shortage caused by recruitment of nurses for wartime military duty. Although the official report of relief operations did not go into detail describing the specific care provided by the registered nurses, the Red Cross did acknowledge the contribution of the nurses' aides who assisted:

> Nurses' aides, in addition to those on regular duty, were assigned on five hour shifts to the hospitals having the greatest number of patients. In the emergency wards, they made and remade beds, listed patients' clothing and valuables, held the patients while physicians gave life-saving blood plasma and intravenous injections, took the temperatures, tirelessly moistened parched lips and mouths, and gave liquid feedings. They applied cold compresses and boric solution to inflamed eyes. They washed glass tubes piled high in ward kitchens, and mopped the floor of blood, cinders, burnt hair, and clothing. They also placed identification tags on the dead.[37]

CARE OF THE INJURED AT MASSACHUSETTS GENERAL HOSPITAL

Across town at MGH, an astute nursing supervisor's instinct became aroused when three patients, admitted with severe burns close to the 11:00 p.m. shift change, described the nightclub fire scene to the emergency ward staff. A hospital-wide alert was called only minutes before 114 casualties started to arrive at the hospital. An MGH nurse later recalled, "At half-past ten our head night supervisor saw three patients, one of whom was a soldier, arrive in quick succession. Sensing from long experience that something unusual was afoot, she called for help before ambulances, taxis and delivery wagons brought their first loads."[38] The hospital had maintained the wartime habit of keeping a full complement of disaster nurses on call, and a large contingent of nurses were either on site or housed nearby.

Responding to the MGH alert were the staff teams for burns and resuscitation. Yet the emergency ward was quickly thrown into chaos. Accurate patient identification was impossible owing to the vast number and critical status of the patients, especially the women who had left their personal belongings behind in the burning nightclub. Many patients were unconscious. Seventy-five brought to MGH were dead upon arrival, and the large number of corpses hindered care in the emergency ward. Grace Parker Follett, an instructor with the MGH diploma nursing school, authored a 1943 article in the *American Journal of Nursing* and described the chaotic MGH emergency ward scene:

> Patients dead on arrival, numbering about twice the living, were placed in that large hall known as the "brick corridor," where their screened and blanketed bodies covered the red tiles which on Ether Day and at graduation receptions swarm with the milling feet of our friends. The careful examination on arrival was repeated until each body had been examined, in all five times, for possible sign of life.[39]

Dr. Cope, MGH's burn expert, noted for the *New England Journal of Medicine:*

> The casualties reached the hospital on an average of one every fifty seconds. It was necessary to dispose immediately of the dead in order to have room for the living. Four medical interns, working in pairs, were stationed at the admitting door to sort out the dead, who were taken along one corridor to a temporary morgue.[40]

The sense of urgency, sheer number of patients, continuous noise, stench of burnt hair and flesh, and horrific wounds were overwhelming to the experienced physicians and nurses.

Burn injuries ranged from minor to severe, but only 29 out of 39 living survivors at MGH suffered from significant burn injury. Most burns seen at MGH were of partial- rather than full-thickness depth.[41] Similar to BCH, the majority of patients transported to MGH manifested respiratory distress. Of the patients admitted to MGH, only three were spared from it: "Two of the patients covered their faces with a sweater and a cloth napkin, while the other had urinated into a napkin and had covered his face."[42]

The large number of persons rescued from the burning nightclub led to a unique observation regarding respiratory status that later contributed to the diagnosis of smoke inhalation injury. Dr. Cope noted:

> It was obvious almost at once that we were dealing with something more than the problem of burned skin; a severe impairment of respiration also existed. . . . It was then clear that no explosion had occurred but that suffocating fumes in addition to flames and hot air, had been inhaled. . . . The picture presented by the Cocoanut Grove patients on arrival was startling. The majority were either maniacal or unconscious. At first the mania was mistaken for hysteria aggravated by pain. Subsequently, it was realized that in many it was due to anoxia and that it was comparable to the restlessness and mania encountered in the anoxia of cardiac insufficiency.[43]

Upon the patients' arrival at the hospital, staff removed wet clothing and covered the injured with sterile towels. Dr. Cope quickly arrived on the scene and directed emergency care while still dressed in his evening tuxedo. Implementing his research protocol that was already in place at MGH at the time of the disaster, Cope ordered that burn surfaces not be cleaned or debrided prior to dressing.[44] He justified his decision at the 1943 annual meeting of the New Hampshire Medical Society:

> Such treatment of surface burns is unorthodox in modern surgery, when one is accustomed to neat wounds. . . . We were unorthodox and did not cleanse the wounds because we doubt that any cleansing other than vigorous scrubbing materially reduces the number of organisms on the wound. Such scrubbing of delicate, unprotected tissue would presumably result in more extensive injury and as much harm would have been done as benefit derived.[45]

At MGH, teams of medical students and interns covered burn wounds first with fine mesh gauze saturated with boric acid and sterile petroleum, followed by an outer bulky dressing and an elastic compression bandage.[46] They splintered injured limbs over the dressing, often using folded newspaper according to Red Cross wartime guidelines.[47] The dressings remained in place unchanged for several days. The radical simplicity of Cope's research protocol for burn wound care was less demanding than other protocols and did not disrupt essential care such as blood transfusions and oxygen therapy. Remarkably, when these dressings were later removed, most of the burns were clean and healing despite the lack of debridement. The topical use of boric acid was controversial owing to the risk of absorption and toxicity, but Cope justified its use on the basis that it would counteract bacterial organisms on the skin and reduce the risk of burn infection.[48] Although boric acid was detected in the urine of the patients, no one manifested signs of toxicity.

Nurses provided all disaster patients at MGH with morphine sulfate (¼ grain) by subcutaneous injection using a large syringe and a single needle for mass administration.[49] After pretesting for allergic response, nurses also administered anti-tetanus serum. Active duty military personnel were considered to be already immunized against tetanus.[50] Nurses monitored body temperature rectally. Diagnostic testing included serum analysis (hematocrit, protein, electrolytes, pro-thrombin), arterial blood gas, aspiration of burn blister fluid for chemistry and bacteria, electrocardiogram, chest X-ray, and pulmonary vital capacity. Blood products (dried plasma, frozen plasma, and whole blood) were administered for indications of shock and/or reduced oxygen capacity.

Two MGH physicians at the time of the disaster described the use of blood products for the victims:

> In the first seven days, 16 whole blood transfusions were used for patients with reduced oxygen capacity of their blood. Three members of the house staff, two student interns, and three nurses staffed the blood bank; three house staff members supervised plasma administration on the ward. Approximately thirty-three of the thirty-nine patients received plasma in quantities of one to twelve units per individual. The largest quantity given to a single patient in the first twenty-four hours was nine units. Low blood pressure was the first indication used for plasma administration.[51]

To reduce the risk of infection, all patients at MGH received 2 grams of sulfadiazine IV every 8 hours for a total of 2 doses. The dose was then decreased to 1 gram every 6 hours and given orally or IV if the patient could not eat or drink.[52] Topical sulfonamide was not used because it was believed to hinder wound healing, and drug toxicity could better be avoided by the use of IV and oral routes. Physicians monitored serum drug levels, but drug-induced nephrotoxicity was rare in these patients. Liberal IV fluid therapy probably helped to provide renal protection against drug toxicity. Aspiration of burn blister fluid later demonstrated similarities between topical and serum drug levels, indicating that systemic administration of the antibiotic drug did result in travel of the drug to the burn wound site. Physicians from the adjacent Massachusetts Eye and Ear Infirmary assessed the eyes of the patients upon admission and then daily; and they ordered administration of 5% sulfathiazole ophthalmic ointment and atropine eye drops.[53]

For the purpose of focused care and infection control, MGH officials opened a temporary burn unit on the sixth floor of the White Building, using an evacuated 40-bed surgical ward, to care for the majority of disaster patients. Local Coast Guardsmen and members of the hospital's Ladies Visiting Committee guarded the doors to the unit—the servicemen for their strength and authority, the ladies for their poise and knowledge of the hospital.[54] They limited visitors to one per day, regardless of patient status. Staff wore isolation gowns and masks.[55] MGH officials converted the adjacent patient solarium into a sterile operating room for wound care and moved portable X-ray equipment onto the burn unit. According to two physicians:

> A solarium has been converted into a dressing room. The floor was scrubbed with a strong anti-septic solution, an operating table installed, and the windows boarded for blackout requirements. Dressings are done with complete aseptic technique.[56]

Sixty nurses were assigned to the temporary MGH burn unit, with 20 nurses working in 8-hour shifts. The unit was divided into three wings, often with a senior student nurse placed in charge of each wing. The unit had its own nursing supervisor and utility room nurse. Nurses and physicians organized themselves into teams for burn wound care, procedures (including

bronchoscopy and tracheostomy), medications (primarily narcotics, seda-
tives, and antibiotics), IV fluids, blood products, and oxygen therapy.
Patients were divided into groups of four for focused care. As elsewhere,
nurses' aides and orderlies played a major role in patient care, freeing up
nurses and physicians for more essential matters. Follett described how the
enhanced role of the nurse aide grew out of necessity during this time:

> On White 6 the aides have taken much of the responsibility for giving hourly
> fluids to every patient not specialed [sic] by a nurse; and as an example of
> how we have used professional and auxiliary nursing together, a nursing arts
> instructor went to the floor to teach the aides by demonstration and immedi-
> ate supervision how to do mouth care.[57]

Follett also described how nursing students from nearby affiliate hospitals,
MGH nursing school alumni, and other organizations supplemented the
MGH nursing staff:

> We have had graduate nurses, too, from many sources and students from
> McLean Hospital. Our own alumnae from Greater Boston have come, out-
> side special nurses have come as individuals after their day's work, [and]
> other hospitals and nursing organizations not only have sent staff members
> but have paid them to come to us.[58]

Disaster patients at both hospitals remained for months, with MGH absorbing the majority of the costs at that facility.[59] Patients often endured numerous surgeries before being discharged, often scarred and disabled, back
to public life. For example, Shirley Freedmann-Harris was transported to
MGH with burns over 80% of her body. Her thoracic cavity was crushed in
her attempt to escape through the jammed revolving door of the nightclub.
Minutes before the final removal of her dressings, she was told for the first
time that the severity of her injuries forced the amputation of the fingers
on her right hand:

> The hospitalization was awful, five months long. I was unconscious for three
> weeks. I had nine surgeries in the hospital, and five plastic surgeries with

another surgeon later. I was pretty discouraged. And then two weeks before I was to be discharged, the nurse told me that . . . the young man from Dorchester that I was with that night at the Cocoanut Grove had died . . . [Later] some people had been terrible to me for the way I looked.[60]

Freedman-Harris married later and named her first son after the MGH physician who compassionately cared for her through her long hospitalization. By a twist of fate, her son eventually worked together with the physician's son as commercial pilots for the same airline.[61]

Still in research development at the time of the disaster, penicillin was in limited supply and under the control of the NRC. The NRC offered some of the precious antibiotic to MGH for treatment of the disaster victims, and it was transported to MGH under police escort. Staff administered penicillin (5,000 units) by intramuscular injection at 4-hour intervals for persistent rectal temperatures above 101.0° Fahrenheit.[62] The NRC did not offer any penicillin to BCH, however, which was struggling to care for the majority of the disaster victims on a public hospital budget. Many interpreted this as a political maneuver manipulated by MGH, but the NRC justified its action by stating that MGH's burn research was more established than BCH's. Of interest, the penicillin dosage used at MGH was later determined to be too low to be effective against burn infection.[63]

CLIFFORD JONES

The most severely injured of the Cocoanut Grove nightclub fire survivors was a 21-year-old U.S. Coast Guardsman named Clifford Jones, who made multiple efforts to rescue victims from the burning nightclub before being injured himself. Jones was one of the first persons taken to BCH. Dr. Stanley Levenson, a former BCH physician who cared for Jones, recalled: "He was a hero. He'd gotten out quickly, he was near one of the few open exits, and then he went back in five or six times, carrying people out, and then collapsed, and was burned severely."[64]

Jones had significant burns over 75% of his body. Only his face, scalp, and anterior chest were spared. The nursing staff could visualize his right kidney, two ribs, part of his right femur, and the jawbone near his chin.

His burns were so charred that the nurses were unable to differentiate between the dark wool of his military service uniform and burn eschar (dead skin tissue). He was unconscious and barely breathing. Staff was unable to assess his blood pressure by inflatable cuff and relied upon pulse rate to estimate the depth of his shock, which was so significant that he required a total of 17 pints of plasma and 4 liters of normal saline within the first 24 hours. His demise was considered to be imminent, but he survived. The media focused on his plight and updated the public daily by both newspaper and radio.[65]

The severity of Jones's injuries challenged the knowledge, skill, and endurance of the BCH nurses and physicians. Jones struggled to overcome infection, dehydration, and an addiction to the narcotic codeine. The appearance of an alert Jones, despite his massive injuries—in addition to the exhausting and continuous demands of his care—was often overwhelming for even the most experienced BCH nurses. Nurses assigned to Jones by themselves would often be found exhausted and crying in a closet or dark corner. To decrease the workload burden, two nurses were then assigned to him each shift, assisted by local Coast Guardsmen for lifting and linen changes. Despite the increase in staff at his bedside, nurse burnout continued to work its way through the BCH nursing staff. The hospital then turned to the Red Cross for relief. The Red Cross arranged for, and funded, a pool of private duty nurses to care for Jones for almost 12 months until his discharge.[66]

Jones was deemed too unstable to tolerate general anesthesia or to be transported off the unit for surgery. Physicians did weekly skin grafting at the bedside under local anesthesia supplemented with oral codeine, and they used the unburned areas of his arms as the initial harvest sites. One of those physicians recalled 50 years later, "Dr. Browder did thousands of pinpoint skin grafts [moving bits of Johnson's skin from uninjured areas to wounds], all of them as I recall with a Gillette® blue blade." Jones required a total of 21 grafting sessions, each lasting 3–4 hours in duration, with physicians stopping only when the patient could no longer tolerate the pain of the procedure. The new graft sites were treated with 75% cod liver oil and exposed to ultraviolet light to stimulate healing. Cocoa butter was rubbed onto the healed sites to promote skin elasticity for joint movement. Certain areas required repeated grafting or surgical release of scar tissue.

In August 1943, Jones was assisted to his feet by the two Red Cross nurses who had cared for him almost daily since Christmas. Within 2 weeks of his first ambulation, he was walking on his own without assistance or supervision. Jones was discharged from BCH 1 year after admission and transferred to nearby Brighton Marine Hospital for continued rehabilitation, where he remained for another 9 months. He was honorably discharged from the U.S. Coast Guard and returned to his Midwest hometown with the nurse bride who helped care for him at BCH. Driving alone one day, he lost control of his vehicle. Jones became trapped in the overturned, burning truck and exposed to fuel leaking from the ruptured gas tank. Having survived massive burn injury 10 years earlier, Jones was burned to death inside his overturned vehicle on a remote rural road.[67] The nature of his demise haunted his former BCH caregivers for years.

ADVANCES IN BURN CARE

The Cocoanut Grove nightclub fire became a turning point in the care of patients with life-threatening burn injury. Lessons learned from this disaster were quickly implemented on the battlefields of World War II, increasing the chances for survival among burn-injured military personnel. Dr. Cope's research burn protocol was recognized as a simpler and more effective alternative to topical tannic acid and triple dye. Liberal IV fluid resuscitation and aggressive nutritional support became routine burn care. Drs. Lund and Browder further refined burn size estimation, which was later used to determine the burn patient's IV fluid requirements.[68] Early debridement of dead skin and skin grafting for wound closure became the primary means of reducing infection risk.

The injuries suffered on the night of November 28, 1942, extended beyond the obvious burn wounds. Psychological distress manifested among the victims included panic attacks, posttraumatic stress disorder, overwhelming grief, and a persistent phobia of enclosed areas. Suicidal ideation was noted among some of the survivors. One survivor, brought back to MGH by concerned family members because of his alarming mental status, threw himself out of a sixth floor hospital window:

> A young man aged 32 had received only minor burns . . . His wife had
> stayed behind [in the burning nightclub]. When he tried to pull her out,
> he had fainted and was shoved out by the crowd. She was burned while he

was saved . . . He complained about his feeling of extreme tension, inability
to breathe, generalized weakness and exhaustion, and his frantic fear that
something terrible was going to happen . . . "I should have saved her or I
should have died too" . . . After skillfully distracting the attention of his
special nurse, he jumped through a closed window to a violent death.[69]

Dr. Erich Lindemann, a MGH psychiatrist at the time of the nightclub fire,
interviewed many nightclub fire survivors and relatives of the deceased.
This experience contributed to his famous research on posttraumatic stress
disorder and grief following catastrophic loss.[70]

The Cocoanut Grove nightclub fire also led to the recognition of
smoke inhalation injury as a component of burn trauma. The many victims
were exposed to hot air, smoke, and fumes inside the burning nightclub
pending their escape, and their respiratory distress alerted physicians to the
possibility of an airway burn injury. In addition to respiratory problems,
these patients presented to the hospital with facial burns, singed nasal hair,
hoarse voice tone, dark sooty sputum, and cherry-red facial skin color.
Although often stable upon admission, respiratory distress with airway
obstruction significantly worsened within hours and became refractory to
standard treatment. Severity or escalation of the respiratory problems did
not correlate with either burn size or depth but did correlate with loss of
consciousness and the length of time spent inside the burning nightclub.

DISASTER INVESTIGATION

The horrifying nature of the Cocoanut Grove nightclub fire led to a public
demand for answers. Investigation findings revealed inadequate emergency
exits, faulty electrical and construction work, inadequate inspections with
bribes to city building inspectors, suspicious tax cuts, underaged nightclub
employees, and a total lack of regard for fire prevention and emergency
escape measures.[71] Following legal proceedings, survivors and families of
the dead received a check for only $150 to compensate for their loss. The
owner of the nightclub, Barney Welansky, whose own nephew barely escaped from the burning nightclub, was convicted of manslaughter for ne-
glect of safety measures and sent to Norfolk Prison for 12–15 years. Less
than 4 years later, however, the governor of Massachusetts, who was the

mayor of Boston at the time of the disaster, quietly pardoned him. Welansky died within weeks from metastatic cancer. Prior to his death, he released a public statement, "I wish that I had died with the others in the fire."[72]

FINAL COMMENTS

Advances in burn care resulting from the Cocoanut Grove nightclub fire were possible only because of the willingness of nurses and physicians to consider innovative measures that effectively utilized limited resources and a nontraditional teamwork approach in the midst of overwhelming disaster for the benefit of hundreds of injured patients. The role of the nurses who cared for the injured still remains outside the primary focus of anniversary reunions, documentaries, and newspaper articles. The nurses quietly carried on with the duties and responsibilities that had been drilled into them during their nurses' training and that were expected of them by American society. With the continuation of World War II, many probably went into military uniform and took their disaster clinical experience with them, caring for military personnel with combat-related burn injury.[73]

Twenty-five years after the disaster, a hospital was established adjacent to MGH for the research and care of patients with life-threatening burn injuries, especially children. It was named Shriners Burn Institute because of its primary charitable funding source. The new hospital's location, and selection of Dr. Cope as its first director, was intentional because of MGH's significant role in care of the nightclub fire victims. Cope remained a medical maverick and later publically challenged the use of radical mastectomy for the treatment of breast cancer, preferring less surgical resection supplemented by chemotherapy and external beam radiation.

The charred remains of the Cocoanut Grove nightclub were quickly demolished by construction crews after the fire. The nightclub was never rebuilt on its original site or on any site in the city of Boston. Per city licensing board mandate, no entertainment facility in the city of Boston can be awarded licensure under the name of the Cocoanut Grove.[74] In recognition, 50 years after the nightclub fire, the local neighborhood association placed a small brass plaque into an inner city brick sidewalk to signify the site of the American disaster that modernized burn care:

In memory of more than 490 people that died in the Cocoanut Grove Fire on November 28, 1942. As a result of that terrible tragedy, major changes were made in the fires codes, and improvements in the treatment of burn victims, not only in Boston but across the nation. "Phoenix out of the Ashes."

STUDY QUESTIONS

1. Discuss the importance of disaster care protocols for burned patients. On the basis of what has been learned about the effects of toxic fumes on the respiratory system, what information should the first people on the scene of a fire be aware of? What are teaching implications for nurses in this area?
2. Of all bodily injuries, few are more traumatic than burns. Discuss the challenges nurses face as they care for these patients. What are the physical, psychological, and social needs of burn patients? What are the physical, psychological, and social needs of nurses who care for burn patients?
3. Health professionals have been continually developing effective means to combat burn injury and promote rehabilitation. With what other groups in the community should they work to protect society from the hazards of fire disasters?

NOTES

1. Samuel E. Cutler, "400 DEAD IN HUB NIGHTCLUB FIRE! Hundreds Hurt in Panic as the Cocoanut Grove Becomes a Wild Inferno," *Boston Sunday Globe*, November 29, 1942. This was the front page headline of the newspaper on the day after the fire.
2. Jeffrey R. Saffle, "The 1942 Fire at Boston's Cocoanut Grove Nightclub." *American Journal of Surgery* 166 (1993): 581–591.
3. M. R. Montgomery, "Recalling Cocoanut Grove," *Boston Globe*, May 25, 1992, 30.
4. David J. Barillo and Steven Wolf, "Planning for Burn Disasters—Lessons Learned From One Hundred Years of History," *Journal of Burn Care & Research* 27 (2006): 622–634.
5. Grace Parker Follett, "The Boston Fire—A Challenge to Our Disaster Service," *American Journal of Nursing* 43 (1943): 4–8.

6. Saffle, "The 1942 Fire."
7. Barillo and Wolf, "Planning for Burn Disasters."
8. David Arnold, "Decades Later, Clues to an Inferno." *Boston Globe*, September 24, 1993.
9. Noted in ibid.
10. Casey Cavanaugh Grant, "Last Dance at the Cocoanut Grove," *National Fire Protection Association Journal* (May–June 1991): 74–86.
11. Jack Thomas, "The Cocoanut Grove Inferno—50 Years Ago This Week, 494 Died in a Tragedy for the Ages," *Boston Globe*, November 22, 1992.
12. Grant, "Last Dance."
13. Thomas, "The Cocoanut Grove Inferno."
14. Grant, "Last Dance."
15. Tom Coakley, "Night of Hell Recalled," *Boston Globe*, November 28, 1992, 13.
16. Grant, "Last Dance."
17. Coakley, "Night of Hell Recalled."
18. Grant, "Last Dance."
19. Thomas, "The Cocoanut Grove Inferno."
20. Ibid.
21. Ibid.
22. American National Red Cross, *Official Report of Relief Operations—Cocoanut Grove Fire* (Washington, DC: National American Red Cross, 1943).
23. Ibid.
24. Coakley, "Night of Hell Recalled."
25. Saffle, "The 1942 Fire."
26. Grant, "Last Dance."
27. "Hospitals Jammed With Dead, Injured," *Boston Herald*, November 29, 1942; "Where Bodies Can Be Found," *Boston Globe*, November 29, 1942.
28. Charles S. Davidson, "The Cocoanut Grove Disaster," *Journal of Infectious Diseases* 125 (1972): S58–S59.
29. Maxwell Finland, Charles S. Davidson, and Stanley M. Levenson, "Clinical and Therapeutic Aspects of the Conflagration Injuries to the Respiratory Tract Sustained by Victims of the Cocoanut Grove Disaster," *Medicine* 25 (1946): 215–283.
30. Davidson, "The Cocoanut Grove Disaster."
31. Maxwell Finland, Charles S. Davidson, and Stanley M. Levenson, "Effects of Plasma and Fluid on Pulmonary Complications in Burned Patients," *Archives of Internal Medicine* 77 (1946): 477–490.
32. Ibid.
33. Davidson, "The Cocoanut Grove Disaster."
34. Montgomery, "Recalling Cocoanut Grove."
35. Davidson, "The Cocoanut Grove Disaster."

36. American National Red Cross, *Official Report*.

37. Ibid.

38. Follett, "The Boston Fire."

39. Ibid.

40. Oliver Cope, "Care of the Victims of the Cocoanut Grove Nightclub Fire at the Massachusetts General Hospital," *New England Journal of Medicine* 22 (1943): 138–147.

41. Saffle, "The 1942 Fire."

42. Thomas M. Cunningham, "Historical Perspective—Fires in Public Assembly Occupancy; Part 1: The Cocoanut Grove," *WithTheCommand.com—Emergency Services' Information Site* (August 10, 2003), http://www.withthecommand. om/2003-Aug/MD-tom-public1html (accessed June 28, 2006).

43. Cope, "Care of the Victims."

44. Ibid.; and Saffle, "The 1942 Fire."

45. Cope, "Care of the Victims."

46. Ibid.

47. N. W. Faxon and E. D. Churchill, "Cocoanut Grove Disaster in Boston— A Preliminary Account," *Hospitals* 17 (1943): 13–18.

48. Cope, "Care of the Victims."

49. Faxon and Churchill, "Cocoanut Grove Disaster in Boston."

50. Ibid.

51. Ibid.

52. Ibid.

53. Ibid.

54. Ibid.

55. Follett, "The Boston Fire."

56. Faxon and Churchill, "Cocoanut Grove Disaster in Boston."

57. Follett, "The Boston Fire."

58. Ibid.

59. Thomas, "The Cocoanut Grove Inferno."

60. Noted in Gloria Negri, "A Wing and a Prayer Reunion," *Boston Globe*, November 14, 1994.

61. Ibid.

62. Faxon and Churchill, "Cocoanut Grove Disaster in Boston."

63. Maxwell Finland, Charles S. Davidson, and Stanley Levenson, "Chemotherapy and Control of Infection among Victims of the Cocoanut Grove Disaster," *Surgery, Gynecology, and Obstetrics* 82 (1946): 151–173.

64. Noted in Montgomery, "Recalling Cocoanut Grove."

65. Ibid.

66. Ibid.

67. Ibid.

68. Charles Lund and Newton Browder, "The Estimation of Areas of Burns," *Surgery, Gynecology, and Obstetrics* 79 (1994): 352–358.

69. Erich Lindemann, "Symptomatology and Management of Acute Grief," *American Journal of Psychiatry* 101 (1944): 141–148.

70. Ibid.

71. Robert S. Moulton, *The Cocoanut Grove Night Club Fire* (Boston: National Fire Protection Association, 1943).

72. Noted in Thomas, "The Cocoanut Grove Inferno."

73. The majority of these nurses are no longer living.

74. Grant, "Last Dance."

CHAPTER 10

The Great Alaska Earthquake
of 1964: Lessons in Leadership

Barbra Mann Wall

Please remain calm. Stay in your rooms. The hospital will stand.[1]

The operator at Providence Hospital, Anchorage, Alaska, spoke these words on the overhead intercom after an earthquake measuring 8.6 on the Richter scale struck Alaska at 5:36 p.m. on March 27, 1964. This earthquake was the strongest ever recorded on the North American continent.[2] Known as the Good Friday Earthquake, or the Great Alaska Earthquake, it had a tremor that lasted approximately 4 minutes and was later upgraded to a magnitude of 9.2. It was so powerful that tremors could be felt over a 500,000 square mile area, with shock waves tearing boats from moorings as far away as the Gulf of Mexico. The ocean floor rose between 2 and 6 feet over a 12,000 square mile area, with the highest uplift of 50 feet, and tsunamis struck all along the western coast of North America and the Arctic. Large waves tossed boats into downtown Kodiak and destroyed the railroad in Seward. Like the state of Alaska's population, the casualties were from a highly diverse group. Its young population, consisting of Whites, Aleuts, Native Americans, and Eskimos, were all affected. Of the 131 deaths, only 9 occurred outside the areas hit by the tsunami.[3] Fairbanks and Juneau, several hundred miles away, were less affected, and those cities provided vital assistance. The earthquake caused damages estimated at $750 million. Numerous aftershocks of lesser magnitude occurred for months afterward.

The nursing and medical activities for this disaster were generally viewed as competent within multiple environments, such as hospitals, mass shelters, and public health programs. At the same time, the context of 1960s Alaska was influential in how people responded to the earthquake.

Alaska had only recently obtained statehood and, as Thomas Birkland asserts, its "infancy as a state attracted federal attention that might not have been shown other states."[4] For example, the earthquake led to landmark federal policy changes, such as the Alaskan Earthquake Assistance Act in 1964 and the Earthquake Hazards Reduction Act in 1977. Furthermore, Alaska's frontier spirit was highly masculine. This cultural symbol tended to marginalize the feminine, but it will be shown that women nurses complicated this mythical stereotype in their actual practices after the disastrous earthquake.[5]

PROVIDENCE HOSPITAL, ANCHORAGE

One of the defining characteristics of a Catholic hospital in the mid-20th century was the way religious, economic, and social boundaries altered the authority within them. Anchorage's Providence Hospital, and indeed, most Catholic hospitals, were owned and managed by Catholic sisters, or nuns. In a position typically assumed by men, sisters maintained a unique hierarchy over their hospitals' administrative and nursing affairs.[6] Nuns' convent and professional training for their work emphasized community, calmness, order, and discipline. Yet their presence was at variance with the frontier setting of Alaska, where people typically saw themselves as individualistic, savoring their isolation from the outside world or the "lower 48" as they called the rest of the country. In this environment, sisters' vows of chastity could allow them access to male-dominated spaces without fear of scandal. Their special clothing, or habits, concealed their physical bodies and helped transcend usual female stereotypes, thereby minimizing gender limitations.[7]

The Sisters of Providence congregation in the Northwest was a missionary branch of a religious community in Montreal, Canada. Led by Mother Joseph Pariseau, four sisters came to Fort Vancouver, Washington Territory, in 1856 and opened hospitals, orphanages, and schools throughout the area. After the discovery of gold in Alaska in 1898, these French Canadian sisters followed thousands of prospectors to Nome in 1902, where they opened another hospital. As they lived and worked in this northern region, they endured the same economic and environmental challenges as miners and other settlers. The sisters came to Fairbanks in 1910 and then opened Providence Hospital in Anchorage in 1938.

At the time of the Good Friday Earthquake, Sister Barbara Ellen Lundberg, SP, had been administrator of the 155-bed Providence Hospital since the opening of its new building in 1962. Prior to that time, she was assistant provincial for the Sacred Heart Province of the Sisters of Providence; administrator of St. Peter's Hospital in Olympia, Washington, and administrator of Mount St. Vincent Home for the Aged in Seattle.[8] When the earthquake occurred, she and four other hospital sisters were attending religious services at St. Anthony Church in Mountain View, Alaska. They left immediately and drove to the hospital, where Sister Stella Marie Kramer, SP, assistant superior, had remained in the nearby convent. As one chronicler described it, "she literally had to dance as she walked along the hall toward the hospital." The earthquake struck at dinnertime and food trays in rooms spilled everywhere. The chronicler noted, "Much plaster is down; not a wall or ceiling seems to be without cracks of some kind" (Figure 10.1). Sister Philias Denis, SP, who at the time was the supervisor of nurses, was a patient on the fifth floor and was recovering from spinal surgery when the building began to shake. It was difficult for her to remain in bed because of the swaying and rolling of the building. As plants and flowers tumbled to the floor, a large window in her room fell out of its frame and hit the floor. The swaying and groaning seemed endless.[9]

The first priority for medical and nursing personnel was the preservation of life, which began immediately and continued throughout the emergency period.[10] Although telephone service was out, the internal broadcast system at Providence was intact. The 2-year-old hospital, the largest private hospital in the state, kept its promise that the hospital would stand, and within a few hours it became the primary medical emergency center for the entire region.[11]

To understand Providence Hospital's response, it is helpful to obtain some background knowledge of the extent of damage in Anchorage. Located 75 miles from the epicenter, the main business district of the city was heavily hit. This included commercial buildings, city hall, the federal building, and the local American Red Cross office. The low-lying areas of Cook's Inlet, including the upscale residential area of Turnagain Bluffs, collapsed. Yet the casualties in Anchorage were minimal, with only seven killed. For several hours after the earthquake hit, however, no one knew the extent of damage or the number of injuries. Although Providence suffered nearly $200,000 in damages, the structural impairment was minimal. This proved to be extremely important in the hospital's response to the

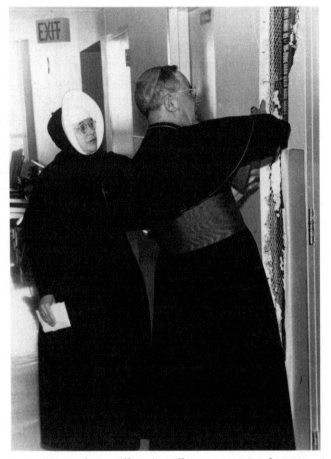

Figure 10.1 Sister Barbara Ellen Lundberg inspects damage, Anchorage, Alaska. Image #160.D51.43. Courtesy: Providence Archives, Seattle, WA.

disaster. It quickly shifted to emergency power, and its lights drew supplies and personnel from all over the city to its facilities.[12]

Two hospitals in the area, the 40-bed Presbyterian and 300-bed U.S. Air Force hospital at Elmendorf, suffered extensive structural damage. The Air Force facility evacuated in 18 minutes after the earthquake subsided, with patients moved into nearby barracks. Others went to the 395-bed U.S. Public Health Service's Alaska Native Hospital (ANH). Presbyterian's patients, along with the majority of the quake's other survivors, went to Providence Hospital.

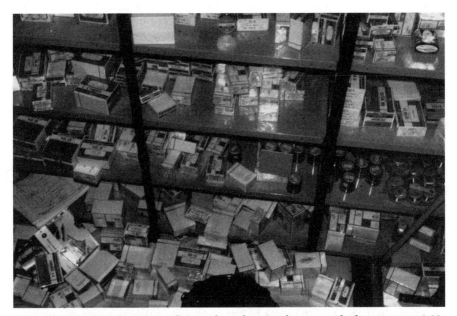

Figure 10.2   Supplies upset by earthquake, Anchorage, Alaska. Image #160. D51.30. Courtesy: Providence Archives, Seattle, WA.

When Sister Barbara Ellen arrived at Providence, there were nine registered nurses on duty with some licensed practical nurses, aides, orderlies, and a regular shift of maintenance and service personnel.[13] Sister Barbara Ellen and her five sister assistants coordinated the task of keeping the hospital in operation. Water was cut off, elevators stalled, the steam plant did not work, sterilizers were useless, toilets did not flush, pharmacy medications spilled all over the floor, and all phone links were dead[14] (Figure 10.2). Nonetheless, damage and destruction did not reduce the hospitals' abilities to provide emergency care, and panic did not occur.[15]

Within a few minutes, an emergency generator restored electricity and heat to vital areas such as the emergency room, surgery areas, nursing stations, and main halls. The U.S. Army provided a generator for the kitchen, and firemen pumped water from a nearby spring into the hospital. Soon, streams of cars, ambulances, and police were making their way to the hospital.[16] The hospital chronicler noted, "Everyone seemed to sense the need for immediate action and responsibility." No nurse left her unit to go to a safer place, and none of the 75 patients in the hospital at the time received injuries from the earthquake.[17] Indeed, a survey of sociologists from the

Disaster Research Center (DRC) observed at the time, "Few if any persons actually abandoned an ongoing organizational responsibility."[18]

Physicians responded with their own action plan, and as the radio broadcast a need for registered nurses, off-duty Providence personnel came. Some doctors and nurses brought their own families to Providence. Additional people were pulled to the emergency room, and within a half hour the first survivors arrived. Many were in a dazed state, and hospital staff provided them coffee and sandwiches from the kitchen. As well, 75 volunteer nurses came, some from the evacuated Presbyterian Hospital. The physical therapy room became a shelter for the homeless, including one Providence physician whose two children had been killed in Turnagain Bluffs. Twenty-two patients from Presbyterian came, and because the elevators were not working, Providence personnel carried the patients up the stairs in chairs and litters. They also hauled portable oxygen tanks up several flights. The Pepsi Cola Company brought water and soft drinks, while other volunteers brought milk, bread, medical supplies, and chlorinators.

Owing to disruptions in communications systems, hospital personnel used amateur and police radios to communicate with civil defense authorities. Because no one knew how many of the injured to expect, physicians and nurses prepared to care for 530 casualties. The military delivered a 200-bed civil defense hospital to Providence, but it was never necessary to use it. Hospital personnel set up other beds and cots in the cafeteria, halls, and business office[19] (Figure 10.3). Providence Hospital did not fill to capacity, however, and not all of the supplies were needed.[20]

Providing Emergency Care

Nurses and physicians set up a triage system in the emergency room and had to improvise to provide care. Emergency room patients went to one of five areas: Area 1, for closed fractures; Area 2, for open fracture cases; Area 3, the operating rooms; Area 4, a row of mattresses in the hallway where less severe cases could be seen; and Area 5, the morgue. By 10:00 p.m., nearly 500 people filled the lobby. Admissions personnel registered 108 the first night, but only a few were critically injured. In the operating suites, flashlights and battery-operated lights were available in addition to the auxiliary power, but one doctor delivered a baby by flashlight early Saturday morning when all power briefly failed. Sterilizers were not operational be-

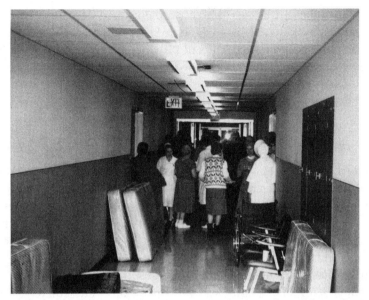

Figure 10.3   Emergency corridor at 9:00 p.m. looking from laboratory toward front entrance, Anchorage, Alaska. Image # 160.F21.2. Courtesy: Providence Archives, Seattle, WA.

cause there was no steam, and a radio call for help resulted in the delivery of a small pressure-cooker type of sterilizer that nurses heated with Bunsen burners. They had to improvise in other ways, with one using snow as a substitute for hypothermia for a patient undergoing a craniotomy. Others heated water for infant formulas in the doctors' coffee urn, and they used distilled water for drinking purposes.[21]

By 8:00 p.m. Friday, the first of U.S. Army and Air Force medical corps-men reported to Providence and worked in various capacities throughout the hospital. They stayed 10 full days after the earthquake. Because of all the volunteers, the hospital did not have a shortage of nursing personnel, and as the emergency situation subsided Friday night, the sisters encour-aged nurses to go home. By Saturday morning, other casualties began ar-riving in the emergency room, most with minor injuries suffered from the cleanup and rescue work. By then, the large autoclaves were operational, and kitchen personnel were able to serve breakfast. Within 48 hours after the earthquake, Providence personnel had treated more than 200 persons. Casualties ranged from adults requiring amputations to children sick from sleeping in unheated homes. Three people arrived dead or died soon after. In addition to the 22 patients from Presbyterian, Providence also received 30 patients from the Sisters of Providence nursing home, St. Mary's Residence, on Easter Sunday because it was located too near the damaged area.

Collaboration and Cooperation

Elmendorf Air Force Hospital, which had been evacuated of patients, was able to provide supplies to Providence. In addition to nurses, Presbyterian Hospital sent food. ANH was not designed to handle large numbers of disaster survivors but did provide typhoid serum to Providence, which, in turn, sterilized ANH's surgical instruments. The Alaska Psychiatric Institute did laundry for Providence.[22]

Prior to the earthquake, the Anchorage Office of Civil Defense (OCD) had changed leadership and was not operational immediately after the quake.[23] Thus the mayor, city manager, and police initially made damage assessments. It was not until 3:00 a.m. that the mayor called a meeting for members of the city council, representatives from city departments and utility companies, military personnel, public health officials, and civil defense personnel.

A newly appointed civil defense director gave first priority to restoration of utility services, particularly providing power to Providence Hospital. The local OCD assessed the needs for food, fuel, medical supplies, equipment, and personnel. Its acting director called in Army personnel, volunteer mountain climbers, and the Alaska Search and Rescue Group to assist in rescue and recovery operations. Water containers and liners and 1,000 chemical toilets were airlifted from Seattle. Elmendorf Air Force Base supplied sanitation kits. By Monday, demolition activity and clearance of debris had begun in earnest.[24]

RED CROSS AND PUBLIC HEALTH NURSING RESPONSES

The Division of Public Health did not begin its response efforts until Saturday, the morning after the earthquake, when city public health nurses began gathering materials needed for massive immunizations. With supplies provided by the Regional Emergency Health Service of Civil Defense and the U.S. Public Health Service, nurses vaccinated over 50,000 people against typhoid and paratyphoid in clinics and schools throughout the city.[25] Nurses also distributed food and diapers for infants; emergency items of oxygen cylinders, electrocardiographs, blood plasma, first aid, and surgical supplies; and household items.[26]

School nurses were active in shelters. Volunteer nurses from Juneau and Fairbanks aided Anchorage school nurses, as did many retired nurses. One opined, "This was a very exciting experience of community cooperation."[27] Other school nurses who were able to leave their families responded over the next 2 weeks, caring for more than 300 evacuated Aleuts from Old Harbor and Kaguyak, where a tidal wave had destroyed their villages. Making formula for babies became a full-time job, and eventually Aleut midwives took over the responsibility from the local school nurses.[28]

One public health nurse was summoned to Anchorage from her post deep in the interior of the state. She noted that, "but for the immediate instigation of previously established emergency routines," the earthquake "would have inflicted a vastly heavier loss of life than that which has been recorded to date." She arrived back in her home base "in a disorganized state of mind and paraphernalia." Eventually, she abandoned her routine and prepared for the unknown.

She also recalled that, like others, the Alaska Natives were numbed by the devastation they witnessed. An 8-year-old boy saw the tide swirling and turning "sideways instead of going back out to the sea." He hurried home and was warned that a large wave was coming:

> Everybody went to the top of the hill except an old man and an old woman. Their house was washed away by the wave. We never saw them again. When the big wave came, it carried away our house too. It was a good house. It was the best one we ever had. It was warm. We had new clothes, too. They were washed away with the house. Only four buildings were left.[29]

Thus, an important nursing activity in shelters was listening to survivors' stories. Other nursing care required taking vital signs and dispensing medications.

Although the natives of Old Harbor and Kaguyak had experienced significant trauma, they organized immediately. Both villages elected new chiefs in the shelter and appointed a rebuilding committee and a committee for sanitation. They continued to hold councils in the shelters where members worked with Red Cross workers and others from the U.S. Public Health Service and the Bureau of Indian Affairs to plan the return to their homes. A nurse praised the evacuees' courage: "These people, who have known a hard way of life, who know how to survive in conditions in which most of us would perish, were stunned by this disaster. . . But they were making plans to return and continue to live near their old village site."[30]

ADDITIONAL SITES OF DAMAGE

Because so much of the Alaskan economy depended on sea industries, its villages and small towns typically crowded the seashores, which became their undoing during the tsunamis that followed the earthquake. The village of Chenega was totally destroyed, 23 people died, and all the survivors had to move. A nurse and a team of physicians and sanitation engineers visited potential evacuation sites to evaluate available housing and water supplies for Chenega's residents.[31]

The damage to the American Red Cross headquarters in downtown Anchorage delayed that organization's response, but within 24 hours it had mobilized. The Red Cross had a long history of work in Alaska. In 1917, the Red Cross Delano Nursing Corps became the state's first public health nurses as they provided services to the most remote regions of the state. The Red Cross also responded to the flu pandemic in 1918 and 1919.[32] After the 1964 earthquake struck, Sigrid Bullard, the Red Cross nursing director for the Alaska disaster, put out a call for volunteers, and 45 registered nurses and 27 trained Red Cross nurses' aides responded. They worked both in Providence Hospital and in outlying areas. Most nurses lived in the general earthquake area and had to face their own personal recovery problems. All of the aides and many of the nurses cared for survivors at Providence Hospital throughout the emergency period. Other Red Cross nurses worked around the clock in shelters and typhoid immunization clinics in Anchorage. One Red Cross shelter housed 166 Aleuts evacuated from Kodiak Island. Aleuts requiring hospitalization went to the ANH. Other Red Cross nurses went in teams to Kodiak, Valdez, and Seward.[33]

The Red Cross spent $1,270,945.95 for aid in Alaska and $79,022 for California families. The incidence of disease turned out to be no higher than in normal times.[34] But Bullard had discovered that the Red Cross chapter in Anchorage did not have an active nursing service committee, and it took days to build satisfactory relationships in some areas. According to her, "preplanning and orientation for nurses in the community as to Red Cross disaster responsibilities would make for far smoother relationships at a time when all in health services are extremely involved with their services to people." On the other hand, after recruiting volunteer nurses, Bullard reported excellent rapport between Red Cross nurses and hospital staffs.[35]

Kodiak Island

Kodiak Island, located off the coast 350 air miles from Anchorage, suffered immense structural damage and listed 19 people dead or missing, despite the fact that enough time had elapsed between the earthquake and the damaging tidal wave to give most people time to seek higher ground. The people killed or missing had been out in boats. This was the area to which the St. Louis, Missouri, Red Cross office assigned Hazel Heywood, then director of nursing services for the Red Cross chapter in Milwaukee, Wisconsin. When notified of the disaster on March 28, Heywood met with 59 other Red Cross nurses from across the nation, and by Monday, March 30, she and another nurse were in Kodiak. No organization existed in the area for such a disaster. Because communications had been knocked out, their only contact with Red Cross headquarters was through the Alaska Communications System, with nurses and others handling the calls as they came through.

As one nurse noted, "It's the job of our disaster teams to supplement local help already on the scene." To this end, their first job was to relieve the fatigued nurse at a schoolhouse shelter where 600–700 people had congregated. Babies needed formula and clean diapers, and someone was able to bring a washing machine into the schoolhouse. There were some colds and minor injuries, and the nurse recalled that "although these Aleuts, Indians, Eskimos and white Americans are a hardy and resourceful lot, there was a great need for tender loving care." The Red Cross set up headquarters in a local church in Kodiak and provided nursing coverage for the schoolhouse shelter until April 7, dispensed groceries and clothes to the needy, helped with housing, fed evacuees waiting for stateside naval flights, and helped answer 60,000 "health and welfare messages" that came from the outside. Red Cross and public health nurses toured the villages to check for survivors. This was a monumental job because there were no transportation facilities, telephones, newspapers, or roads to reach outlying villages on the island.[36]

Valdez

American Red Cross volunteers went to other badly damaged areas. The greatest death toll was in Valdez, where 32 men, women, and children were killed when huge sections of land slid into the sea. As in Kodiak, there was no existing Red Cross chapter structure, and the response initially was un-organized. A local public health nurse and physician gave emergency care. In addition, a Red Cross nurse from San Antonio, Texas, worked with the local health agents in caring for 103 people with injuries, 52 of them seri-ous. Nurses also assisted sheltered survivors, and with a medical unit from the U.S. Army helped arrange for air evacuation of some cases.[37]

At Fairbanks' St. Joseph's Hospital (also sponsored by the Sisters of Providence), the local Red Cross nursing chairwoman helped screen Valdez evacuees for communicable diseases and other problems.[38] In her final summary, she noted that further orientation was needed for the state health department and staff nurses in Valdez regarding disaster preparedness.[39]

Nurses and Army workers also evacuated 55 patients from the Harborview Nursing Home, a mental health institution in Valdez that in-cluded some children, to the Alaska Psychiatric Institute in Anchorage. One Harborview nurse recalled that on the first night, "We packed everyone into the few cars we had and drove over dangerously damaged roads with our overloaded cars." They returned the next day, only to find out that the pa-tients could not stay at the damaged hospital and had to be airlifted to An-chorage.[40] The patients arrived at the Alaska Psychiatric Institute before most of their trained staff, and volunteer nurses from Juneau helped care for them. One lamented that her nursing education did not include experience with people with mental disabilities, and she felt lost when working with them. She noted, "The difference in the skill in handling the patients demonstrated by the personnel from Harborview, who arrived later, was marked." Over the next several days, the Juneau nurses set up an immunization clinic in the hospital's lobby. Because of poor communications, however, there were long periods of waiting for assignments, vaccines, food, and transportation.[41]

Seward

Seward, located on the west coast, had been designated as a wartime evacuation area. As a result, it had large amounts of supplies of food and bedding that were used extensively after the earthquake damaged the town. It was here that the railroad terminal was destroyed and 13 people died. One nurse reported that, as she was evacuating her home with her family, she realized that she would be needed at the hospital. She left her children with friends and went to Seward General Hospital, where she cared for homeless survivors.[42] The hospital suffered only minimal damage and became the headquarters for city offices, civil defense, and police stations. According to a report in the *Alaska Nurse*,

> All of the nurses in the Seward area were "on duty" somewhere . . . herding children, gathering families together, setting up first aid stations. . . .
> The nurses did everything, scrubbed, cooked, set up trays, washed dishes, answered lights, comforted the hundreds who swarmed about the Hospital that first night and all the next day.[43]

While much of this work involved typical caretaking activities, nurses also dealt with disrupted health and sanitation facilities and the dangers of communicable diseases.

OTHER NURSING RELIEF WORK

Red Cross survey teams made daily trips into the remote, mountainous Alaskan countryside.[44] In speaking of her fellow nursing colleagues, Heywood noted, "So far as standing up to the strain of disaster jobs, women do it just as well as men." While Red Cross male case workers scoured the rugged mountains and remote villages, "a woman is supervising their work. In fact, the Red Cross has more women case workers than men."[45]

Division of Public Health nurses worked with U.S. Public Health Service physicians, the Regional Emergency Health Service, and sanitary engineers as they visited sites in Prince William Sound and Kodiak Island. Nurses provided care for acute injuries, preventive measures, health teaching, and further assessments of sanitary conditions. They worked with agencies responsible for the care of evacuees, and as they returned to the areas badly damaged or destroyed, they helped arrange temporary facilities. The Regional Emergency Health Service reported complete support from other individuals and agencies for its work:

> It is largely due to this high degree of cooperation that it has been possible to overcome difficulties which have arisen in relation to health, and to expect that reconstructive efforts will result in a health climate superior to that existing at the time of the disaster.[46]

"PEOPLE RIDE WITH A WINNER"

Accolades went out to many of the responding agencies. After the earthquake struck, Major General R.L. Bohannon, Surgeon General of the U.S. Air Force, wrote, "The operational readiness of our military forces in the Alaskan earthquake was a shining example of the wisdom of a realistic program for the effective control of emergency situations."[47] Providence Hospital also received positive publicity for its work during the disaster. Three months later, Ed Fortier, Providence's current public relations director and the former director of civil defense in Alaska, wrote that the hospital seemed to be busier than ever. Indeed, the hospital was a "big winner when the quake was over," and "people ride with a winner."[48]

Other organizations recognized Providence's success. The Catholic Hospital Association provided Providence Hospital with a special recognition plaque. The American Medical Association's Committee on Disaster Care commended Sister Barbara Ellen and her staff. The Department of Defense disaster experts and the American Hospital Association both asked her for a copy of her staffing patterns.[49] Sister Barbara Ellen even heard from a hospital in Auckland, New Zealand, another earthquake-prone area, asking for information on Providence's disaster plan and in-service education, and the National Safety Council requested that an article in *Hospital Progress*, "How Providence Hospital Withstood Quake Ordeal," be reprinted in the *Hospital Safety Newsletter*. The editor of the *Newsletter* wrote, "My sincere congratulations on an excellent article, but primarily on the calmness and fortitude with which the earthquake was met."[50]

In November 1964, Sister Philias, who had been a patient at Providence Hospital on the day of the disaster and who by November had become its director of nursing, spoke at a national operating room nurses' meeting in California. Ever the booster for her hospital and adopted state, she showcased "Spotlight Anchorage, 1964" as part of her presentation. She also emphasized "three Cs" in disaster response: "competence, calmness, and courage." Trained, competent physicians and nurses responded to the disaster immediately, and they had the ability to improvise as needed. Calmness prevailed throughout the hospital, led by Sister Barbara Ellen, who never lost control of the situation. Indeed, her authority and her maintenance of control in the crisis helped maintain stability throughout the emergency. This courage persisted, despite rumors of an imminent tidal wave, warnings of typhoid, and threats of uncontrolled fires due to lack of water.[51]

While obviously meant to be complimentary, the following descriptions illustrate the way gender was used to categorize thoughts and actions of women and men. In a memo to Sister Philias, Fortier noted that Sister Barbara Ellen "was firm but flexible. Achieving this is a rare art. . . . She guided and directed calmly, quietly, and effectively without shouting or brandishing her authority."[52] In a communication to a physician, he praised Sister Barbara Ellen's "patience and understanding" and the nursing supervisors' "quiet competence" compared to physicians' expertise that prevented "shouting" and arguments.[53] Because shouting and flaunting authority are more commonly masculine characteristics, in essence, Fortier suggested that Sister Barbara Ellen and the nursing supervisors acted skillfully while simultaneously maintaining their stereotypical feminine identities.[54] Even though by modern standards some might criticize this conformity to traditional gender roles, the bottom-line result was that it worked and worked well.

Fortier reported seeing a disciplined health care team composed of doctors, nurses, and assistants who worked tirelessly in the aftermath of the earthquake. Adding to the stability was the reduced tension when Sister Barbara Ellen decided not to close Providence to nonpatients. Most disaster plans prohibited admittance of nonworkers and noncasualties to hospitals, but by remaining open to the public Providence had ready access to both skilled and unskilled workers. In addition, Sister Barbara Ellen allowed dependents of hospital personnel to stay in the hospital, which greatly reduced employees' worries about their families.[55]

THE IMPORTANCE OF "PLACE"

The situation of Alaska in the 1960s affected the disaster response. The estimated population of Anchorage and its suburbs at the time was 84,000.[56] The fact that Alaska was sparsely populated was a primary reason for fewer casualties. Because of their isolation from the mainland United States, Alaskans chronically experienced problems in food service and other provisions owing to distance from suppliers. As one nurse noted, "Alaska is far from its hospital supply companies and there is no such thing as a 'medical emergency,' it seems. Therefore it is necessary that we have a larger supply on hand in the storeroom." Because Providence had a vast amount of supplies on hand for normal use, its own operating room and pharmacy stores were sufficient during the disaster.[57] Alaska also had in place a wide availability of two-way radios, small planes that moved emergency equipment and personnel all over the state, mountain rescue teams, and heavy construction equipment, all of which were valuable assets during the emergency.[58] In addition, U.S. military facilities and personnel were of immense value during the earthquake. During World War II, owing to its strategic location, Alaska had been the site of many military bases, and large numbers of servicemen and women had stayed in the area afterward. In 1964, these military personnel helped in all phases of the response to the earthquake.

Sister Barbara Ellen elaborated on Alaska's distinctiveness: "Our first general reaction on [our] arrival was that Alaskans tend to exaggerate in considering their way of life different. After a year, however, we are inclined to agree that the management of a hospital in Alaska presents problems not common to the average hospital in the South 48." In a 1964 article in *Hospital Topics*, she described Anchorage's unique location as the transportation, communication, population, and medical center of Alaska. Providence Hospital typically admitted patients from more than 50 towns and villages throughout the state, from other states, and from Europe and Asia. Although other hospitals had been built in smaller communities, none had the equipment, medical and nursing personnel, and facilities that were available at Providence. Staffed by 60 physicians and surgeons, many were recognized specialists in their fields. The hospital had a 10-bed intensive care unit, a real innovation in Alaska's private hospitals in 1964. Significantly, the surgical, laboratory, and radiology departments were all on the first floor, enhancing the ability of personnel to treat survivors of the earthquake when the elevators were not in operation.[59]

Many Alaskans believed their frontier spirit of self-reliance and independence helped them to recover rapidly after the earthquake. Radio announcements and newspapers discussed it often during the emergency period, but social scientists dispelled this myth. They argued that an altruistic spirit generally prevails after any disaster, one that "breaks through previous class and status barriers to provide help to anyone who needs it." Second, it is not unusual to see self-reliance and innovation after disasters. "Local heroes emerge who exercise leadership at crucial control points; and afterward they are lauded in the press." Despite the fact that the Alaskans responded quickly to the disaster, they did ask for help from the military for manpower, vehicles, supplies, food, and water. Later, they requested state and federal money to deal with their economic problems. Still, although federal help did come to Alaska, the people did not wait for it before responding on their own.[60]

Ultimately, the government's response to the earthquake owed much to the place itself, Alaska, as the country's "last western frontier."[61] Alaska's economy, which was still in its early development, relied heavily on timber and fisheries and on federal aid. Afterward, President Lyndon Johnson formed the Federal Reconstruction and Development Planning Commission, which guided not only recovery from the earthquake but also development of Alaska itself.[62]

This disaster became one of the most studied natural disasters in U.S. history. The National Research Council did a large report on its engineering, social, and scientific aspects.[63] In addition, the nationally recognized DRC sent a team of social scientists to the scene 28 days after the Alaska earthquake hit. They showed how the Alaskan experience refuted basic assumptions about disaster preparedness. Sociologists E.L. Quarantelli and Russell R. Dynes from the DRC noted that, typically, community officials with limited disaster experience assumed that panic and pandemonium would occur during disasters. There would be social disorder and increased dependency on voluntary helping organizations outside the region. Another assumption was that "while individuals may cope well with a disaster, human service organizations often stumble."[64] Quarantelli and Dynes argued that, in contrast to these assumptions, "in a typical disaster, there is relatively controlled behavior, order, and personal initiative." Under unusual circumstances, such as limited access to escape routes during fires or explosions, people may flee in panic, but in most disasters, they generally "rise to the occasion and deal rather effectively with the personal challenges presented by the disaster."[65] This occurred with nurses and other health care personnel at Providence Hospital and public health facilities after the Anchorage earthquake.

Quarantelli and Dynes also noted that popular images of disaster behavior assumed personal and social chaos among organizations and survivors:

> The assumption is that many persons are so emotionally disorganized that they need outsiders to do the most elementary tasks for them such as being fed, housed, and clothed. In line with this, certain kinds of aid and supplies should be sent unsolicited to large-scale disaster areas since it is almost certain they will be needed.[66]

Chaos, however, did not occur in Anchorage. A variety of community organizations, including local hospitals, city departments, public health officials, and other state and local groups, responded and took control of the situation. Despite the severity of the quake, no epidemics occurred, and little looting was reported.

Several factors helped reduce injuries in Anchorage and enhanced Providence Hospital's ability to respond effectively. The quake occurred shortly after 5:30 p.m., so that, for most people, the workday was over. In addition, schools were not in session due to the Good Friday holiday. In spite of the convergence of patients on the hospital, it never had more than 123 admitted patients, although its bed capacity was 155. Another important factor was that disaster plans were already in place in area hospitals and nursing homes. At the height of the Cold War, with Alaska separated from Russia by only a few miles, Alaskans were particularly keen on military and civil preparedness. Thus, places like Providence Hospital had a disaster plan in operation for several years, which changed from time to time as conditions warranted.[67] Primarily, however, disaster plans were geared toward nuclear attacks and airplane crashes. Indeed, the earliest civil defense plans were for evacuation from Anchorage to Seward, but this changed to a "remain in place" plan because the highway and railroad to Seward were destroyed by the quake. Significantly, on March 25 and 26, Providence Hospital personnel had watched a film on a revised emergency fire plan. It demonstrated correct actions to take during emergencies and emphasized the need for maintaining calmness and order. These meetings proved helpful when the earthquake struck the next day.[68]

In many organizations, the fatigue factor affected the efficiency of their personnel,[69] but this did not occur at Providence, which was accustomed to operating around the clock. As the emergency tapered off Friday night, Sister Barbara Ellen sent the nurses home as others came in to replace them. In this way the hospital always had an adequate number of nurses who were rested. Fortier wrote, "My experience at Providence has resulted in a new respect for the medical and nursing professions. I spent many years in disaster work and planning, but not until March 27 did I really appreciate the meaning of the words 'duty,' 'professional dedication,' and 'courage.' Any break which could lead to panic never came." Indeed, "doctors, nurses, and other workers . . . performed as though they had been preparing all their lives for the March 27 disaster test."[70]

During the emergency response, many agencies cooperated in relief operations. The Red Cross worked with the Salvation Army; the Office of Emergency Planning in Washington, DC; the Alaska Survey for Reconstruction; the American Legion; and the AFL/CIO representatives to the Central Labor and Building Trades Councils.[71] Military corpsmen went to Providence Hospital and assisted on all shifts. The Air Force helped evacuate patients from St. Mary's Residence to Providence on Easter Sunday. The Army and Air Force provided needed generators, temporary beds, mobile mass feeding kitchens, and water purification units to local hospitals. More than 800 military personnel assisted in these activities, along with guarding devastated areas; serving survivors in Valdez and other outlying places; and assisting the Corps of Engineers in clearing slides, opening roads, and repairing railroads.[72] In addition, Air Force rescue units flew over 1,300 sorties and airlifted 374 people to safety.[73]

LESSONS LEARNED

Although her hospital had won praise for its performance in serving as Anchorage's major medical emergency center after the earthquake, Sister Barbara Ellen listed several lessons they had learned. First, the hospital needed a larger power plant for emergency power. Even though an emergency generator supplied power to key areas, such as the emergency room and surgery, the X-ray department, laboratory, pharmacy, Central Supply, and kitchen suffered serious operational problems owing to lack of electricity. Second, the City of Anchorage provided pumps to move nearby spring water into the hospital, and Sister Barbara Ellen believed that a permanent pump should be established at the spring site to ensure an adequate supply of drinking water. Third, it was the consensus of doctors and nurses that a system was needed to identify the vehicles of medical and nursing personnel to prevent the delays that occurred when they could not provide acceptable identification to guards. Fourth, some of the emergency supplies delivered to the hospital were outdated, including needed transfusion kits and blood substitutes. Last, the lack of a reliable communication system was problematic. Initially, Providence Hospital did not know how many patients to expect, and the medical facility was not notified of the demands that might be placed on it. The OCD had provided the hospital with a small radio unit with which to contact emergency operations centers, and Sister Barbara Ellen asked that this be permanently assigned to Providence Hospital.[74]

Sister Mary Elisa Lavoie, SP, Providence's pharmacist, also made recommendations for future preparedness. The pharmacy should be included on the auxiliary generator circuits or at least be provided with large extension cords that could quickly be plugged into emergency power outlets. She also recommended a ready supply of flashlights and reserve batteries. Because most of their drugs were locked in closed shelves, breakage was minimal; however, some were in gallon bottles that broke because they were located on smooth stainless steel shelves. The sisters had since ordered 3-inch lips installed across the bottom of all open shelves as a protective measure. They also were moving to replace glass gallon bottles with plastic. Importantly, the fact that Providence had a reserve supply of essential drugs enabled Sister Mary Elisa to provide prescribed medications for the general public and the 200 casualties that presented to Providence Hospital in the first hours after the earthquake.[75]

In 1969, the DRC summarized the inadequacy of disaster plans in Anchorage. It focused on the lack of communication to hospitals about the nature and extent of the initial damage, the damage to telephone facilities, and insufficient radio contact that hampered communication. In addition, an emergency coordinating center did not exist before the earthquake owing to lack of adequate planning. Finally, Anchorage had planned for a nuclear catastrophe, not an earthquake, and although Providence Hospital's disaster plan proved helpful, the city's existing disaster plan, which that called for evacuation to Seward, was inappropriate.[76]

FEDERAL POLICY CHANGES

The Alaska earthquake was one of the first disasters to directly lead to policy legislation when the Alaskan Earthquake Assistance Act (PL 88-451) passed in 1964.[77] As Birkland argued, "It rekindled interest in earthquake engineering nationally . . . and began a process in the federal government that eventually led to the enactment of the Earthquake Hazards Reduction Act in 1977 (PL 95-124)."[78]

Furthermore, in 1964 the Alaska earthquake was the beginning of a deadly occurrence of natural disasters over the next 18 months: Hurricanes Hilda and Betsy in the Southeast, a flood in the Northwest, and tornadoes throughout the Midwest. In all, over 500 people died during that time period. Thus, it was in the 1960s that the federal government began paying more attention to providing relief to people after disasters. Ted Steinberg asserted that "It was not so much the death toll or the exorbitant property damage as the fact that so many Americans felt the effects of natural catastrophe during a relatively brief period that distinguishes this chapter in the annals of calamity."[79] In 1969, the Disaster Relief Act (PL 91-79) passed; it placed management of federal assistance under a presidential appointee. Additional Disaster Relief Acts passed in 1970 (PL 91-606) and 1974 (PL 93-288). Congress established the Federal Emergency Management Agency in 1979 under President Jimmy Carter.[80]

CONCLUSION

The 1964 Alaska earthquake reveals key leadership requirements for nursing personnel. It also shows how such a dramatic event could act as a vehicle for policy change. After the earthquake, priorities included preservation of life, restoration and maintenance of utilities and communication, and reestablishment of order. In the first and third of these, nurses were active in both inpatient and public health facilities. In the process, their actions demonstrated a nuanced aspect of the role that gender plays during a disaster. Regarding Providence Hospital's response, Sister Philias pointed out a key skill needed during a disaster: leadership. She asserted that the "entire operation required leadership and control. . . . The fact that key people knew the hospital well and their co-workers and that Sister

[Barbara Ellen] would support them, resulted in the development of a rapidly improvised team."[81] Sister Barbara Ellen earned her authority by exercising judgment that commanded respect and obedience. In addition, women nurses participated in the hard physical and psychological work of providing relief to survivors. While male Red Cross case workers did search and rescue operations in Alaska's rugged mountains, Red Cross female nurses supervised their work.

This disaster experience also shows that even though emergency systems were damaged, nurses' overall capacity to respond to the emergency was not compromised. As one school nurse noted, "It should be repeatedly emphasized that these clinics and their success were only possible with the labor of many nurses."[82] On the other hand, to enhance future preparedness, Bullard, who had encountered an unorganized Red Cross nursing service in the local chapters, recommended that more disaster nursing conferences be held.[83]

Any disaster plan must be based on systematic knowledge about disaster responses, which historical evidence can provide yet no universal disaster plan can be carried out without an understanding of the influence of time and place on disaster responses. Indeed, much can happen that disaster planning may not anticipate. As the Anchorage experience showed, the plan needed to address all types of disasters that the state would likely face, not just nuclear calamities. At the same time, while providing basic instructions, any plan had to be flexible enough to allow for on-the-spot creativity.

STUDY QUESTIONS

1. As a nurse working in a disaster, how can you prevent panic in others and in yourself?
2. After a disaster, it is not unusual for on-duty personnel to experience conflict between their hospital responsibilities and their family obligations. We do not know if nurses had a choice to immediately leave the disaster area to care for their families or whether or not single nurses stayed while married nurses with families left. Discuss nurses' "duty" to care.

3. How can you plan for an earthquake? Where should efforts go? How would one teach disaster planning?
4. What do professionals need to do to take a leadership role? What aspects of the leadership role are critical to disaster management?

NOTES

1. Noted in Ed Fortier to Dr. Elizabeth Tower, editor, *Alaska Magazine*, n.d. (160) EQ Reports, Providence Alaska Medical Center (hereafter PAMC), Providence Archives, Mother Joseph Province, Seattle, WA (hereafter SPA).
2. Ed Fortier, "How Providence Withstood the Quake Ordeal," *Hospital Progress* (May 1964): 8. The Great Chilean Earthquake in May of 1960 was the most powerful ever recorded, rating 9.5 on the moment magnitude scale. See http://en.wikipedia.org/wiki/Great_Chilean_Earthquake (accessed October 8, 2009).
3. "Here's Official Quake Result," *Daily News*, November 3, 1967, box 32, 1964 Earthquake; and "Alaskan Quake," *Plastichrome Travel Series*, Special Event Edition, Series C, vol. 315, B9116 (160) PAMC, box 33, 1964 Earthquake, SPA. See also http://www.anchorage.net/822.cfm (accessed October 2, 2009).
4. Thomas A. Birkland, *Lessons of Disaster: Policy Change After Catastrophic Events* (Washington, DC: Georgetown University Press, 2006), 132.
5. Maureen P. Hogan and Timothy Pursell, "The Real Alaskan," *Men and Masculinities* 11, no. 1 (2008): 63–85.
6. Barbra Mann Wall, *Unlikely Entrepreneurs: Catholic Sisters and the Hospital Marketplace, 1865–1925* (Columbus: Ohio State University Press, 2005).
7. Carol K. Coburn and Martha Smith, *Spirited Lives: How Nuns Shaped Catholic Culture and American Life, 1836–1920* (Chapel Hill: University of North Carolina Press, 1999); Wall, *Unlikely Entrepreneurs*.
8. Sister Barbara Ellen was born and reared in Portland, Oregon, and graduated from St. Joseph's Training School in Vancouver, Washington. My thanks go to archivist Loretta Greene for this information. Only 3 years earlier, in 1959, Alaska had become the country's 49th state.
9. Providence Anchorage Medical Center, *Chronicles, 1952–1968*, March 27, 1964, SPA.
10. Daniel Yutzy and J. Eugene Haas, "Disaster and Functional Priorities in Anchorage, Alaska," draft prepared for use the Geography Panel at the National Academy of Science's Committee on the Alaska Earthquake, April 1967. Disaster Research Center, University of Delaware, Newark (hereafter DRC).

11. Fortier, "How Providence Withstood the Quake Ordeal," 8.

12. J. Eugene Haas, "Some Preliminary Observations on the Responses of Community Organizations Involved in the Emergency Period of the Alaskan Earthquake," Working Paper 2, 1964, DRC.

13. Frank B. Norton and J. Eugene Haas, "Disaster Narratives," Working Paper 9, 1967, DRC.

14. Special Report, "Hospitals and the Alaskan Earthquake," *Hospitals: Journal of the American Hospital Association, 38* (1964): 23A–24A.

15. Haas, "Some Preliminary Observations."

16. Providence Anchorage Medical Center, *Chronicles.*

17. Ibid.

18. Haas, "Some Preliminary Observations," 26.

19. Ibid. Sister Philias Denis, SP, "Three C's for an Operating Room in Disaster;" (160) PAMC, box 32, 1964 Earthquake, SPA; and Dr. Don Val Langston, "A Hospital in a Disaster Area," *Journal of the American Medical Association, 189* (1964): 306–307.

20. Haas, "Some Preliminary Observations."

21. Denis, "Three C's."

22. Ed Fortier, "Providence Hospital Employees Unshaken by Earthquake Crisis," *Anchorage Daily Times*, March 31, 1964.

23. Haas, "Some Preliminary Observations."

24. Office of Civil Defense, "The Alaskan Earthquake" (Washington, DC: Office of Secretary of the Army, Department of Defense, May 1964).

25. Thomas R. McGowan, "Emergency Health Service in an Alaskan Disaster," *Alaska Medicine 6*, no. 2 (1964): 36–38.

26. Office of Public Information, Western Area, American Red Cross, "Nurses Answer Call Quickly for Alaskan Disaster Duty," American Red Cross Office, Anchorage, Alaska. Quotation is on p. 37. Located in SPA. See also Haas, "Some Preliminary Observations."

27. Arne Beltz, "Greater Anchorage Health District," *The Alaska Nurse XIII*, no. 4 (1964): 8.

28. Elva Scott, "School Nurses—Anchorage," ibid., 3, 6. By the 1950s, commercial milk formulas were available for all social classes.

29. Ibid., 9.

30. Ibid.

31. Beryl A. Bonehill, "Prince William Sound Area as Seen by a PHN After Alaska's Disaster," in ibid., 10.

32. American Red Cross of Alaska, "A Brief History of the American Red Cross of Alaska," http://www.alaska.redcross.org/index.php?pr=History (accessed October 25, 2008).

33. Office of Public Information, "Nurses Answer Call Quickly." See also Thomas G. Hays to Richard F. Gordon, "Medical Narrative Summary, Alaskan Earthquake," RG 200, National Archives Gift Collection, Records of the American National Red Cross, 1947–1964, box 1772, folder DR810.08, Statistical Highlights; National Archives Building, College Park, Maryland (hereafter NABCP).

34. Hays to Gordon, NABCP.

35. Sigrid H. Bullard, "Summary Nursing Services from March 28-May 5, 1964," RG 200, National Archives Gift Collection, Records of the American National Red Cross, 1947–1964, box 1772, folder DR810.08, Final Reports Alaskan Earthquake, NABCP.

36. Jane Mary Farley, "Alaskan Earthquake Jolts Nurse's Schedule," *The Milwaukee Journal*, April 26, 1964.

37. Catherine Blasena, "Nursing Narrative Report," RG 200, National Archives Gift Collection, Records of the American National Red Cross, 1947–1964, box 1772, folder DR810.08, Final Reports Alaskan Earthquake, NABCP.

38. Ruth Benson, "Fairbanks Reports," *The Alaska Nurse XIII*, no. 4 (1964): 11.

39. Blasena, "Nursing Narrative Report."

40. Grace Anderson, "Harborview Nursing Home," *The Alaska Nurse XIII*, no. 4 (1964): 3.

41. Helen Hartigan, "Juneau Reports," *The Alaska Nurse XIII*, no. 4 (1964): 13–14. Quotation is on p. 13.

42. Lillian Thorn, "Impressions From Seward Nurses," *The Alaska Nurse XIII*, no. 4 (1964): 5.

43. Elsie Blue, "Seward General Hospital," *The Alaska Nurse XIII*, no. 4 (1964): 1, 5. Quotation is on p. 1.

44. Office of Public Information, "Nurses Answer Call Quickly."

45. Farley, "Alaskan Earthquake."

46. Ibid., 38.

47. R. L. Bohannon, Letter to All Medical Service Personnel, *Medical Service Digest XV*, no. IX (1964).

48. Ed Fortier to Sister Benedict, June 3, 1964; (160) PAMC, Box 321964, 1964 Earthquake Correspondence, SPA.

49. Sister Barbara Ellen Lundberg, SP, to Mr. Jack Collins, California Medical Association, April 27, 1964; (160) PAMC, box 32, 1964 Earthquake, Misc., Letters, Contributions; and Ed Fortier to Sister Barbara Ellen, April 10, 1964; (160) PAMC, box 32, 1964 Earthquake, Accounts, Resolutions; SPA. See also "Nurses' Group to Hear Talk on Earthquake," *Daily News*, November 13, 1964.

50. Helen Bernstein to Ed Fortier, June 4, 1964; (160) PAMC, box 32, 1964 Earthquake, Accounts, Articles, SPA.

51. Haas, "Some Preliminary Observations;" Denis, "Three C's."
52. E. J. Fortier, "Observations for Sister Philias on Providence Hospital and Earth-quake Prepared Exclusively for Sister Philias by E.J. Fortier, Last Territo-rial and First State Civil Defense Director," (160) PAMC, box 32, 1964 Earthquake, SPA.
53. Fortier to Tower.
54. For further discussion on gendered language, see Kristina Minister, "A Femi-nist Frame for the Oral History Interview," in *Women's Words: The Femi-nist Practice of Oral History*, eds. Sherna Berger Gluck and Daphne Patai (New York: Routledge, 1991), 35.
55. Fortier to Tower; Denis, "Three C's."
56. Office of Civil Defense, "The Alaskan Earthquake."
57. Ibid.
58. Haas, "Some Preliminary Observations."
59. Sister Barbara Ellen Lundberg, SP, "Alaska's New Providence—Serving a New State," *Hospital Topics* (April 1964): n.p.
60. Yutzy and Haas, "Disaster and Functional Priorities."
61. Thomas A. Birkland and Regina G. Lawrence, "The Exxon Valdez and Alaska in the American Imagination," in *American Disasters*, ed. Steven Biel (New York: New York University Press, 2001), 399.
62. Birkland, *Lessons of Disaster*, 133.
63. Ibid. See also National Research Council, Committee on the Alaska Earth-quake, *The Great Alaska Earthquake of 1964* (Washington, DC: National Academy of Sciences, 1968–1973); http://www.dggs.dnr.state.ak.us/pubs/pubs?reqtype=series&abbrev=P&abbrevID=217&seriesname=Profession al%20Paper&publisher=USGS; http://www.dggs.dnr.state.ak.us/webpubs/usgs/p/text/p0543i.PDF; and http://www.pnsn.org/HIST_CAT/1964.html (accessed August 14, 2008).
64. E.L. Quarantelli, "Organizational Behavior in Disasters and Implications for Disaster Planning," Disaster Research Center Report Series 18, 1985, DRC. See also E.L. Quarantelli and Russell R. Dynes, "Images of Disaster Behav-ior: Myths and Consequences," Working Paper 37, 1971; DRC.
65. Quarantelli, "Organizational Behavior," p. 8. An earlier study was authored by Charles E. Fritz and Harry B. Williams: "The Human Being in Disaster: A Research Perspective," *Annals of the American Academy of Political and Social Science*, 309 (January 1957): 46.
66. Quarantelli and Dynes, "Images of Disaster Behavior"; 4, DRC.
67. Denis, "Three C's."
68. Ibid., 3.
69. Haas, "Some Preliminary Observations."
70. Fortier, "Observations for Sister Philias."

71. Letters to agencies located in RG 200, National Archives Gift Collection, Records of the American National Red Cross, 1947–1964, box 1772, folder DR–810.02, "Cooperation With Other Agencies," NABCP.

72. Office of Civil Defense, "The Alaskan Earthquake," 14; "Mighty Earthquake Took Tragic Toll in Alaska," *Anchorage Daily Times*, April 14, 1964, 3–4.

73. Col. Herbert H. Kerr, "Medical Disaster Operations in the Alaskan Earthquake," (160) PAMC, box 32, 1964 Earthquake, p. 13, SPA.

74. Sister Barbara Ellen Lundberg, SP, to Mr. Warren Griffin, May 14, 1964; (160) PAMC, box 32, 1964 Earthquake, SPA. Griffin was a member of the Greater Anchorage Health Mobilization organization.

75. Sister Mary Elisa Lavoie, SP, "Alaska's Great Earthquake: Operation of Providence Hospital's Pharmacy," *Journal Mond. Pharm.* 3 (1964): 213–216.

76. Arnold L. Parr, "A Brief View on the Adequacy and Inadequacy of Disaster Plans and Preparations in Ten Community Crises," June 1969. DRC, Working Paper 17.

77. Rutherford H. Platt, *Disasters and Democracy: The Politics of Extreme Natural Events* (Washington, DC: Island Press, 1999), 13.

78. Birkland, *Lessons of Disaster*, 133.

79. Ted Steinberg, *Acts of God: The Unnatural History of Natural Disaster in America* (New York: Oxford University Press, 2000). Quotation is on p. 175.

80. Platt, *Disasters and Democracy*, 13.

81. Denis, "Three C's," 6.

82. "Nurses' Group to Hear Talk on Earthquake," *Daily News*, November 13, 1964.

83. Bullard, "Summary Nursing Services."

Part II

CHAPTER 11

Gendered Notions of Expertise and Bravery: New York City 2001

Julie A. Fairman and Jonathan Gilbride

Nurses and physicians working in hospitals respond to disasters on a daily basis. From hemorrhage in the operating room to cardiac arrest at night in the intensive care unit (ICU), from the respiratory arrest of a baby in the nursery to the utter chaos of scale on the general floors, disasters occur on many levels, both natural and human made. Health professionals are trained to be prepared for the unexpected, whatever that may be. But one can undertake as much training as possible and still find oneself in situations where policies and protocols no longer apply, where the traditional boundaries between health professionals vanish and emerge according to expediency and patient need. These are the gray areas where the typical, and highly gendered, notions of expertise and role become fluid, emotionally charged.

This, then, is a "hospital tale," the kind of story not always at the forefront of the news, and usually highly gendered.[1] The stories are the telling of tales, usually by women caring for relatives or within the boundaries of, in this case, the nursing profession. As Prue Chamberlaine and Annette King described it, "hospitals form a politically salient meeting ground of public authority and personal intimacy."[2] They are a place of continuous nurturing, and cycles of grief and joy—unlike wars, the stories of hospitals are not single events.

Outside of the Civil War, our country has never seen a disaster to the extent of the destruction of the Twin Towers in New York on September 11, 2001. Although New York health care personnel, both in the fire department and in its many hospitals, routinely practiced disaster drills, no one expected a disaster of this scale at this time. One nurse recalled the following:

> I went to work at New York-Presbyterian Cornell Medical Center in New York City on September 11th as a critical care nurse in the William Randolph Hearst Burn Center, the nation's largest and busiest specialized inpatient center for the treatment of traumatic burn injuries. The morning of September 11th was beautiful; it was a cool, clear day in Manhattan and I remember wishing that I had the day off.
>
> In recent weeks, the Burn ICU had become busy. Typically, the fall season is characterized by an increased incidence of burn injuries, and our census had been on the rise . . . I began the day precepting a new nurse who was approaching the end of her orientation period. We were taking care of a critical care patient who had suffered thermal burns and a smoke inhalation injury. I anticipated a busy but typical day in the Burn Center.[3]

During conflicts and crises, such as the destruction in New York on September 11, 2001, people involved in rescue and relief work tend to break down traditional boundaries in order to respond to the emergency. There is no time to argue about professional prerogatives or roles. "Getting the job done," whether putting out fires or preparing a hospital for a large-scale admission of casualties, blurs categories such as gender, class, race, and ethnicity—if only temporarily.

In health care, where crises of multiple layers occur daily, people respond as they believe they are morally obligated and tend to rise to the level of intensity required by the situational crises. The nurse working in the Cornell Burn Unit noted:

> If you're a health care professional, you know what supplies and equipment you need in preparation for major emergencies. It doesn't matter what you were trained as. First, you need empty rooms and space for patients. Second, you need countless numbers of IV fluid bags and IV lines along with mechanical ventilators and emergency medical supplies.[4]

The height of the polio epidemic in Denmark in the early 1950s offers one such example: "At one time during the epidemic when 900 polio patients had already been admitted, 75 patients were under manual artificial ventilation on the same day. For this, it was necessary to employ 250 medical students to do the ventilation, 260 nurses to attend to patient requirements, and 27 hospital workers to change [ten-gallon] cylinders and attend to the machines."[5] In this example, roles are well demarcated—medical students hand-ventilated patients, nurses provided personal care, and anesthesiologists directed the care.[6]

The ICUs of the 1950s provide a different example of fluid, informal strategies both nurses and physicians used during times of crises. When a patient's condition changed rapidly and the time needed to follow protocols did not exist, then neither did the protocols; fluid expertise jurisdiction was necessary. Situational credentialing—giving nurses the unspoken authority to respond to particular patient care situations—allowed nurses and physicians to temporarily discard traditional patterns of communication and behavior. For example, nurses diagnosed and initiated treatment at night when physicians were unavailable. As one nurse noted, "I was there, he wasn't, and some decisions had to be made right then. If you found the physician [at home and waited] it might be too late. . . . I didn't want to lose the patient."[7]

In so many ways, the 9/11 disaster was on a different level during a different time and context. From the time the first plane hit, trauma units all over the city prepared for the victims who, for many medical centers, never came. The Cornell Burn Unit, however, received most surviving victims. There, as in the other medical centers, the health care professionals in the unit prepared for a large admission of patients:

> The second big event of the morning immediately altered Burn Unit activity. Our multidisciplinary staff of nurses, physicians, physical and occupational therapists, respiratory therapists, and ancillary personnel prepared for what would turn out to be the most memorable day in Burn Unit history. In response to the alarming events near Wall Street, our staff started the process of transferring our current patients to our step-down unit in anticipation of the arrival of burn victims from the World Trade Center. The nurse orientee was prepared to be fully responsible for her current patient so that I could accept the admission of a second patient, who would be arriving from the World Trade Center site.[8]

At this point, a sort of triage already had occurred—the less experienced nurse took over the care of a less critical patient so that the experienced nurse could accept a more critically ill patient. From their previous experience, the more seasoned nurses believed they knew what to expect of newly burned patients in terms of complexity of care, or thought they did:

The patient I admitted on 9/11 arrived at approximately 10:30 in the morning. She was a middle aged woman . . . She had been near an elevator in World Trade 1, somewhere between the 50th and 60th floors when the first plane hit. A fireball traveling through the elevator shaft engulfed her in flames. She managed to climb down 50 or 60 floors with the aid [of] kind strangers to an Emergency Transport vehicle, which brought her to New York Hospital. She was already intubated upon her arrival to her room in our Burn Center, being ventilated via an Ambu bag. Her clothes and accompanying pocketbook were charred. Initially, we did not know her name. We gave her the name "Urgent 12" to temporarily identify her. I hooked her up to an EKG monitor and placed her on a ventilator.

She was responsive, occasionally opening her eyes sluggishly and weakly moving her arms and legs. I reassured her as best as I could by talking calmly to her and telling her that I was going to take good care of her. My initial assessment of her found that she had suffered deep 3rd degree burns to both her arms and legs, face, abdomen and 2/3 of her back. She had been burned over 65% of her body, and suffered smoke inhalation. One of my colleagues admitted a patient who had 3rd degree burns over 100% of his body.[9]

In his 15 years in burn nursing, he had never before seen a patient who suffered a 100% total body surface area burn involvement. "Even the soles of his feet had been burned."[10]

The care of a patient with extensive burns requires exquisite and highly specialized knowledge of the physiology of the skin, fluid and electrolyte balance, and cardiac and renal functions. Both physicians and nurses must be experts in these areas, as well as be highly proficient in resuscitation. The nurse continued the story:

After completing my initial assessment, I placed my patient on rapid fluid resuscitation. It is not uncommon for burn patients with large burns to receive 24 liters of fluid during the first day of hospitalization in order to counteract the [shock] state typical during the initial emergent phase of burn injury. My patient was set to receive an initial rate of 1/2 a liter of IV fluid an hour in order to maintain her blood pressure in normal ranges.[11]

In this burn unit, as in most critical care units, the personnel at all levels were prepared to care for large-scale casualties and for different types of providers to merge into a highly competent team.

From this point on, our multidisciplinary team divided into 1 nurse/1 physician teams in order to meet the needs of our victims. I worked with a 4th year resident for most of the day. In the room with my patient, I was the "charge nurse" and N. was the "charge doctor." These "titles" were not meant to represent a hierarchy, rather to represent some sort [of] structured order during a time of extreme chaos and disorganization.

Included in my room were 1–3 nurses at different times of the day, a handful of physical therapists [who] functioned as nurse's aide[s], and 2 or 3 other doctors to aid N. in the placement of chest tubes and other medical interventions requiring more than 2 hands. N. and I relied on each other heavily throughout the morning and afternoon, supporting each other emotionally.[12]

Each team member had a specific function, but over several hours the boundaries between them were more porous and melding:

Thinking back on my experience, I recall with interest the central role that the nursing staff played during this initial preparation period. We immediately asked many of the physical therapists to begin the process of priming intravenous fluid bags so we could tend to other more pressing concerns. I also recall how the responsibilities of medical professionals during this period converged: It was difficult to discern a physician from a nurse from a physical therapist. Our roles and responsibilities, often well demarcated, lost their boundaries during this period of crisis. The theoretical and practical knowledge common to health care professionals like nurses, physicians and therapists became more translucent. Traditional responsibilities of each health care professional, often defined in the context of a professional's scope of practice, state laws, and hospital policy and procedure manuals, became irrelevant during the morning of September 11th.[13]

The work was made more difficult by the emotions and fears the staff experienced:

It's difficult for me to describe the emotions I was feeling during the first day of the crisis because there were so many of them. First and foremost, I was scared. Rumors were being spread around the Burn Unit that there were potentially more hijacked planes in the air around the city. I think the fact that all of us were too busy to look at CNN or fully hear news reports contributed to the hearsay that I recall from the early part of the day. I was scared to be in Manhattan but fortunately didn't have much time to think about my safety. In addition to fear, at various times throughout the day I felt sadness, anger, surprise, reassurance, disappointment, loss, and confusion.[14]

When we think about 9/11, we perhaps think primarily about the heroes and heroines who tried to save the people and the buildings. In many ways, theirs are narratives of war. As Alessandro Portelli notes, "war embodies history; having been to war is the most immediately tangible claim for having been in history. Even in peacetime, the military is the most immediately accessible experience of the public sphere."[15]

The stories included here, the "hospital tales," were told by a nurse who is male, thus providing an extra degree of complexity to our traditional gendered assumptions. He speaks from the vantage point of a profession traditionally considered female, but his language is decidedly scientific, technical, and infused with a great deal of expertise similar to another highly gendered profession, that of medicine. His stories also embody an almost militarist sense of preparation for a war—that of a war against death, while at the same time, promising to take "good care" of the patient and talking with her to try to soothe at least a little of what must have been tremendous fear and pain. During the long hours he spent in the unit during the disaster, it must have become clear to him that he was doing something heroic, although this was a job he was trained to do without hesitation. But what he remembers is the bravery of his patients and their families, visiting daily for weeks and months.

This oral history shows how disasters test gendered notions of expertise and bravery. His is a story that brings together images of wars and hospitals. By hearing about both, we may begin to reformulate our sense of suffering and the skills and strength needed to deal with the suffering either through emotional support or battle-ready technical know-how. This is the part of the story that sometimes goes unacknowledged and untold. In *Necessary Targets*, Eve Ensler wrote, "When we think of war, we think of it as something that happens to men in fields or jungles. We think of hand grenades and Scud missiles . . . But after the bombing, after the snipers, that's when the real war begins."[16] By bearing witness through his stories, the nurse featured in this chapter brings this point home to us in poignant detail.

While his story reveals the personal trauma of a single case, it can also illustrate how the masculinization of heroism can be a complicated issue. Gilbride's and other nurses' stories provide a different look to journalist

Cathy Young's argument that "it's overwhelmingly men who put their lives on the line in dangerous jobs," referring to the firemen and police officers who were "the heroes of the World Trade Center" and "the male passengers of United Airlines Flight 93 who foiled the highjackers' plan to use the plane as a missile."[17]

This story also provides another lesson. As Nancy Tomes asserts, more recent stories have documented how lack of trust, communication, and coordination impeded the response of fire and law enforcement personnel after the 9/11 disaster. This chapter, then, offers insights into how other responders to disasters could benefit by observing in ICUs where nurses, physicians, and other health care workers cooperate and communicate daily under extreme pressure.[18]

STUDY QUESTIONS

1. How did the 9/11 catastrophe break down traditional distinctions between physicians' and nurses' areas of expertise?
2. How does this chapter add to understandings about the gendered attributes of heroes?
3. Has the war on terrorism ushered in a restoration of traditional gender roles, that is, the "manly man" and "feminine woman"?

NOTES

1. Alessandro Portelli, *The Battle of Valle Giulia: Oral History and the Art of Dialogue* (Madison: University of Wisconsin Press, 1997), 7.
2. Prue Chamberlaine and Annette King, "Carers' Narratives as Genre: An East–West German Comparison," *International Yearbook of Oral History and Life Stories,* vol. 5 (unpublished volume), quoted by Portelli, *The Battle,* 8.
3. Jonathan Gilbride, unpublished manuscript, April 19, 2002.
4. Ibid.
5. "Preliminary Report on the 1952 Epidemic of Poliomyelitis in Copenhagen," *Lancet* (1953): 1, 37.
6. Mark Hilberman, "The Evolution of Intensive Care Units," *Critical Care Medicine* (1975): 3, 159–165.

7. Cheryl Larson, telephone interview with Julie Fairman, September 7, 1989, as quoted by Julie Fairman and Joan Lynaugh, *Critical Care Nursing: A History* (Philadelphia: University of Pennsylvania Press, 1998), 74.

8. Gilbride, unpublished manuscript.

9. Ibid.

10. Ibid.

11. Ibid.

12. Ibid.

13. Ibid.

14. Ibid.

15. Portelli, *The Battle*, 7.

16. Eve Ensler, *Necessary Targets* (New York: Villard, 2001), as quoted by Nancy Franklin, "War Stories: Revisiting the Ruins of Bosnia," *New Yorker,* March 11, 2002, 91.

17. Cathy Young, "Feminism's Slide Since Sept. 22," *Boston Globe*, September 16, 2002, A-15.

18. Nancy Tomes, "Reflections on September 11: A Symposium," *Journal of the History of Medicine and Allied Sciences* 58, no. 4 (2003): 428–432; and Jim Dwyer, Kevin Flynn, and Ford Fessenden, "Fatal Confusion: A Troubled Emergency Response," *New York Times,* July 7, 2001, I-1.

CHAPTER 12

A Tale of Two Shelters:
A Katrina Story, 2005

Teresa M. O'Neill and Patricia M. Prechter

On August 29, 2005, Hurricane Katrina hit the city of New Orleans and crushed more than 150 miles of coastline along the Gulf of Mexico. While not comparable to the 1900 Galveston hurricane in terms of deaths, the death toll was still high at more than 1,800. Eighty-one billion dollars in damages occurred and one million people were displaced. With winds of 150 miles per hour, the hurricane caused a storm surge of 25 feet. When New Orleans' levees and floodwalls were breached, 80 percent of the city flooded and remained so for weeks.[1]

The following is an account from two nurses who experienced Hurricane Katrina first hand as they provided care and support to the survivors of this disaster. Patricia M. Prechter is a professor and chair of Nursing at Our Lady of Holy Cross College in New Orleans and was a colonel in the Louisiana National Guard: she retired in February 2008. Teresa M. O'Neill is a nurse and professor at Our Lady of Holy Cross College in New Orleans. These are their personal stories and are not meant to tell the complete saga of Katrina; indeed, the Katrina historiography will be written for many years. Rather, this is a tale conveying a portion of elements reflecting conditions at two shelters: one, the shelter of last resort, the Superdome, where Colonel Prechter was deputy commander of the Louisiana Medical Command; and the other, a shelter located west of New Orleans in Gonzales, Louisiana, where Professor O'Neill volunteered after evacuating to that area. This story does not represent all nurses, nor can it ever represent all those delivering health care or maintaining the health of the population affected by Katrina. Rather, it is a tale of two shelters.

Much has been written about the Superdome (otherwise known as the Dome), but less if anything has been written regarding the Lamar-Dixon Expo Center in Gonzales, which sheltered as many as 1,900 people in a building designed for 1,200. In both the Superdome and Lamar-Dixon, nursing care was given to help those within its confines. Though not as dramatic as conditions in the Dome, the care given to those at Lamar-Dixon reduced or eliminated the need for additional medical care in the Gonzales–Baton Rouge area, and in so doing reduced the impact of stressors placed on the local medical infrastructure.

SETTING THE STAGE

Teresa M. O'Neill

The 2005 hurricane season was notable for its numbers: 28 named storms, with 15 reaching hurricane status. Of these, four were Category 5 storms, and four of the major hurricanes hit the United States.[2] Hurricane Ivan gave New Orleans a scare in 2004, resulting in the municipal authorities calling for a voluntary evacuation of the city. Ivan veered east, making landfall by Gulf Shores, Alabama, and devastating that area. New Orleans, however, had dodged the bullet.

The last major hurricane to hit New Orleans was Hurricane Betsy in 1965, a Category 4 hurricane still in the consciousness of those who lived through it. Though landfall with Betsy actually occurred 95 miles southwest of New Orleans, storm damage to the city resulted from its location in the northeast sector of the hurricane zone, where the most intense winds and rain typically happen. Gusting winds of 125 mph hit New Orleans, causing the worst flooding in decades, most notably in the city's Ninth Ward.[3] Still, the major damage had been to property and, while regrettable, loss of life in Louisiana was limited to 58 people.

It was in 1965, in response to Betsy's flooding, that the Orleans Levee Board raised the levees to 12 feet to safeguard life and property.[4] Another hurricane in 1969, Hurricane Camille, was a Category 5 storm that caused property damage to New Orleans, but its major impact and devastation were to the Mississippi Gulf Coast, where it made landfall. Thereafter, complacency regarding hurricanes slowly wove its way into the city's fabric. Those who experienced Betsy grew older or died, and as the years progressed the terror of that storm faded from public consciousness.

Hurricane season spans June 1 to November 30. During that time, people in hurricane-prone areas are exhorted to have a "hurricane plan."

Gathering nonperishable food items and having sufficient batteries, lanterns, and charcoal in the case of electrical failure are among the tasks one completes during hurricane season. Buying "hurricane food" is a common ritual in New Orleans and surrounding areas in summer, when stores advertise specials on canned foods such as chili, red beans, spaghettios, and other foods that do not need special preparation to eat.

Evacuation in the event of a storm prior to Katrina was not considered a serious component of hurricane preparation. After all, New Orleans had not had serious flooding or damage from a hurricane since Betsy, and many in the city deemed New Orleans safe. Others looked at folk wisdom: Because the New Orleans Saints football team was a perennial poor finisher in the NFL, it provided the trade-off to hurricane protection. Also, the power of prayer had worked in the Battle of New Orleans in the War of 1812, and thus far it had worked for hurricane protection.

The 1990s saw a slight upsurge in hurricane activity in the area, but not much. In 1992, Andrew caused a run on plywood to protect windows, but it had its worst impact on Florida and the southern part of Louisiana in Plaquemines Parish, not as far north as New Orleans. The public's concern about hurricanes and their impact on New Orleans resurged in 1998 with Hurricane Georges as its projected path showed a heading toward the city. A slow-moving storm, Georges's winds created a storm surge and damage to camps located outside the levee protection areas along Lake Ponchartrain, causing some flooding that did more damage than the actual storm in New Orleans. At what seemed the last minute, however, Georges moved east and made landfall in Biloxi, bringing only wind and some rain to the New Orleans area. The city had dodged another bullet.

Yet the threat from Georges alarmed municipal authorities sufficiently to call for a voluntary evacuation of the New Orleans population. The Superdome opened as a storm shelter, and an estimated 14,000 people went there for protection. Afterward, the Superdome management reported widespread vandalism and property theft, causing them to state that never again would it be used as a shelter of last resort.[5]

Hurricane Georges highlighted the city of New Orleans' vulnerability in many areas, most notably in levee protection and, more importantly, the safety of the citizens who lived in low-lying areas. Contrary to accepted wisdom, New Orleans does not lie totally below sea level; many areas are slightly above it. The levees surrounding the city are higher than the existing land they protect. Prior to levee construction, natural flooding from the Mississippi in certain areas served to build up the land. The levees removed that natural rebuilding, and as the 20th century progressed, areas that had formerly been swamps were drained or filled in to enable building construction.

Hurricane Georges underscored the need for an evacuation program because, as noted earlier, the Superdome management stated that the facility would never again be used as a hurricane protection shelter. A city with a poor population dependent on public transport, however, was a city that was dependent on a centrally located facility that could shelter a population with no other place to go. As time passed after Georges, the Dome management agreed to let its building be the shelter of last resort but with caveats: Those using the Dome had to bring their own food and water. It was a shelter to be used only for protection; it was not one that would provide food or other supplies.

Hurricane Ivan in 2004 posed the most serious threat to New Orleans since Betsy in 1965. Again, a voluntary evacuation was called for residents of the metropolitan area as Ivan's westerly path showed a likely impact on New Orleans. Improved hurricane tracking and forecasting and the strengthening of this storm to a Category 5 (later lessening to a Category 4) resulted in over 1 million people evacuating the area, which caused unanticipated massive traffic jams. A 70-mile trip from New Orleans to Baton Rouge, usually less than a 90-minute journey, stretched to eight hours as vehicles crept along the interstates. Those without transportation had to find local shelters. The Superdome opened as an agency of last resort, but with cautions to people coming to provide their own supplies as none would be provided for them. As it turned out, Ivan did not strike New Orleans, and the people heaved a sigh of relief as they dodged the bullet yet again. It was only a matter of time, however, before their luck would run out.

HURRICANE SEASON 2005

Teresa M. O'Neill

In 2005, New Orleans had already been affected by a hurricane when Cindy, the season's third tropical storm, hit on July 5. Winds and rains from Cindy, a Category 1 storm, caused minimal damage, though they also caused the largest blackout since Betsy. By August 23, the twelfth tropical storm of the season had formed and, in keeping with the alphabetical naming of storms, became Katrina. Initially a mild storm, Katrina rapidly intensified and appeared to be headed to the Florida panhandle until the evening of August 26, when its path changed and put it on a trajectory toward New Orleans. With its projected path, this was the storm feared by all—similar to Betsy but with a higher category of intensity, bearing down on a city that had not truly tested its official hurricane plan for safeguarding its populace. On Sunday, August 28, New Orleans Mayor Ray Nagin ordered a mandatory evacuation for the first time ever. Having learned the lessons from the traffic debacle of Ivan the previous year, contraflow traffic patterns were initiated to facilitate evacuation away from the area. It is estimated that between 80% and 90% of the metropolitan area evacuated.[6] The remaining populace, however, including many of the sick and poor, did not have the transportation to leave. Again, the Superdome was opened as a shelter facility, with the same dictates as in Ivan: shelter only. Those evacuating to the Dome had to bring their own food and supplies.

THE START OF THE STORY: SATURDAY, AUGUST 27, 2005

Colonel Patricia M. Prechter

On Saturday, August 27, the Louisiana National Guard called 4,000 troops into service, including the medical unit at Jackson barracks in New Orleans. I was State Chief Nurse and Deputy Commander of the Louisiana Army National Guard. I must admit I did not hurry to the barracks because in the back of my mind I thought it was another one of "those alarms." I actually went by the bank and got some cash.[7] When I got to the barracks to attend the operations meeting regarding the storm, I could sense the tension in the room.

My assignment was to call in at least 71 people to go to the Superdome on Sunday. Like other hurricane missions, I thought it would not be a difficult one. I thought it would be another one of those times when we went to the Dome and, in a couple of days, went home. I returned to my house and prepared to report to the Dome on Sunday morning, August 28, at 8:00 a.m. I had not heard the news all day, and, upon arriving at home and hearing about the intensity of the storm, I became concerned. The National

Hurricane Center had raised the hurricane watch to a warning. The news was very bad, and so then not only did I begin to think about myself, but I worried a lot about my husband and my son, because they were going to have a lot to do Sunday without me to get ready to go, and then I began to think, "Where were they going to go?"[8]

Teresa M. O'Neill

At the same time, the local Red Cross for the Baton Rouge area began plans to open a shelter at Dutchtown High School (HS) in Prairieville, Louisiana. Local Red Cross chapters typically plan for a 3-day shelter oversight until the national organization takes control.[9]

SUNDAY, AUGUST 28

Colonel Patricia M. Prechter

By Sunday, August 28, Katrina had been rated as a Category 4 hurricane. That morning at Jackson Barracks, the expected buses to transport the medical detachment had not been ordered, requiring the National Guard unit to be convoyed by personal vehicles to the Dome, a decision that, later, became a benefit for some. All they had left when the storm was over was the car they had with them.

The Guard's mission was to set up a special medical needs unit in the Superdome. Special-needs considerations included requiring help with daily activities. To be admitted to the special-needs area, one had to be accompanied by a caretaker because we did not have enough staff to take care of the person. That caretaker, would administer the medications or change the dressings, whatever was needed. In addition, those coming to the special-needs unit had to bring all their supplies. We had no equipment. We would just be there to help if needed.

Thousands of people had already come to the Dome for shelter that Sunday morning when the detachment arrived. An area was provided for the detachment on the second floor to serve as a medical command area. Detachment personnel were organized to work in 12-hour shifts, dispersing doctors, nurses, medics, and administrative personnel between the shifts. Some physicians in the detachment were emergency room (ER) doctors, and they were assigned to the day shift because we believed the needs would most arise during these hours. The special-care patients checked in on the loading dock on the ground floor of the Dome, where New Orleans Health Department (NOHD) personnel determined who needed special care. After being checked in, they were sent to my National Guard detachment area. This check-in procedure, however, quickly broke down.

Around 1:00 p.m., a sergeant came to me and said, "They're sending up the wrong kind of patients here." I then realized that we did have patients in the area who required dialysis and oxygen. We were not prepared to care for those types of patients. Then I went to the loading dock to survey what was happening. I was overcome. I will never forget the feeling, because the loading dock area in the Dome was like mass chaos. It was jammed with people in no particular order, and the NOHD group became overwhelmed. They told me they had run out of check-in slips and so were just sending everyone upstairs to the medical-needs unit. People with intravenous infusions (IVs), tracheostomies, those needing suctioning—all were being directed to the special-needs unit.

I quickly set up an Army-system triage with two ER physicians and some medics. Those being triaged were divided into two groups: (a) those who could not stay at the Dome because of their conditions and needs and (b) those who could remain for shelter. No tags were available to delineate these groups, so sections of the loading dock area were designated for the various groups.

As the population coming to the Dome grew to nearly 10,000, security was required at the general population check-in area. The medical detachment had no security people attached to it, and while there were some Guard security agents at the Dome, they were needed elsewhere. As nighttime came, patients continued to come to the medical-needs area; many were those for whom we had not planned on caring. While the Guard's mission was to provide personnel, another agency was supposed to provide medical supplies; however, I learned that there were no medical supplies available. One of the Guard physicians who worked at the ER at Charity Hospital went over to Charity and brought back what supplies he could.

Later Sunday evening, a Federal Emergency Management Agency (FEMA) representative arrived and told me that a FEMA hospital would be set up at Tulane University Hospital and Clinic located a few blocks from the Dome. Tulane was already open with routine staff and patients. The FEMA representative said some of the more acute-care patients could be sent there, and eventually ambulances came to transport 60–75 patients to Tulane, as many as I could fit in, and I sent the most acute. The downside to sending those patients was that they required nurses and medics to be sent with them. Once the appropriate staff at Tulane arrived, the plan was for my nurses and medics to return to the Dome. Even though I sent two of my nurses and two of my medics with those patients, FEMA never went to Tulane. Conditions there worsened, and eventually, under gunfire, a SWAT team rescued the nurses and medics from Tulane. The group did not return to the Dome until Wednesday, September 1.

MONDAY, AUGUST 29

Colonel Patricia M. Prechter

As the weather worsened Sunday night, people never stopped being accepted into the Dome. It was obvious when the storm hit Monday morning, because the electricity went out around 3:00 or 4:00 a.m. The Dome had some emergency generators available in certain areas but not throughout the facility, so it was very dark. Loss of electricity also meant loss of sanitation, and even as early as Monday morning, a half-inch of wastewater was accumulating on the floor of the restrooms.

After the worst of the storm passed on Monday, I went outside and saw people still making their way to the Dome. I could look out on the interstate and see people walking, I mean, way out. I followed one guy on a crutch. He looked so old. I watched him, and it took him all day to get to the Dome. Patients not meant for the special-needs area continued to stream in. There were patients with IVs, patients needing medications that we did not have. The new patients were kept in the loading dock area, which became a makeshift emergency room. We would put any of the patients who had to be bagged (for ventilation) there. All day Monday, people came to a Superdome with no sanitation, no air conditioning, and no lights. Water and Meals Ready to Eat were available, but some of the special-needs patients were not able to eat them, as it required chewing, which some could not do. Babies in the special-needs area had no formula or bottles. At some point on Monday, the NOHD received some supplies that included formula and baby bottles. Other supplies started coming in on Monday.

Security problems worsened on Monday, the day of the hurricane, as darkness and minimal security affected the general population's behavior. As other Guard members arrived at the Dome, they brought radios and M16 rifles. I requested soldiers with M16s in my area for security, because theft became an issue as the general population started to come to the special-needs area on the mistaken belief that this group had drugs.

Among other problems was sanitation, not only for those capable of using overflowing Dome restrooms but also for the many special-needs patients who were in adult diapers with no replacements. Food for the special-needs patients who required certain diets remained a concern as well. There was drinking water, not chilled, but available.

Once the National Guard security came, my fears eased. Still, after Sunday night I never slept in the Dome but rather in my car until the medical detachment moved into an area in the parking garage. I was afraid. Darkness brought fear of the present and fear of what was to come.

Teresa M. O'Neill

In Prairieville, Louisiana, the Dutchtown HS Red Cross shelter contained evacuees who had driven out of the New Orleans metropolitan area. News regarding the storm was sparse because the storm-generated winds had downed trees and electrical lines. There were reports of flooding in St. Bernard Parish and parts of Orleans Parish, but most believed it was from the rain. There were no reports of levee collapses. Plans were being made to close down this shelter so school could resume within a few days. A new shelter at the Lamar-Dixon Expo Center in nearby Gonzales was being readied for those who continued to need shelter.[10]

TUESDAY, AUGUST 30

Colonel Patricia M. Prechter

The situation in the Dome medical area was slightly better organized by Tuesday, August 30, but the crowds continued to swell. With the electricity still out, the interior Dome temperature had risen, and it was very hot. As the command person of the Guard medical unit, I attended all the command meetings with various personnel in the Dome, which met two or three times a day. I constantly advocated for our patients for diapers and other items, and the need to relocate them, and I held out hope that electricity would soon be restored.

Around 1:00 p.m., I went to the loading dock and found myself standing in water.[11] We still had no communication with the outside, so we had no knowledge of the severity of the levee collapses or of the extent of the storm area beyond New Orleans. As I started receiving communication from the outside, I realized it was not going to get better. What had happened in the city was becoming more known to those in the Dome.

The Guard mission now became a double one. Many in the Guard unit lived in the Ninth Ward, an area hard hit by the floods. In addition to the logistical meetings regarding the special-needs unit and the general population, I began regular meetings with my staff to reassure them that the Guard would take care of them. It was hard to tell them that they could not leave to see what had happened to their families. I remember saying to them, "You're on orders. It would be desertion if you go home. You'll be AWOL."

Those patients on the ground floor were moved to higher floors in a Dome that had lost part of its roof, and finding an area that wasn't wet was impossible. It became obvious that the special-needs patients needed to be moved. The mission to care for them now became the mission to get them out of the Dome. From an original plan to care for 300 patients, the special-needs unit had swelled to 1,500 people. The decision was made to move them to the New Orleans Arena, another large facility located next door to the Dome. While separate buildings, there was a walkway connecting the two. The move to the Arena occurred on Tuesday and Wednesday.

Teresa M. O'Neill

In the meantime, the Dutchtown HS shelter had closed and evacuees were redirected to nearby Gonzales, Louisiana. Local Red Cross officials were transitioning for the national office to have oversight, but the local authorities remained in charge at Lamar-Dixon. This Expo Center had been founded as a multiuse facility primarily designed for agricultural and trade events. It had many buildings on its site; the Trade Mart building had the capability of housing approximately 1,200 people. Additional smaller buildings could house other administrative services.[12]

WEDNESDAY, AUGUST 31

Colonel Patricia M. Prechter

By Wednesday, August 31, the Dome had closed to all other evacuees.[13] It was a challenge to transfer the special-needs patients because many could not walk and wheelchairs were nonexistent. In addition to the special-needs patients, the unit now included pregnant women and children. FEMA came to the Arena and set up a hospital with an entire pharmacy, operating room, and additional equipment. FEMA hospitals are operated by contracted civilians: pharmacists, physicians, even a dentist. With the security situation in the Dome worsening on Wednesday and Thursday, however, FEMA pulled its people out of the Arena, leaving the hospital and its supplies. A newly acquired pharmacy now became part of the medical needs area, which was an advantage, but the close proximity to drugs added to the security problems.

Teresa M. O'Neill

Arriving at Lamar-Dixon late Wednesday morning, August 31, I spoke with the Red Cross manager in charge at the facility, stating that I had been requested by Jan Jaeckle, the Red Cross Health Disaster Services official in charge, to help organize the medical unit there. No designated person was yet in charge, but a nurse from the national Red Cross would be coming within a few days.

Donations from the local Gonzales and Ascension Parish area had been delivered to the Lamar-Dixon Trade Mart building to help those who had come for shelter. Preliminary sorting at the back of the building involved separating toiletries and other items from medical supplies, and I pitched in to help. We sorted medications according to type and classification and arranged them on rows with paper labels on the few tables in this area. A rudimentary special-needs area had also been set up in this back area, with some cots already occupied (see Figure 12.1).

By late afternoon, when the donated medications were fully organized, I told the shelter manager I would return the next day. Jaeckle had designated me in charge of the medical area until the national Red Cross nurse arrived. At this time, Red Cross medical services were restricted to handling

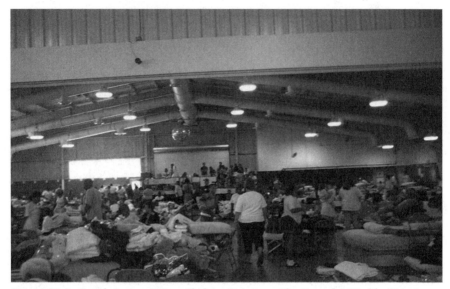

Figure 12.1   Inside Lamar-Dixon Shelter. Courtesy: *The Gonzales Weekly Citizen.*

first aid and other basic health-related matters. In an emergency, obtaining medical treatment or replacing essential prescription medications and equipment could also come under Red Cross jurisdiction, according to its most recent report on disasters.[14] I wondered how well delivering only first aid to a large population that had probably lost everything would play out in the larger arena of this disaster.

THURSDAY, SEPTEMBER 1

Colonel Patricia M. Prechter

By Thursday, September 1, SWAT teams had been flown to the Dome and convention center, the site of another shelter problem. I sent a small group of my unit to the convention center and also went myself to see what was happening. Many people were collapsing owing to dehydration from lack of water and outdoor heat. Because IVs were not plentiful, I cautioned the unit at the Convention Center not to start intravenous fluids unless the situation was life threatening. Unlike the convention center, the Dome population was never without water or Meals Ready to Eat. It was necessary to stand in line to receive them, but they were available.

I characterize Thursday, September 1, as "Showdown Day." The NOHD left the Dome because of the worsening security situation. I didn't blame them, because the violence in the Dome was increasing. People who had been attacked came to our unit for first aid. FEMA civilian contractors and NOHD personnel felt unsafe, even with the presence of military security. The Emergency Medical Services (EMS) group evacuated with the NOHD, but they left their ambulances. The only security that now remained for all areas was the military.

Officials from various state agencies, including the governor's office, continued to have meetings. It was obvious that there was no set plan to deal with the chaotic security situation in the Dome. Military teams came by helicopter, resulting in scenes that looked like they were from "Apocalypse Now" (see Figure 12.2). I have pictures of these helicopters coming in; soldiers are hanging out the sides with their weapons. The scene has to intimidate you. Had the military not taken over security by Thursday, I think more would have died. People had knives; they brought weapons into the Dome. Adding to the intimidation, the military had M16s.

Once the security teams arrived, people were restricted to their areas of the Dome. Armed guards were posted on the ramp leading to the Arena with orders not to let anyone through. As I traveled to the Dome meetings in a golf cart, I had to ignore the begging for help. I had to totally ignore

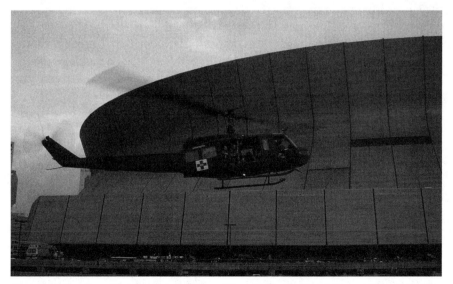

Figure 12.2 Outside the Superdome, New Orleans, Louisiana. Courtesy: Patricia Prechter.

human need, because they weren't the people I could help at that time. So I would ignore old people who looked like your mama begging for help. But I had to keep my eyes on my mission. And certainly I was not used to ignoring such pleas for help.

By Thursday, ground and air evacuation started to take place, and the ambulances left behind by the EMS now demonstrated their worth. The patients in the Arena were loaded into ambulances and high water trucks and taken to the top parking area of the Dome where the airlift operation occurred. Getting to certain areas, though, meant going through the general population still sequestered, and security had to maintain order. Evacuations continued until nighttime, when they were halted because of the danger of the area.

Teresa M. O'Neill

By Thursday, September 1, while special-needs people were being evacuated from the New Orleans Arena, the influx of evacuees to Lamar-Dixon increased. Many people were in the Trade Mart building and outside with their pets as no provision had been made for those evacuating with animals. (A barn was later opened for pets and other animals rescued from the storm.) Going in the back Trade Mart entrance, I saw more tables with volunteers set up. After introductions were made, I saw people coming up and asking for medications for headaches and other minor ailments. It was obvious that some type of documentation needed to be created in order to keep track of what was occurring. We established protocols for dispensing these medications along with a record form for the person requesting and the person dispensing them.

More medications were being donated, so further organization was needed. By this time, Janice Springer, the national Red Cross Disaster nurse, had arrived at Lamar-Dixon to be in charge; she concurred that I was to be her assistant. Springer negotiated with the shelter manager and other officials, and soon more tables, storage cabinets, and other equipment arrived to store the medications in a locked area. A refrigerator was requested because evacuees with insulin were bringing their medications to this medical area for refrigeration. A cooler came from somewhere with ice in it, and this is where we placed the insulin. Individuals' insulin was put into plastic bags with their names on the bags to prevent confusion.

Local volunteers began to come to the shelter and offered help. Along with them came some additional medical equipment. Glucometer supplies for glucose testing arrived, and a donation of a nebulizer for treating asthma attacks appeared. Local nurses and physicians came to donate their services and were assigned to duties in the medical area. As evacuees realized that a medical unit was in place that dispensed more than just acetaminophen for headaches, they began to come to ask for medical help. I realized there needed to be some record keeping started regarding this, and we wrote triage and medication protocols and put them into place. A cardboard box served as the file for the triage and treatment records with alphabetized folders to streamline record keeping.

Two physicians from the New Orleans area came daily to see the evacuees seeking medical attention. These physicians had the authority to dispense the medications, and the local volunteer physicians followed their leads. Medical supplies were limited, however. Physicians were instructed to dispense only enough medication for 24–48 hours, not for an entire week or more as there was not enough to go around. Treating these evacuees and their medical needs at Lamar-Dixon prevented the overuse of the local EMS service, and it lessened the work for the overwhelmed local area hospital ERs. Technically, anything beyond first aid was to be referred to local ERs according to the Red Cross. A quick realization that existing Red Cross first aid protocols would not suffice in this situation made those volunteering at the medical area determined to resolve what could be done within the Lamar-Dixon area.

FRIDAY, SEPTEMBER 2, AND BEYOND

Teresa M. O'Neill

At Lamar-Dixon, the population grew each day, with Friday's numbers determined to be 1,700 people in a shelter designed for 1,200. At one point, the population soared to 1,900. Every available inch of floor was occupied by cots. People carved out their niches within the building (e.g., family groups that had evacuated together), and small communities formed within the overall structure. With the large grouping of people, there also were the attendant responsibilities for long-term shelter, housing, health, and sanitation.

By the end of the first week, the Southern Baptist Disaster Relief group had a trailer in place at Lamar-Dixon, with people cooking lunch and dinner for those at the shelter, and other national relief groups came to offer help. The local Ascension Parish School Board assigned students to local schools and sent buses for them each day. Local churches sent buses on Sundays for various services.

Two male and female restrooms, each housing four stalls, initially served for sanitation purposes. Outside, portable toilets were in place by the end of the week with plans made to arrange for portable showers on trucks to come. These were in place by the end of the second week, and designated times were posted for male and female showers.

HEALTH CHALLENGES

Teresa M. O'Neill

Medical needs and health challenges result when a population is relocated, whether voluntary or mandatory. In the Dome, the medical needs unit had shortages of equipment and medications, though the FEMA hospital pharmacy had supplies. Many people at the Dome did not bring their medications with them. At Lamar-Dixon, while some evacuees had their medications, they needed prescriptions refilled. The challenge in refilling prescriptions was identifying what specific pills corresponded to what specific medication, as often pills were in bags or unlabeled bottles. This took careful questioning and assessment of the pill and the reason the person took it. "The white pill for my blood pressure," "the blue pill for my fluid" were not uncommon responses.

Local physicians wrote new prescriptions at Lamar-Dixon, but many evacuees utilized the Charity Hospital pharmacy in New Orleans to fill their prescriptions. The larger store pharmacies, such as Wal-Mart and Walgreen's, would not fill these prescriptions as these evacuees were not part of their overall system. Only a local Gonzales pharmacy, Landry's, filled as many prescriptions as possible, with Mr. Landry, the pharmacist, absorbing the expense.

Congregate living as seen in shelters has potential concerns for group health, most notably respiratory problems and issues with cleanliness. By the weekend, through the efforts of Springer and the Red Cross, large gallon-size sanitizer dispensers were in place throughout the Trade Mart, with periodic exhortations over the system announcements to "wash your hands."[15] The Trade Mart building had a facility-sized kitchen, which was put to use as a baby bottle cleaning and sanitizing station. Another protocol was written as a guideline for cleaning these bottles. Those with baby bottles came to the kitchen area at daily predetermined times with the dirty bottles, returning with cleaned and sanitized ones in Ziploc bags with their name and their shelter section number along with the "dirty" bag.

Unlike the conditions in the Dome, basic sanitation challenges were addressed and resolved at Lamar-Dixon, but other medical issues created real concerns. A sizable group of evacuees had psychiatric illnesses with no access to their medications, leading to breakdowns in behavior for some. They needed special monitoring by local health care workers and, later, Red Cross mental health workers in the overall facility, because this group was not placed in the special medical-needs area. Another group of approximately eight had no access to their methadone, and withdrawal symptoms emerged among some. It took more than a week for their needs to be addressed.

HIV-positive evacuees needed their medications, which were available only through a (Louisiana) state-funded program administered at Charity Hospital. It was flooded and out of service, however, so how would their medications be obtained? A mechanism was finally set up, but not until 2 weeks after the storm occurred.

As Lamar-Dixon became a long-term shelter, health concerns for residents in these types of facilities could not be ignored. Pregnant women resided in the Trade Mart building, some close to term. Prenatal care and delivery arrangements needed to be made for these women, in addition to addressing the implications of a newborn infant residing in a shelter. Several evacuees needed chemotherapy. In addition to determining specific chemotherapy protocols, challenges were complicated by the implications of immunosuppression in an emergency shelter environment. Several evacuees were in hospice care, and their oxygen was running low. How were we to obtain it?

At Lamar-Dixon, the abundance of volunteer nurses helped to organize and staff the medical unit. The specialized expertise of the nurses helped with the diverse group of medical conditions of the shelter population. Diabetic evacuees could speak with diabetic nurse educators and be counseled by them. Pediatric nurses could effectively evaluate children needing nebulizer treatments for asthma. Assessment skills were put into use for triaging for the medical area.

In the end, Lamar-Dixon reflected Florence Nightingale's dictums in action. Nurses facilitated the evacuees' health through listening to their stories, providing nutrition and other health services, and ensuring a clean and sanitary environment. Ultimately this population remained healthy. Potential concerns of urinary tract infections, gastrointestinal diseases, and infant illnesses were averted through aggressive protocols and campaigns of handwashing and infant bottle cleaning.

LESSONS LEARNED

Teresa M. O'Neill

By Sunday, September 4, all special-needs patients in the New Orleans Arena were gone. The general Dome population was being evacuated by bus to other areas, and the National Guard completed its mission. The unit left together on Tuesday, September 6, driving to Carville, Louisiana, its relocated base 65 miles west of its flooded Jackson Barracks home. In all, as many as 25,000 evacuees, 400 National Guard members, and other facility and medical personnel had been in the Dome at one time or another.[16] Lamar-Dixon served as a shelter until November 2005, when it closed.

Several lessons were learned from this disaster. First, disaster plans are just that—plans. Until implemented, the disaster plan is an uncertain document, no more demonstrated than in the Dome, where the overall general deterioration of conditions contributed to further chaos. In a disaster, it is imperative to have a strong command to organize those who are there and to maintain order so that the natural chaos that occurs can be minimized. Equipment and personnel do not just show up, and when they do, organization and collaborative efforts ensure that their use is maximized. Every organization involved must be responsible for its own component. The National Guard's mission was to help the special-needs unit. The NOHD was to provide the necessary equipment. Without the latter, the former's mission was compromised. In the wake of Hurricane Katrina, all state disaster plans have been reworked, and all Louisiana residential health care facilities are mandated to have a plan on file where a specific evacuation location is identified.

But even with a plan, what makes it work and succeed is having all involved be aware of their jobs and responsibilities. Knowing who is helping and what their skill sets are can result in effective delegation of responsibility. Yet, as the common saying goes, "the road to hell is paved with good intentions,"[17] and this is often borne out in a disaster. Although they have good intentions, unsolicited help can become more of a burden than blessing. Patricia Prechter recalled non-Louisiana Guard units calling her, "Col. Prechter, this is the Iowa State Guard . . . Where do you want us to go?" Another responsibility added to an already burdened job becomes a liability. At Lamar-Dixon, unsolicited volunteer groups had to be politely told that their services could not be utilized at that point. Too many offers of help can serve to confuse and undermine the basic purpose of shelter and aid.[18]

A second lesson is that in a disaster, the goals must be flexible. While the Guard's initial mission at the Dome was to see to the medical needs of a specific group, it changed to safeguarding this group's safety in moving it to another location. At Lamar-Dixon, the Red Cross regulations for medical care in shelters were quickly revised to become workable in a fully staffed medical unit that provided care for shelter residents. In so doing, this prevented the overloading of an already overwhelmed medical infrastructure in the closest urban area to New Orleans.

Flexibility and organization are hallmarks of experienced nurses. The nursing process is so ingrained that it kicks in automatically. As Prechter notes, "I could not praise the nurses in my unit enough regarding their ability to function without complaining. . . . You give a nurse a job and I'm telling you, they do it. I never had a nurse complain, 'I'm tired of seeing urinating in the corner . . . and pooing in the red bag.' . . . Nurses, they're flexible, they work systematically, and they're not complainers. And they think on their feet. The nurses . . . got us through."[19]

A third lesson revolves around what determines how a person acts in a disaster? What prepares someone for being in a disaster situation? For Prechter, her Guard training and experience prepared her for the Dome. Previous deployments to Iraq in Desert Storm, continued training, and other experiences prepared her to carry out the mission. What defines a person in a disaster? For Prechter, it was her faith, her military background, and her trust in the military order. For me at Lamar-Dixon, my previous experience supervising students in a pediatric emergency room and a recent medical mission to Nicaragua helped me develop triaging protocols and be creative in medication administration. For both of us, the automatic nursing process response guiding nursing practice helped us organize, delegate, and deliver care to diverse populations.

Fourth, nurses who volunteered had to have ingenuity and organization. As an example, at Lamar-Dixon the ability to improvise was seen in the dispensing of medications. Many people developed mild itching, perhaps as a response to stress or as a result of allergies. In any event, nurses had hydrocortisone ointments and topical Benadryl ointments, but certainly not enough to distribute to everyone in the building. We did have Ziploc bags, however, which became lifesavers. We would squeeze a small amount in to the Ziploc bag (sandwich or snack size works best) and give them a few days' supply to use. The Ziploc would keep the contents contained, and it was easy to squeeze and access it.

Fifth, nurses also had to have the ability to see what was needed to become the advocates for the client population served. They viewed their work as an opportunity to use their skills for those in need. Prior to the Red Cross coming to staff the medical unit at Lamar-Dixon, the nurses and physicians who got the unit up and running under the supervision of one Red Cross nurse were volunteers; some, like me, were also displaced by the hurricane, but many others who lived in the surrounding area came to help on their days off, or after their workdays were finished, because they saw a need. Some were uncertain if they could be effective or not, but others were confident in their skills. One nurse, who was a graduate of Charity Hospital in New Orleans, had vast experience and felt that she could do anything.

Nurses often say that they are "just doing their jobs" or that they are "*just* nurses." In doing so, they do themselves a disservice. Suzanne Gordon addressed this very issue when she eloquently conveyed how tongue tied nurses are in articulating what it is that they do.[20] Katrina provided a wonderful example of how nurses can say that this is what they do. Gordon notes that the public is aware of nurses' kindness and compassion, but they need to know that nurses, not just those in advanced practice, constantly participate in diagnosis, prescription, and treatment, therefore making a real difference in medical outcomes. That is unequivocally what the nurses did during the Katrina disaster.

Finally, nurses who worked in the Dome and Lamar-Dixon did not stop to reflect on whether or not they were making history. Rather, their primary goal was to maintain the health of the group being served. Responding to a need, whether dictated by military command or through human compassion, nurses providing care in the Dome and Lamar-Dixon provided a necessary component of skills for survival and continuation amidst a background of unprecedented turmoil.

STUDY QUESTIONS

1. Elaborate on the essential skills for a nurse who helps in a disaster.
2. This chapter points out that unsolicited assistance could cause as much harm as the disaster itself. Do you agree or disagree, and why?
3. Should public facilities be used as shelters for pending weather disasters? What responsibilities should these facilities have with regard to the population sheltering there?

NOTES

1. http://www.hhs.gov/disasters/emergency/naturaldisasters/hurricanes/katrina/index.html (accessed March 24, 2010). Although not as devastating as the 1900 Galveston hurricane, Katrina became the nation's deadliest hurricane since the storm of 1928, when more than 4,000 people in Florida and the Caribbean lost their lives.
2. National Oceanic and Atmospheric Administration, "2005 Hurricane Season: Water Vapor With SST Gray Scale IR Satellite." http://sos.noaa.gov/datasets/Atmosphere/2005hurricane.html
3. D.A. Goodeau & W.C. Conner, "Storm Surge Over the Mississippi Delta Accompanying Hurricane Betsy, 1965," *Monthly Weather Review* 96, no. 2 (1968): 118–124. http://docs.lib.noaa.gov/rescue/mwr/096/mwr-096-02-0118.pdf (accessed March 21, 2010).
4. P.F. Mlakar, "The Behavior of Hurricane Protection Infrastructure in New Orleans," *The Bridge* 36, no. 1 (2006). Retrieved from http://www.nationalacademyofengineering.com/publications/thebridge/archives/v-36-/theaftermathofkatrina/thebehaviorofhurricaneprotectioninfrastructurein neworleans.aspx. See also B. Handwerk, "New Orleans Levees Not Built for Worst Case Events," *National Geographic News* (September 2, 2005). http://news.nationalgeographic.com/news/2005/09/0902_050902_katrina_levees_2.html (accessed March 21, 2010).
5. http://web.mit.edu/12.000/www/m2010/teams/neworleans/hurricane%20history.htm (accessed March 28, 2010).
6. B. Wolshon & B. McCardle, "Temporospatial Analysis of Hurricane Katrina Regional Evacuation Traffic Patterns," *Journal of Infrastructure Systems* 15, no. 1 (2009): 12–20. http://www.nationalacademyofengineering.com/Publications/TheBridge/Archives/V-36-1TheAftermathofKatrina/EvacuationPlanningandEngineeringforHurricaneKatrina.aspx (accessed March 21, 2010).

7. Interview with Patricia Prechter, July 1, 2009, by T. M. O'Neill [tape recording].
8. Col. Prechter's husband and son went to Dallas, Texas. Dr. O'Neill evacuated with her family to Gonzales, Louisiana. She stayed with Jan Jaeckle at her home in Gonzales.
9. Jan Jaeckle, personal communication with T.M. O'Neill, March 19, 2010.
10. Ibid.
11. The storm surge had sent water over the Industrial and 17th Street Canals and flooded the lower Ninth Ward and St. Bernard Parish the previous day.
12. "Lamar-Dixon Exposition Center" (n.d.). http://www.lamardix onexpocenter. com/schedule-event.php (accessed March 21, 2009).
13. Douglas Brinkley, *The Great Deluge: Hurricane Katrina, New Orleans, and the Mississippi Gulf Coast* (New York: HarperCollins Publishers, 2006).
14. American Red Cross, "America's Disasters 2004: Meeting the Challenge." http:// www.redcross.org/www.files/Documents/pdf/corppubs/amdisasters2004. pdf (accessed March 21, 2010).
15. Janice Springer, personal communication, March 2, 2006.
16. Brinkley, *The Great Deluge*, 237, 275, 632. The population in the Superdome grew from 10,000 during the storm to 25,000 by Monday night.
17. Although many people credit this quotation to Samuel Johnson, others say he should not get credit. See http://forum.wordreference.com/showthread. php?t=116365 and http://www.samueljohnson.com/road.html (accessed March 26, 2010).
18. S.B. Hasenmiller, "Bioterrorism and Disaster Management," in *Public Health Nursing: Population-Centered Health Care in the Community*, 7th ed., eds. M. Stanhope & J. Lancaster, 453–478 (St. Louis, MO: Mosby-Elsevier, 2008).
19. Interview with Patricia Prechter.
20. Suzanne Gordon, *Nursing Against the Odds: How Health Care Cost Cutting, Media Stereotypes, and Medical Hubris Undermine Nurses and Patient Care* (Ithaca, NY: Cornell University Press, 2005).

CHAPTER 13

Striving for the "New Normal": The Aftermath of International Disasters

Audrey Snyder, Fusun Terzioglu, and Arlene W. Keeling

Two recent earthquakes—both disasters of great magnitude—were met with worldwide attention and international response. The 1999 Marmara earthquake in northwestern Turkey caused massive human losses and damages estimated to be in the billions of dollars, and thus achieved worldwide attention.[1] The most recent, 2010, earthquake in the Caribbean island of Haiti garnered headline news because of its devastation. In both cases, medical and nursing response teams crossed international borders to help.

In both cases, many people were left homeless, and tent cities that housed hundreds of thousands of people were set up either by the government, private agencies, or the survivors themselves. The following excerpts give some insights into life in these camps and the role that nurses had in gathering data and practicing their profession. The first includes a report by Fusun Terzioglu on the impact of Turkey's Marmara earthquake on family health. The second examines the work of a nurse practitioner and other health care workers through a faith-based organization in Haiti.

This chapter contributes to theoretical understandings of "the new normal," a term used to describe many aspects of uncertainty in today's world, from health care, to the economy, to the aftermath of disasters. The earthquake devastation, particularly in Haiti, was so great that it is highly unlikely that this country will ever return to what it was in the past. The disaster forced deep changes in all aspects of life, and practical solutions have yet to be found.[2] Nurses have important roles to play in helping survivors through the grieving process to accept "the new normal" in an uncertain world.[3]

THE 1999 MARMARA EARTHQUAKE—TURKEY

On August 7, 1999, one of the worst natural disasters in recent decades occurred when an earthquake struck northwestern Turkey around the Izmit region. Known as the Marmara earthquake, it registered 7.8 on the Richter scale. It caused approximately 17,000 fatalities and 32,000 injuries, left an estimated 20,000 collapsed buildings, and displaced more than 250,000 people.[4] Thus, the earthquake has had a huge social impact. The fatality rate of approximately 14.3 per 1,000, depending on different provinces, was five times the usual death rate in Turkey. In addition, according to the Ministry of Education, 114,000 school-aged children were left homeless. Unemployment rates were estimated to range from 20% to nearly 50%.[5] Assessing health care needs became a primary concern.

Although tent cities in Turkey provided much-needed shelter and food, they did not offer psychosocial support, and mental health needs surfaced that could not be adequately met.[6] Terzioglu and volunteers from the Turkey Family Planning Association in Ankara, Turkey, investigated family needs at Mehmetçik Dernekkırı Tent City, established by Land Forces Command in Adapazarı Province in Turkey after the 1999 earthquake. This camp housed 2,500 people in 600 tents. It was selected as the study area because people staying there had already overcome the initial shock of the earthquake and their basic physical needs for housing, nourishment, clothing, and cleaning were being met. Land Forces Command established a well-organized system in this tent city. Tents were of two-room types that were provided with electricity and catalytic heaters. Facilities such as a library, tailor, cafe, youth center, and a health center were provided. Still, during visits to tent cities in Adapazari, the Turkey Country Office of the World Bank found that survivors identified uncertainty about their future as their heaviest psychological burden.[7]

In assessing the impact of the Marmara earthquake on family health, Terzioglu and volunteers undertook a descriptive pilot study using a 30-item questionnaire that investigated married females ($n = 117$), married males ($n = 23$), and single young people ($n = 59$) living in Dernekkırı Tent City who had volunteered to take part in the study.[8] The questionnaire was designed to gather demographic data and participants' opinions about post earthquake life in areas such as sexual problems experienced after the earthquake, nutrition and hygiene habits in the camps, and contraception.[9]

Interesting findings came from the adolescents in the camp. More than three-fourths explained that they could not continue their education because of physical impossibilities because their schools had been destroyed. Other reasons listed were absence of teachers and earthquake fear. Significantly, the young participants emphasized that they did not have any job to occupy their time; excess idleness led to an increase in sexual intercourse among them.

While food was sufficient and facilities provided the means to meet hygiene needs, residents' general hygiene habits suffered, as people could only bathe once a week, seldom brushed their teeth, and did not wash their hands before and after meals. Regarding sexual and urinary disorders experienced after the earthquake, one-fourth of female participants complained about painful urination, some had vaginal itching, and one-fourth of the men had an odorous and discolored discharge. More than half of the female and male participants stated that they used contraception for birth control after the earthquake, with the most commonly used methods being withdrawal and condom use.[10] Nearly a fourth of the women stated that they had sexual intercourse just because their husbands demanded it. While both women and men explained that their partners appreciated it when they did not want to have sexual intercourse, one-tenth of the women in the study reported violence associated with sexual intercourse.[11]

A central point of this study is that proper housing, adequate nutrition, safe environments, and stable occupations are important for satisfying sexuality needs to be met.[12] While the study investigated only a small number of people and thus has limitations, it highlights concepts and themes for future grounded theory or phenomenological studies.[13]

As rescue operations shift from finding survivors and meeting physical needs to giving attention to people as they resume daily activities, nurses can be helpful in many ways. Awareness about reproductive and sexual health matters should be raised among those who dwell in tent cities. Training programs should be prepared for the prevention of reproductive organ infections and the improvement of general hygiene habits. Importantly, young people should be provided with positive activities to occupy their time. Indeed, activities and programs should be developed for all survivors to create income for them and to develop their problem-solving skills as they struggle to resume their lives after such a disaster.

THE 2010 HAITIAN EARTHQUAKE

Three weeks after Haiti's earthquake in January 2010, the country remained in shambles. Damaged and collapsed buildings and government offices in Port-au-Prince, destroyed communications services, and disrupted or ruined water and sewage lines wreaked havoc in the poverty-stricken country. Shelter needs were unprecedented. Thousands of homeless Haitians set up refugee camps in tent cities, where food and water were scarce and grief-stricken survivors wandered aimlessly among the wreckage. According to the U.S. Agency for International Development, by mid-February 230,000 people had died, 700,000 were displaced, and 511,400 refugees had departed the capital city. Altogether, over three million people had been affected.[14] Many had sustained major wounds, amputations, and blunt trauma. Thousands had lost everything.

The country was indeed desperate for help, both from within and outside its borders, and local people as well as emergency response teams from all over the world took action. Among these were advanced practice nurse Audrey Snyder and emergency medicine physician Scott Syverud from the University of Virginia. The two left Charlottesville on February 4, 2010, to join a group organized by the Lutheran Church (Missouri Synod) to aid a Haitian group working in Jacmel, a small, quaint, historic Caribbean port city about 25 miles from Port-au-Prince and not far from the epicenter of the earthquake. Like Port-au-Prince, Jacmel had been devastated.

Scenes from Jacmel were much like those shown on the news from Port-au-Prince. The center of town bore a swath of destruction. Makeshift cloth tents lined the streets, providing limited shelter for the survivors—some of whom had walked for days to find a place with more food and water than Port-au-Prince. A pervasive odor of human decomposition hung over the city; citizens covered their noses with bandanas to block out the smells. Throughout the rubble-strewn countryside, walls of houses crumbled and floors collapsed, destroying homes and lives.

By the time Snyder and Syverud arrived at the improvised clinic in the Lutheran church in Jacmel, the townspeople and international volunteer response teams were dealing with the aftermath of the disaster, trying to restore some semblance of normalcy for the citizens and refugees who had fled there. During the night, the church provided a place for people to sleep; during the day, it served as a temporary medical clinic. It also was a

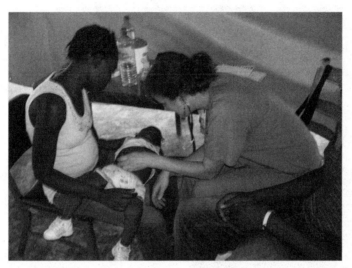

Figure 13.1   Audrey Snyder, PhD, RN, ACNP, with patient. Courtesy: Audrey Snyder Collection.

source of food: During the day, patients and their families were fed lunch; later, they were given bags of food to take with them.

Collaboration between locals and international relief workers was essential to the clinic's success. The faith-based organization, firmly rooted in the community prior to the earthquake, spontaneously acted to provide organization for patient flow as well as Haitian (Kreyól) language interpretation for the visiting medical team. Charter flights bringing medical and nursing staff and supplies to Jacmel also brought in 50-pound bags of food for the community.

Working out of the church, the health care team (consisting of a physician, nurse practitioner, physician assistant, pharmacist, team leader, and other nurses, along with their interpreters) saw more than 120 patients a day, over half of whom were children. Common concerns were wound infections from injuries sustained during the earthquake. Other commonplace diseases included cold, bronchitis, pneumonia, malaria, and dengue fever, along with issues of malnutrition, dehydration, worms, lice, and scabies. Some were typical diseases of tropical developing countries; others were complications developed because of the squalid living conditions and the lack of water and shelter after the quake.

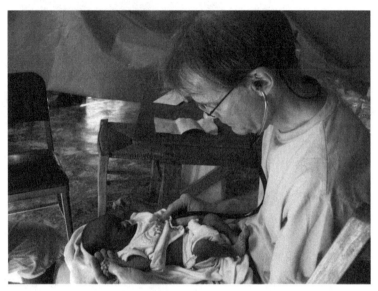

Figure 13.2   Scott Syverud, MD, with infant. Courtesy: Audrey Snyder Collection.

Of particular concern was the lack of access to normal care or pharmacy services. One patient with Parkinson's disease was without medication, and another patient who had been receiving treatment for breast cancer needed her maintenance prescriptions. The pharmacy had been destroyed, and the local medical team had been unable to obtain the medications from elsewhere in the country. Supplies were scarce, and destroyed roadways as well as a devastated infrastructure delayed the delivery of critical medicines and other basic necessities to areas where they were desperately needed. In the Jacmel church clinic, collaboration with medical teams in the United States ultimately resulted in the commitment for the needed medications to be delivered to the church pastor who would in turn ensure the patients received them the next week. It was international collaboration at the grassroots level a situation where locals and international volunteers worked together to accomplish disaster relief.

Lack of access to routine medical follow-up for wound care, as well as the lack of water, led to other challenges for both patients and medical and nursing personnel. Using bottled water and improvised dressing equipment, Snyder and other nurses cleaned wounds, applied Premetherin for scabies, administered medications, and provided psychological first aid.

They also gave patients bandages and taught them how to not only clean and dress their own wounds but also prevent dehydration in the 90° heat. In addition, nurses and physicians fitted crutches for those needing them and taught them how to use them.

In all these situations, the visiting nurse/physician teams had to learn to work within the context of the local culture. In this case, the Haitians relied on verbal rather than written communication. Nurses and physicians accustomed to written orders and documentation were thus at a disadvantage; often local nurses would provide appropriate care, yet not document that care in writing. Moreover, the language barriers and need for translators further complicated communications, as did the fact that makeshift paper medical records quickly curled with the humidity. Working within these constraints, local and international relief personnel learned to make daily rounds in the morning and evening to improve communication. In some instances, in the absence of patient charts, the time of the last pain medication was written on the patient's forehead. Other barriers related to timing arose. In the United States, medical orders are executed in a precise sequence at precise times. Haiti is a Caribbean island, and locals often operate on "island time," which is more laid back. Once this cultural difference was recognized and discussed, communication among the international teams improved. Cooperation was key.

In addition to providing medical and nursing care for injuries and illness following the earthquake, giving prenatal care for pregnant women was a challenge. In Jacmel, a military group from Sri Lanka had set up a camp on a fenced soccer field, where an estimated 3,500–4,000 displaced evacuees, including 130 pregnant women, were housed in canvas tents. Concerned that these women would go into labor during the night when the gates were closed and they were unable to get to a hospital, a self-proclaimed camp leader rose to the occasion. She was a Haitian woman displaced from Port-au-Prince, and she toured the camp with a megaphone, identifying Haitian women who were midwives or who had delivered babies in the past. She also acquired medical supplies so that the seven midwives who volunteered to be on call could assist with deliveries after hours. She then arranged for a small medical team to provide education to the expectant women in their last trimester, screen them for preeclampsia, and provide them with prenatal vitamins. In this case, ingenuity, leadership, and innovation were essential to meeting the challenges that the team faced.

Physical needs were only part of the problem for those who had survived the earthquake. Psychological care was also important, as the survivors were grief stricken with the loss of multiple family members, their homes and businesses, and their former way of life. Three weeks after the earthquake, many presented with blank stares as evidence of their distress. Without sufficient numbers of social workers and psychologists to meet the need, both local and visiting health care teams had to intervene. Nurses often were the primary support. According to nurse practitioner Snyder, nurses worked with patients to help them "(1) identify what they liked to do before the earthquake and to focus on their ability to do that activity again, (2) to create a good dream to replace the nightmares and flash backs [sic] they were experiencing, and (3) to create a plan to do one thing each day that would help them the next."[15] In short, the nurses helped patients focus on the future and look for a "new normal," and for that the Haitians were grateful.

Working in a foreign country following a widespread disaster required nurses to rely on basic nursing skills, to be flexible, creative, and collaborative. Snyder and Syverud drew on their experiences working at a Remote Area Medical Clinic in the United States to clarify roles, provide feedback on clinic flow for efficiency, and anticipate needs. The nurse practitioner, physician assistant, and physician each saw the next patient waiting; specifically, Snyder completed assessments, diagnosed conditions, performed procedures, and prescribed medications. The close proximity of examination areas made consultation or the sharing of unusual presentations with each other easy.

Assessing what resources were available in the community and local hospitals was key. Cooperation and collaboration were evident as nurses working in makeshift clinics negotiated with local hospitals for needed supplies. They traded medical supplies that were in excess for those that were needed. Baby bottles were in short supply, and rinsed gloves creatively became both nipple and bottle.

The challenge of providing wound care in hospitals was great. Decontamination of water was the first test. Impregnated gauze, which is frequently used as wound dressings in the United States, "became a soupy mess in the heat."[16] Instead, over a period of 10 days of treatment with just old-fashioned soap and water for cleaning, wounds began to granulate and improve. Instructing patients to provide their own wound care had its own challenges. For example, patients had to be taught to avoid contaminating the cleaning water with dirty gauze. In the outpatient setting, patients needed coal or wood to heat water, a pot to heat it in, and help from someone else to get the water to heat at home. "Home" was often a refugee camp or makeshift lodging in a church or other community building.

Although many international nurses who went to Haiti volunteered with altruistic spirits, many found conflict between their duty to survivors and their own family obligations. The need for nursing help was so great that many volunteers did not want to leave when their committed time was over. Recommendations from early health care teams to those that followed included, "Stick to the date your team has set to leave. You can always come back."[17] Nurses also encountered emotional distress when patients needed to be discharged from the hospital. In the United States, a patient would be discharged to home, a nursing home, or a rehabilitation center. In Haiti, nurses often had to discharge patients from the hospital with no place to go and often with no family to help care for them. Once refugee camps were in place, the patients were discharged there but often without the means to get around. Crutches and wheelchairs were scarce early in the early disaster response.

Working in teams with colleagues one had worked with prior to the disaster experience often helped with communication, as did making daily rounds as a team and ensuring on and off shift reports. These daily debriefings provided an opportunity for team members to share their experiences and identify concerns for group discussion and problem solving.

As the world population grows, people will continue to live in danger zones where earthquakes, storms, and floods—indeed, all natural disasters—will continue. It is important for the world community of nurses to learn from previous disaster responses and be prepared to assist.

STUDY QUESTIONS

1. How have men, women, boys, and girls been affected differently by disasters and displacement from their homes? How have specific events, such as the destruction of schools and sanitation facilities, affected survivors?
2. How do culture and ethnicity influence the different coping mechanisms used by women, men, and young people?
3. What are specific threats or risks facing survivors in tent cities?

NOTES

1. Charles Scawthorn, "The Marmara, Turkey Earthquake of August 17, 1999: Reconnaissance Report." http://mceer.buffalo.edu/publications/Reconnaissance/00-0001/default.asp?sH2=-1&oH0=-1&oH1=-1&oH3=-1&oH4=-1 (accessed October 8, 2009). See also International Recovery Platform, "Marmara Earthquake, 1999." http://irp.onlinesolutionsltd.net/countries_and_disasters/disaster/26/marmara_earthquake_1999.

2. Vickie Taylor and Sybil Wolin, *The New Normal: How FDNY Firefighters Are Rising to the Challenge of Life After September 11* (New York: Fire Department Counseling Service Unit, 2002); Eric Dinallo, *The New Normal: Everything Old Is New Again After a Decade of Quick Fixes, Fake Money, and Made-Up Rules* (New York: John Wiley and Sons, 2010); Scott Anthony, "Constant Transformation Is the New Normal," http://blogs.hbr.org/anthony/2009/10/constant_change_is_the_new_nor.html (accessed April 12, 2010).

3. Michael Turpin, "Getting Over the New Normal," http://www.thehealthcareblog.com/the_health_care_blog/2010/04/getting-over-the-new-normal.html (accessed April 13, 2010); Louise K. Martell, "Heading Toward the New Normal: A Contemporary Postpartum Experience," *Journal of Obstetric, Gynecologic and Neonatal Nursing* 30, no. 5 (2006): 496–506.

4. Scawthorn, "The Marmara, Turkey Earthquake." See also International Recovery Platform, "Marmara Earthquake, 1999."

5. The World Bank, "Turkey: Marmara Earthquake Assessment," http://siteresources.worldbank.org/INTDISMGMT/Resources/TurkeyEAM.pdf (accessed October 8, 2009); U.S. Technical Reconnaissance Team, "Initial Geotechnical Observations of the August 17, 1999, Izmit Earthquake," http://nisee.berkeley.edu/turkey/report.html (accessed October 8, 2009).

6. For similar problems after other earthquakes, see A.N. Nasrabadi et al., "Earthquake Relief: Iranian Nurses' Responses in Bam, 2003, and Lessons Learned," *International Nursing Review* 58 (2007): 13–18; and Erum Burki, "The Pakistan Earthquake and the Health Needs of Women," http://www.odihpn.org/report.asp?id=2809 (accessed April 6, 2009).

7. The World Bank, "Turkey: Marmara Earthquake Assessment."

8. Researchers would like to have reached all family persons, but they were not able to succeed; thus they selected only persons who volunteered to take part in the study. Before the study started, people were informed via announcement system that a meeting was going to be held on family health. People who attended this meeting and willingly agreed to take part in this study were included. Participants then came to family health meet-

ings, where field experts made speeches and answered participants' questions. For those who could not read, a face-to-face interview method was adopted.

9. Results were analyzed with the SPSS 11.0 package program using percentage values in data analysis. Female study participants ranged in age from 25 to 34; male participants ranged from 35 to 44; and young participants ranged from 15 to 24. The majority of females (97.2%) and males (86.9%) were married and primary or secondary school graduates, while 95% of the young participants were single and high school graduates. Most (97.3%) of the study participants lived in their tents with more than five people, and generally one person in the family held employment.

10. Turkey Demographic and Health Survey (TDHS), 2008; Hacettepe University Institute of Population Studies, Republic of Turkey Prime Ministry State Planning Organization, European Union, Ankara, Turkey. http://www.hips. hacettepe.edu.tr/eng/tdh508/TDH2008_Main_Report.pdf. This was consistent with other findings. In Turkey, for example, 26.2% of every couple (i.e., one of each four couples) used withdrawal methods, and 14.3% used condoms. Note that the level of pregnancy with the withdrawal method is still high, at 38.1%.

11. This was consistent with another study in Turkey, which found that 9 out of every 100 married women stated that they were forced to have a sexual relationship. See T. C. Prime Ministry, General Directorate of the Status of Women, "Domestic Violence Against Women in Turkey, Ankara, 2009," Pres in Elma Teknik, p. 50.

12. S. Correa, R. Petchesky, and R. Parker, *Sexuality, Health, and Human Rights* (New York: Routledge, 2008).

13. Margarete Sandelowski, "Focus on Research Methods: Whatever Happened to Qualitative Description?" *Research in Nursing & Health* 23 (2000): 334–340.

14. http://idh.cidi.org:808/ofda/Haiti-earthquake-fs2010, p. 1.

15. Audrey Snyder, personal communication, March 15, 2010.

16. Kathy Butler, personal communication, March 1, 2010.

17. Audrey Snyder, personal communication.

Conclusion

Barbra Mann Wall and Arlene W. Keeling

Sociologist J. Eugene Haas has noted that rates of recovery after disasters are related not only to the extent of the damage and available resources but also to prevailing trends in prior disasters, the personal quality of leadership, and how communities plan and organize for reconstruction.[1] While it is impossible to conflate all disasters today to direct parallels of the past, and it is no easy task to extract common elements from the wide-ranging stories recorded in this book, certain themes do stand out and can alert nurses, academic scholars, and policy makers to elements that can enhance a successful response to disasters. In fact, nurses and others who are faced with planning for disasters have few points of references except the past.[2]

The case studies presented in this book show that nurses responded with improvised activities at the local and national scenes. As nurses dealt with massive destruction and death, they did so in ways that restored a sense of order in the aftermath of a chaotic tragedy. Spontaneous community participation consistently occurred. From Mississippi to Texas, Boston to Halifax, Monongah (West Virginia) to Tulsa, and New York to New Orleans, nurses and others offered to help in any way they could. They participated in not only the initial response but also the recovery efforts afterward as they helped prevent disease, dealt with grieving families, and educated the public.

Yet some conflicts did occur among health care workers and other authorities. After the 1906 earthquake and fire in San Francisco, complaints surfaced that the Red Cross was withholding relief at key times. Many people continued to live in temporary structures and were impoverished for some time. In Tulsa after the riot of 1921, the political and racial situation made it extremely difficult for the Red Cross to administer disaster assistance using routine procedures. City leaders were ineffective in caring for the needs of Blacks, making it necessary for the national Red Cross office to take greater control of the relief activities. Conditions were eventually alleviated when, under the guise of "disaster relief," the Red Cross stayed over a longer period of time and established a hospital for Blacks. Another example is, of course, the Katrina catastrophe: Local government authorities were largely ineffective and untrained in disaster procedures. The National Guard stepped in with nurses and other forces and helped evacuate thousands of patients at the Superdome, and volunteer nurses worked in shelters throughout the region. Yet tensions and blame persist to this day.

This book builds upon other scholarly literature that examines disasters. The case studies reveal that very few problems associated with disasters are entirely new. Historians and sociologists have been saying for decades that little panic occurs after a disaster and that health care workers and survivors are resilient in the face of disasters.[3] Furthermore, while deviant behavior, including looting, occurs after disasters, some of it is not the result of criminal activity. Rather, it is a consequence when normal citizens try to obtain the basic necessities of life that are in short supply.[4] Lessons also have been learned about disaster policies and the implementation of disaster practices. These have led to advocacy efforts that ultimately result in policy changes that can prevent future disasters.

This book also enhances our understanding of human responses to disasters. From the case studies, we see that the affected populations needed to make sense of the disasters in order to cope with what seemed senseless. Kevin Rozario theorizes that "stories reveal the meaning of events," and they help survivors cope with calamities.[5] To deal with adversities and chaos, people constructed healing stories, or narratives, that reflected heroism, and they cannot be discounted. Certainly, the events called for acts of extreme bravery. In addition, when disasters strike, there often is a sense of helplessness regarding the inability to stop or control the enfolding catastrophe. The human psyche needs affirmation that individuals are not totally helpless, that they still can make choices and exercise control in defined areas. It is for these reasons that heroism becomes important, and it frequently emerges when people give personal accounts of disaster events. These are therapeutic narratives that help survivors, including nurses, to cope with the trauma.[6] At the same time, we need to resist overly simplistic notions of heroism. After the 2001 terrorist attack in New York City, a nurse remembered not his own bravery but that of his patients and their families.

In addition to heroism, people constructed narratives that reflected Edward T. Linenthal's categories. Progressive narratives deal with making sense of the horror through reassuring language of civic rebuilding and could be seen with the 1900 Galveston newspaper notation that "Galveston shall rise again."[7] Redemptive narratives include calling upon religious traditions as a means of healing, as demonstrated in New London, Texas, in 1937. Toxic narratives reveal the persistence of deep mourning and strained relations, as seen after Hurricane Katrina.[8] A major point is that whether of the optimistic kind, religious, or ones of disillusionment, these narratives endure. Nurses can better comprehend or even challenge their own interpretations of human events by studying the variety of ways in which other people view their personal experiences.[9]

Along these lines, nurses need to educate professionals and survivors about life after disasters. This involves survivors telling their own stories from a first-person perspective so that all voices are represented and the mainstream media are not the only source of the story 100 years from now.[10] Our findings also support the need for continuing care that includes long-term mental health care policies. In addition, women have special needs relating to pregnancy, nursing infants, and safety.

It is important to reiterate that disasters can have constructive outcomes. The San Francisco earthquake of 1906 led to significant structural changes in the way nurses organized formal disaster relief efforts. Disasters also unraveled stable geographical boundaries as people responded with improvised activities at the local and national scenes in collaborative efforts with others. For example, nurses from Boston, Massachusetts, assisted in Halifax, Nova Scotia, after the ship collision and explosion in 1917. They were rewarded a year later, when Canadian nurses went to Boston to help during the flu pandemic. More recently, rescue teams, including nurses, once again crossed international boundaries to provide assistance for survivors of the 2010 Haiti earthquake.

History also reveals leadership strategies that are needed after disasters. Witness the case of Sister Barbara Ellen Lundberg, SP, administrator of Providence Hospital in Anchorage, Alaska, during the 1964 earthquake. She made difficult decisions, acted with confidence and certainty, inspired and calmed others, and had strong collaborative relationships with key city leaders. She also provided a place for workers' families so that the employees could be available to work without concern for their relatives. In the end, she proved to be a person of great skill and competence, and she was not afraid to use her authority as she operated under trying circumstances.

Sister Barbara Ellen's case and others show how disaster responses disrupt assumptions about gender norms. Women overturned society's accepted gender roles that viewed women as "protected" and men as "protectors." Women were not powerless in times of crises brought on by disasters. While heroic narratives often emphasized calmness that implied control over one's fears, gendered terms such as "calmness" and "actions" could play off one another. "Calmness" connotes temperament, and focus and discipline connote "action." For most people, "calmness" carries a feminine connotation, like a mother who calms her crying child. It is assumed that women who remain calm will not run away, cry, or get hysterical. By contrast, men in similar situations are more often said to act in a disciplined and highly focused manner. As often is the case, however, there is a disparity between gender stereotypes and gender realities.

This book also has important implications for understanding nurses' work. Nurses turned disasters into opportunities, and they showed pride in their work. As Mary Beard said in 1918, "the universal need for nurses during the [flu] epidemic . . . brought a great volume of understanding" of their work.[11] What nurses' texts did not reveal is also interesting; they did not talk about fear or lack of control. Whether they actually experienced these emotions is unknown; they might have been trying to protect relatives or other loved ones from worry. Alternatively, nurses valued being emotionally strong, disciplined, and skilled. Historical accounts and the more recent memoirs of nurses working during the Katrina disaster revealed this firsthand. As Tener Goodwin Veenema notes, "Caring for patients and the opportunity to save lives is what professional nursing is all about, and disaster events provide nurses with an opportunity to do both."[12] What is often omitted from most contemporary caring models is the personal fulfillment that the nurses and other health care workers find in actively using their knowledge and skills and being present for patients and their families in times of great need.[13]

This historical study on disasters also offers insights into how issues of race, class, and ethnicity operate in U.S. society. The featured disasters occurred in contexts of inequalities that existed long before the specific disaster happened. For example, Black women and men were crucial to the nursing response during the yellow fever epidemic in Mississippi in 1878, yet, as representatives of a marginal group in nineteenth-century society, Black nurses received the lowest of all salaries for their work. In addition, racial and ethnic minorities were more vulnerable to disasters in areas such as San Francisco in 1906, West Virginia in 1907, Tulsa in 1921, and New Orleans in 2005 owing to employment patterns, housing construction, racial segregation, and cultural insensitivities. By presenting these case studies side by side, one can see patterns of racial and ethnic inequalities that may not have been as visible if studied individually. It is also important to note that many gaps exist in studies on race and ethnicity during disasters. We need more research on the perceptions of minorities in terms of risk and more studies on older people as subjects of disaster research.[14]

More research is also needed on nurses as practitioners in the field during disasters. That work should take into account the historical and cultural context of each disaster and be careful about over-generalizing. It is important that nurses be ready for contingencies. While preparation is important, events occur that disaster planning could never prevent. Nurses have to gear up for the unexpected and quickly adjust. Policies and protocols may no longer apply as expediency and patients' needs take priority. Traditional boundaries between health care workers often blur as professionals focus on getting the work done.

Finally, as this book has provided views into many different disasters at different times and places, it has given voice and visibility to nursing. The cases have uncovered what nurses experienced, the conflict-riddled nature of disaster responses, and what many shared when faced with such calamitous events. The nurses' stories reflect what Steven Biel called "concerns of contemporary politics, society, and culture."[15] No doubt those concerns will resonate as nurses strategically plan for disasters in the future.

NOTES

1. J. Eugene Haas et al., *Reconstruction Following Disaster* (Cambridge, MA: MIT Press, 1977).
2. Lawrence J. Vale and Thomas J. Campanella, eds., "Conclusion: Axioms of Resilience," in *The Resilient City: How Modern Cities Recover From Disaster*, 335–356 (New York: Oxford University Press, 2005).
3. E.L. Quarantelli, "Organizational Behavior in Disasters and Implications for Disaster Planning," Disaster Research Center Report Series 18, 1985, 11, Disaster Research Center, University of Delaware, Newark (hereafter DRC); E.L. Quarantelli and Russell R. Dynes, "Images of Disaster Behavior: Myths and Consequences," Working Paper 37, 1971, DRC; Steven Biel, ed., *American Disasters* (New York: New York University Press, 2001);

Thomas A. Birkland, *Lessons of Disaster: Policy Change After Catastrophic Events* (Washington, DC: Georgetown University Press, 2006).

4. For further discussion on looting, see Sandra K. Schneider, "Governmental Response to Disasters: The Conflict Between Bureaucratic Procedures and Emergent Norms," *Public Administration Review* 52, no. 2 (1992): 138.

5. Kevin Rozario, "Making Progress: Disaster Narratives and the Art of Optimism in Modern America," in Vale and Campanella, *The Resilient City*, 35.

6. Ibid., 27–53.

7. "Galveston," *Galveston News*, September 13, 1900, n.p.

8. Edward T. Linenthal, *The Unfinished Bombing: Oklahoma City in American Memory* (New York: Oxford University Press: 2001).

9. Barbra Mann Wall, "Healing After Disasters in Early Twentieth-Century Texas," *Advances in Nursing Science* 31, no. 3 (2008): 211–224.

10. Jamaal Bell, "Social Media Activism: Adding to the Haitian Narrative." http://www.huffingtonpost.com/jamaal-bell/social-media-activism-add_b_509609.html (accessed April 6, 2010).

11. Mary Beard, Instructive District Nursing Association Board of Managers Minutes, December 4, 1918, Howard Gottlieb Archives, Boston University, N 34, box 11, folder 5.

12. Tener Goodwin Veenema, *Disaster Nursing and Emergency Preparedness* (New York: Springer Publishing, 2007), 17. See also Denise Danna and Sandra E. Cordray, *Nursing in the Storm: Voices from Hurricane Katrina* (New York: Springer Publishing Co., 2010).

13. Julia Hallam, "Ethical Lives in the Early Nineteenth Century: Nursing and a History of Caring," in *New Directions in the History of Nursing: International Perspectives*, eds. Barbara Mortimer and Susan McGann (London: Routledge, 2005), 25.

14. These issues are noted in Alice Fothergill, JoAnne DeRouen Darlington, and Enrique G.M. Maestas, "Race, Ethnicity and Disasters in the United States: A Review of the Literature," *Disasters* 23, no. 2 (1999): 156–173; Marian Moser Jones, "Confronting Calamity: The American Red Cross and the Politics of Disaster Relief, 1881–1939," PhD Diss., Columbia University, 2008, Proquest Dissertations and Theses, Publication #AAT 3317567; and David Dante Troutt, ed., *After the Storm: Black Intellectuals Explore the Making of Hurricane Katrina* (New York: The New Press, 2006).

15. Steven Biel, "Unknown and Unsung: Feminist, African American, and Radical Responses to the *Titanic* Disaster," *American Disasters*, ed. Steven Biel (New York: New York University Press), 305–338. Quotation is on p. 333.

Index

Italic numbers indicate photos

access to care, lack of, 258
accidents, xi
Adapazari Province, 254
adolescents, 255
advanced practice nurse, 256
Aedes aegypti, 2
AFL/CIO, 213
Africa, 1
African–American, xxii, xxiii, 6
Africville (Halifax, Nova Scotia), 90
Aftermath, xxiv, xxv, 11, 32, 61, 100, 120,
      157, 158, 189, 256
airway burn injury, 188
Alabama Great Southern Railroad, 7
Alaska Communications System, 205
Alaska earthquake, description of, 197–198
Alaska Native Hospital, 198, 202
Alaska Nurse, 207
Alaska Psychiatric Institute, 202, 206
Alaska Search and Rescue Group, 202
Alaska Survey for Reconstruction, 213
Alaskan Earthquake Assistance Act, xii,
      xxiv, 196, 215
Alaska, population, 195
alcohol, 30
Aldrich, Robert, 178
Aleuts, 195, 203, 204, 205
Alpert, Mickey, 171
American Hospital Association, 208
American Journal of Nursing (AJN), 43, 49,
      55, 134, 180
American Legion, 153, 213
American Medical Association's
      Committee on Disaster Care, 208

American Nurses Association (ANA), xii,
      xxi, 61
American Nurses Foundation, xvii
Americana Histories, 160
amputation, 184, 201
Anchorage, Alaska, xxiv, 195, 203, 206,
      212, 267
Anchorage Office of Civil Defense, 202
angels of mercy, xxiii, 3, 127, 136
Ankara, Turkey, 254
Antibiotics, ix
appendicitis, 56
Arkansas, 4
armory, 133
Army, 213
      Hospitals, 137
      Nurse Corps, xxi, 112
      system triage, 237
arsenic, 78
Ascension Parish, 241
Ascension Parish School, 246
Ashe, Elizabeth, 55, 60
assess the situation, 92
assessing needs, 29, 254
assessing resources, 260
assessing the situation, 92
assessment of damage, 202
assessment of needs, 202
atomizers, 30
Auckland, New Zealand, 208
Austin, Ida Smith, 24
avian influenza, x

babies, 136, 203, 205, 238, 259
babies, premature, 130
baby, 57, 116, 200, 223

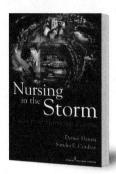

Nursing Interventions Through Time
History as Evidence

Patricia D'Antonio, PhD, RN, FAAN
Sandra Lewenson, EdD, RN, FAAN, Editors

Nursing has a rich history that consistently informs contemporary practice and standards. This book, by examining pivotal historical interventions across the spectrum of clinical care, allows nurses of today to incorporate the wisdom of the past into their own daily work. Maternal-child health programs, palliative care, tuberculosis, medications, pediatric care, diabetes care are included, and more.

This invaluable resource documents how and why specific nursing interventions came about, what aspects of these interventions remain today and why, and how nurses of the past have addressed and solved the challenges of practice, from adapting to new technologies to managing the tension of the nurse-physician relationship.

Learn how nurses throughout history combated the challenges of:

- Providing care to victims of pandemics, such as yellow fever, tuberculosis, and influenza
- Integrating cultural sensitivity into clinical care for special populations and underserved communities
- Adapting to new medical practices and technologies throughout the 20th century
- Bringing public health services to rural communities
- Fighting for public health policies that support hospice services in the United States

September 2010 · 192 pp · Paperback · 978-0-8261-0577-6 · $45.00

11 West 42nd Street, New York, NY 10036-8002 • Fax: 212-941-7842
Order Toll-Free: 877-687-7476 • Order Online: www.springerpub.com

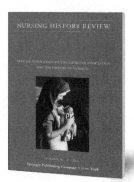